ATLAS OF
HISTOLOGY

SECOND EDITION

by

C. Roland Leeson, M.D., Ph.D.
Professor of Anatomical Sciences
College of Medicine
University of Illinois
Urbana, Illinois

Thomas S. Leeson, M.D., Ph.D.
Professor of Anatomy
Department of Anatomy
University of Alberta
Edmonton, Alberta, Canada

and

Anthony A. Paparo, Ph.D.
Professor of Anatomy
Department of Anatomy
School of Medicine
Professor of Zoology
Department of Zoology
College of Science
Southern Illinois University
Carbondale, Illinois

A companion volume to **Textbook of Histology**
also by
Leeson, Leeson, and Paparo

1985
W. B. Saunders Company
Philadelphia □ London □ Toronto □ Mexico City □ Rio de Janeiro □ Sydney □ Tokyo

W. B. Saunders Company: West Washington Square
Philadelphia, PA   19105

1 St. Anne's Road
Eastbourne, East Sussex BN21 3UN, England

1 Goldthorne Avenue
Toronto, Ontario M8Z 5T9, Canada

Apartado 26370—Cedro 512
Mexico 4, D.F., Mexico

Rua Coronel Cabrita, 8
Sao Cristovao Caixa Postal 21176
Rio de Janeiro, Brazil

9 Waltham Street
Artarmon, N.S.W. 2064, Australia

Ichibancho, Central Bldg., 22-1 Ichibancho
Chiyoda-Ku, Tokyo 102, Japan

Library of Congress Cataloging in Publication Data

Leeson, C. Roland (Charles Roland), 1926–

Atlas of histology

1. Histology—Atlases. I. Leeson, Thomas Sydney. II. Paparo,
Anthony A. III. Title.

QM57.L42   1985   611'.018   84–13893

ISBN 0–7216–1202–4

Cover photography courtesy of the authors.

Front cover: Large bronchiole, plastic section. (Methylene blue, basic fuchsin, oil immersion.)
Back cover: Endochondral bone formation, plastic section. (H and E, medium power.)

Listed here is the latest translated edition of this book together with the language of the translation
and the publisher.

Japanese *(1st Edition)*—Igaku Shoin Ltd., Tokyo, Japan

Spanish *(1st Edition)*—Nueva Editorial Interamericana, Mexico City, Mexico

Portuguese *(1st Edition)*—DISCOS CBS Industria e Comercio Ltda., Rio de Janeiro, Brazil

Atlas of Histology   ISBN   0–7216–1202–4

Last digit is the print number: 9   8   7   6   5   4   3   2

PREFACE

The format of this edition remains unchanged, closely following that of our companion book, *Textbook of Histology*. In each chapter, as before, there is a brief introduction, often with a diagram and/or an electron micrograph or scanning electron micrograph, followed by a series of color plates, each figure with a brief description on the opposite page and with labeling where this is deemed necessary. All the color photomicrographs are from our own material and illustrate a variety of staining techniques. Often, an organ, tissue, or cell is shown at different magnifications and using different staining techniques. Many of the illustrations are new, mostly replacing those in the first edition, but many are additions. The increased number of figures has resulted in a change in the title, the adjective "Brief" being dropped. These new figures mostly are of plastic-embedded material. Such sections, embedded in either methacrylate or epon, are only 0.5 to 2 micrometers (μm) in thickness, compared with the 8 to 10 μm of paraffin sections. They provide better detail, show less distortion or artifact, and aid the correlation between light and electron microscopy. Such material has been introduced into the slide collections of many histology departments in recent years, as it has in ours.

The greatest problem facing the authors of an atlas such as this is selection of material, perhaps more in the sense of what to omit rather than what to include. Often, we grieved at rejecting slides of high quality because they did not illustrate exactly what was required. Selection is necessary to keep the book at a reasonable size, and at a moderate price. However, we believe that our efforts to improve the quality and to increase the comprehensiveness of the illustrations have been successful.

In no sense should this atlas be regarded as a substitute for the use of the microscope. It is intended as an aid in laboratory courses, and we are gratified by the acceptance of the first, briefer edition by both students and faculty, an acceptance that encouraged us to embark upon this larger edition. We hope, too, that it will continue to be of value in those histology courses where the bulk of the material is presented by lectures and lecture demonstrations and in pathology courses, where it has been used to review normal tissue compared with diseased tissue.

In addition to changes in both text and illustrations, other changes should be noted. This edition has been prepared simultaneously with the fifth edition of our textbook. This has obvious advantages, with the major disadvantage being an increase in the workload for both the authors and the publishers. However, it is a decision we do not regret and we thank our publishers for their support and encouragement. It has ensured that the two books are compatible in content, accuracy, and pertinency and, in several instances, that the atlas color and the textbook monochrome figures are of the same material.

As with the text, the senior authors are pleased to welcome Dr. Anthony Paparo. His considerable background and experience in biology and histology has resulted in a valuable contribution to this edition and we look forward with pleasure to his increasing participation in future editions.

Finally, we are pleased that a selection of the color photomicrographs will be made available as 35-mm transparencies, together with a brief description booklet, through an agreement between our publishers and the Carolina Biological Supply Company of Burlington, North Carolina.

As always, our association with our publisher has been exemplary and we particularly wish to thank Dana Dreibelbis for his assistance with this edition and Brian Decker, who originally provided the stimulus for the first edition.

THOMAS S. LEESON
C. ROLAND LEESON
ANTHONY A. PAPARO

CONTENTS

Introduction

The color illustrations in this book are light photomicrographs of routine histological sections prepared principally from surgical or autopsied human material. In certain instances, to illustrate a particular point, a species other than man has been used.

In order to interpret the photomicrographs adequately, it is important that the student understand how the specimens were prepared. It must be appreciated that tissues undergo a number of alterations during their preparation; for instance, water-soluble materials are lost when the specimens are in aqueous solutions and lipids are removed while in lipid solvents. Also, the method of fixation employed will determine the type and quality of tissue preparation and often the subsequent choice of stains that may be employed.

For routine light microscopy, the tissue is first placed in a *fixative* to preserve protoplasm with the least alteration from the living state. Fixatives coagulate protoplasm, thus rendering it insoluble, and harden the tissue so that sectioning is facilitated. After the tissue has been fixed, it is *embedded* in a hard substance to provide rigid support to the tissue blocks so that they may be cut into thin sections. Prior to embedding, the fixed tissue is *washed* to remove excess fixative and *dehydrated* by passing it through increasing strengths of ethyl alcohol or some other dehydrating agent. The tissue then is "cleared," a process that involves the removal of the dehydrating agent and its replacement by some fluid, such as xylol or benzene, that is miscible both with the dehydrating agent and with the embedding medium. After clearing, the tissue is infiltrated with the embedding agent, usually paraffin or celloidin. The embedding agent then is made to solidify so that a firm homogeneous mass containing the embedded tissue is obtained. The embedded tissue is sectioned with a *microtome*, and each section is transferred to a glass microscope slide on which a little egg albumen has been smeared to serve as an adhesive. The mounted section now is ready for *staining*.

The purpose of staining is to enhance natural contrast and to make more evident various cell and tissue components and extrinsic material. Since most stains are employed in aqueous solution, to stain a paraffin section it is necessary first to remove the paraffin by placing the section in a paraffin solvent and then to rehydrate the tissue. After staining, the tissue section must be dehydrated again and then transferred to a clearing agent. The clearing agent is removed, a drop of mounting medium is added, and the preparation is covered with a coverslip and allowed to dry.

Stains in general use are considered to be either *acids* or *bases,* but in fact they are *neutral salts* having both acidic and basic radicals. When the coloring property of the dye is in the basic radical of the neutral salt, the stain is referred to as a basic dye and structures that stain with it are termed *basophil.* In most instances, the basophil substances that attract the basic dyes are themselves acids, for instance, the nucleic acids of the nucleus and the acidic components of the cytoplasm such as ribonucleic acid (RNA). Similarly, when the staining property is in the acidic radical of the neutral salt, the stain is spoken of as an acid dye and the structures stained, for instance, the general cytoplasm, as *acidophil.* Most histological sections are stained with both a basic stain and an acidic stain. The most common combination is *hematoxylin and eosin* (H and E), in which nuclear structures are stained dark purple or blue and practically all cytoplasmic structures and intercellular substances are stained pink. Trichrome methods, such as Mallory's connective tissue stain, Masson's staining procedure, and the Mallory-Azan method, possess the advantage that they differentiate between cytoplasmic structures and intercellular materials. It must be appreciated that special methods of staining are necessary to demonstrate certain constituents of cells and formed extracellular fibers and that a single staining method does not suffice to demonstrate everything present within a section. Numerous examples of these special methods are found throughout this book.

It should be noted that the method of preparation of sections for electron microscopy in general is similar to that employed for light microscopy, although there are some important points of difference. Much smaller pieces of tissue are used, since preservation and fixation of cellular fine structure is more critical and requires rapid interaction with the fixative. Current procedures of fixation generally involve the use of glutaraldehyde, which maximally retains protein constituents of the cell, and of osmium tetroxide, which retains the lipid components. Since paraffin is not suitable for very thin sectioning, it is replaced as an embedding medium by some agent, usually a plastic material such as Epon or Araldite, which produces a firm block. The sections, cut upon a special microtome with glass or diamond knives, are minute and they are mounted on perforated copper grids for viewing in the electron microscope. Thicker sections, about 0.2 to 1.0 micron, or micrometer (μm), thick, of such plastic-embedded material can be mounted on glass slides, stained, and examined by light microscopy. In the past few years, many institutions have introduced such material into their slide collections, since it provides better detail than that found in paraffin-embedded material and it facilitates correlation between light and electron microscopy. Many of the photomicrographs depicted in this text are of sections of plastic-embedded material because the clarity of detail generally is much better than with paraffin-embedded material.

The Cell

The body is composed of three different elements: (1) cells, (2) intercellular substance, and (3) body fluids. Body fluids include blood, lymph, and tissue (intercellular) fluid. Intercellular substance is the material that lies between and supports cells. It includes formed fibers such as collagen and elastin and amorphous material, or ground substance (please see Chapter 3). The obvious feature of most tissue sections is the presence of cells, although their entire outlines are not always seen easily. Cells consist of *protoplasm,* including a *nucleus* and *cytoplasm,* bounded by a delicate *cell* or *plasma membrane.* Cells vary greatly in size, shape, and function. Many are highly specialized or differentiated—e.g., the muscle cell is designed for contraction and the nerve cell for conduction—but cells often have multiple functions.

In most preparations, cytoplasm appears homogeneous; in fact, however, it contains two types of small bodies: *organelles* and *inclusions.* Organelles are permanent, living, structural components of the cell, each with a specific structure (usually seen only on electron microscopy) and function. Inclusions comprise metabolic products and ingested substances, many only temporarily present in cytoplasm, and, while often regarded as nonliving, many probably are essential for normal cell metabolism. A brief description of the elements found within the cytoplasm and nucleus follows, but students are advised to consult a textbook of histology for details.

CYTOPLASM

Cytoplasmic Organelles

In many cells, the cytoplasm is specialized regionally; i.e., organelles are located in different regions. For example, centrioles and the Golgi apparatus often are found near the nucleus; in cells that secrete protein, granular endoplasmic reticulum (cytoplasmic basophilia) lies toward the base of the cell (i.e., it is subnuclear), with secretory droplets or granules in apical cytoplasm. Each cell is bounded by a *plasma membrane* or *plasmalemma,* considered as one of the organelles.

Plasma (Cell) Membrane

The plasma membrane is very thin, basically only 7.5 nanometers (nm) thick, and may not be resolved by light microscopy. Associated material on its external surface may increase the apparent thickness, and this may make it visible by light microscopy. The plasmalemma differs from other membranes of the cell in that it has a cell coat, or *glycocalyx.* The cell coat varies in thickness and is composed of sialic acid containing glycoproteins that are firmly anchored in the plasma membrane. It is formed in the Golgi apparatus and can be stained, e.g., by the periodic acid–Schiff technique.

On electron microscopy, the plasmalemma has a trilaminar appearance with two outer densely staining leaflets separated by an electron lucid interval; chemically, it is believed to be two layers of lipid covered on both outer and inner surfaces with layers of protein. However, some membrane proteins are located within the lipid layers and probably even protrude from it.

Small molecules pass through the plasma membrane readily. Larger molecules are carried across the membrane and into the cell by a process of pinocytosis, small vesicles being pinched off to form cytoplasmic vesicles. A similar process with respect to particulate material is called phagocytosis. The reverse—extrusion of material—is termed exocytosis.

Some modifications of the plasmalemma are visible by light microscopy. For example, in cells specialized for absorption, at the luminal border are a series of regular, closely packed, finger-like processes (microvilli) forming a brush or striated border. In a few cells, e.g., ductus epididymidis, long branching microvilli are present. These are called stereocilia.

At the base of some cells, e.g., those in kidney tubules, deep invaginations of the plasmalemma divide the cytoplasm into pockets in which elongated mitochondria are present. The plasmalemma also shows specializations for cell contact (see Chapter 2).

Basophilic Component (Chromidial Substance)

Present in the cytoplasm of cells, particularly those that actively synthesize protein, are regions that stain with basic dyes, for example, blue with hematoxylin. On electron microscopy these areas correspond to *rough-surfaced,* or *granular, endoplasmic reticulum,* consisting of a three-dimensional network of membrane-limited channels in the form of cisternae, or flattened sacs, tubules, and vesicles, and the membranes are studded on their outer (cytoplasmic) surfaces with ribosomes. The membranes are 6 to 7 nm thick. Ribosomes also occur freely in the cytoplasm. They are 15 to 25 nm in diameter, each formed by two subunits, and are composed of ribonucleic acid (RNA) and protein. The role of granular reticulum and ribosomes in protein secretion is discussed in textbooks of histology.

Agranular Endoplasmic Reticulum

Smooth-surfaced, or *agranular, endoplasmic reticulum* is not demonstrated by light microscopy, but on electron microscopy it is seen to differ from granular reticulum in that its membranes are smooth-surfaced tubular and vesicular elements unassociated with ribosomes. The membranes are 6 to 7 nm thick and enclose a tubular lumen of about 50 nm. Agranular reticulum is particularly prominent in many steroid-secreting cells, such as the adrenal cortex; in interstitial cells of the testis and corpus luteum, where it is involved in steroid biosynthesis; in liver cells associated with glycogen formation and storage and cholesterol synthesis; and in intestinal epithelial cells, where probably it is concerned with neutral fat synthesis.

Golgi Apparatus

The Golgi region or complex may be visible on light microscopy as either a "positive" or "negative" image. Special techniques, such as silver impregnation or prolonged treatment with osmic acid, demonstrate the Golgi complex as a reticular network of canals and vacuoles or as an irregular mass lying near the nucleus. This is a positive image. Sometimes it is multiple. It is prominent in protein-secreting cells, where it appears as a "negative" image or unstained area in the region of basophilic cytoplasm, e.g., in osteoblasts and plasma cells. On electron microscopy, it consists of a stack of membrane-bound cisternae or saccules with associated vesicles and vacuoles, the stack of membranes being curved with convex (immature) and concave (mature or secreting) faces.

The Golgi apparatus constantly changes, with vesicles passing to the immature face and condensing vacuoles leaving the mature face. Thus, there is "movement" of membrane through a Golgi stack. The Golgi apparatus receives secreted protein from the granular reticulum and condenses it, sometimes adding a carbohydrate moiety, the material leaving the Golgi as secretory granules. It also forms the glycocalyx and lysosomes. Thus, it plays a major role in the transport and release of secretory materials from the cell.

Mitochondria

While usually not visible in H and E preparations, mitochondria can be demonstrated by iron hematoxylin and after supravital staining with Janus green B. They are thread-like, ovoid or spherical in shape, about 0.5 micron or micrometer (μm) wide and 2 to 5 μm long, and vary in number with cell activity—that is, the higher the metabolic activity of the cell, the larger the number of mitochondria. On electron microscopy, they all have a double limiting membrane, with the inner membrane infolded into the center of the organelle as a series of plate-like projections, the cristae mitochondriales. Some cristae are of tubular or vesicular form. Mitochondria synthesize adenosine triphosphate (ATP) from adenosine diphosphate (ADP), the ATP being utilized as an energy source by the entire cell. They contain enzymes of the tricarboxylic acid cycle—the electron transport system and phosphorylating enzymes—and show a functional distribution within the cell; that is, they are found in regions of metabolic activity, for example, in relation to contractile elements in muscle cells and near basal infoldings of kidney tubule cells for active transport.

Lysosomes

Lysosomes are small, membrane-bound bodies of pleomorphic size and shape that contain lytic enzymes for intracellular digestion. They can be demonstrated, e.g., by a Gomori technique for acid phosphatase. Generally, they are of two types: (1) primary lysosomes, which contain newly formed enzymes yet to be active in the cell; and (2) secondary lysosomes, which are bodies formed by fusion of a primary lysosome with some other body arising within or outside the cell and in which enzymatic digestion is occurring or has occurred. The "granules" of neutrophilic leukocytes, for example, are lysosomes. Primary lysosomes are relatively small, usually spherical bodies of 25 to 50 nm in diameter but they may be as large as 0.8 μm. The results of enzymatic digestion in a lysosome may leave in the cell a "residual body," such bodies containing silica or cholesterol. For example, lipofuscin granules, found particularly in aging cells, are residual bodies. Lysosomes play an essential role in cellular defense mechanisms.

Centrioles

Centrioles are seen as short rods or granules lying near the nucleus, usually as a pair in interphase cells, and usually in or adjacent to the Golgi region. On electron microscopy, they have a characteristic structure. Each is a hollow cylinder about 150 nm in diameter and 300 to 500 nm long, with a wall composed of nine sets of triplets, i.e., three microtubules. Centrioles are self-replicating and prominent in mitosis.

Cilia and Flagella

Cilia are motile processes protruding from the cell surface; they are usually multiple, but do occur as single elements. Flagella are similar but longer; for example, the motile tail of a spermatozoon is a flagellum and may be 70 μm long. Cilia usually are 5 to 15 μm long and 0.2 μm in diameter. In the shaft, on electron microscopy, are nine peripheral doublets (pairs of microtubules), with two central, single microtubules (singlets). The regular arrangement of microtubules is lost near the tip. At the base of a cilium, within the apical cytoplasm of the cell, is a basal body that is very similar to a centriole in structure, with nine peripheral triplets. Strands of fibrous material pass from the basal end of each triplet into apical cytoplasm as "striated rootlets." Cilia contract with a wave-like motion to propel fluid material, such as mucus, on the surface of the cell.

Fibrils

Many cells contain fibrillar material, usually invisible by light microscopy. In many cells, the fibrillar or filamentous material is composed of contractile proteins. In muscle cells, the bundles of filaments or myofibrils are of such a size as to be clearly visible by light microscopy.

Other organelles are present in cytoplasm that are invisible by light microscopy. They include *microbodies,* or *peroxisomes,* which are similar to lysosomes.
These organelles are found in kidney tubule cells, bronchioles, liver cells, and
odontoblasts and contain catalase and urate oxidase. *Microtubules* are slender,
tubular structures only 25 nm in diameter, with an electron-lucent core of 15 nm
and a wall thickness of 5 mm; the wall in turn is composed of 13 longitudinal
subunits. Microtubules occur in many cells and are found in cilia and centrioles.
They serve as a type of cytoskeleton, are involved in change of cell shape, and in
mitosis form the mitotic spindle. *Annulate lamellae,* usually found near the nucleus,
consist of parallel double membranes with numerous pores or annuli. These
organelles are found particularly in rapidly dividing cells (embryonic and neoplas-
tic) and in male and female germ cells; functionally, they may carry information
from the nucleus to the cytoplasm.

Cytoplasmic Inclusions

While formerly considered nonliving accumulations of metabolites resulting
from synthesis of materials brought into a cell from outside, many inclusions in
fact participate in the normal functioning of the cell. They include materials such
as *stored foods, pigments,* and some *crystalline materials.* Bodies such as secretory
droplets or granules were formerly considered inclusions, but are actually membrane-bound packets of enzymes.

Stored Foods. Fat, apart from its storage as adipose tissue, is present in many
cell types and is seen as clear vacuoles and droplets containing neutral fats, fatty
acids, and cholesterol. Usually fat is removed in tissue preparation, leaving clear,
spherical deficiencies, but it can be preserved and stained, e.g., by osmium
tetroxide. *Carbohydrate* is stored in cells as glycogen. Glycogen is water soluble
and also is removed by ordinary preparative methods, leaving irregular, ragged
spaces in the cytoplasm and thus giving a "moth-eaten" appearance. It can be
retained and stained specifically.

Pigments. Pigments are materials with natural color and are classified as
exogenous (formed outside the body and later taken into it) or *endogenous*
(formed within the body). Exogenous pigments include carotenes (lipochromes),
dust, and minerals. Endogenous pigments are mainly of two types: (1) melanin,
and (2) hemoglobin and its breakdown products.

Crystalline Materials. Crystals and crystalloids occur in a few cell types and
usually are proteinaceous in nature.

THE NUCLEUS

Only erythrocytes and platelets of the blood lack a nucleus or nuclei. Nuclei
vary greatly in shape, but usually are spherical or ovoid. They are usually 3 to 14
μm in diameter, except in a few cells—in which they are much larger. Characteristically, the nucleus is basophil; i.e., it stains blue with H and E.

The nucleus is bounded by a *nuclear envelope* or membrane and is filled with
lighter-staining nuclear sap *(karyoplasm).* The nuclear envelope may show small

irregular, densely staining masses of chromatin and a nucleolus. Basically, the nuclear envelope is formed by two membranes 7 to 8 nm in thickness separated by a perinuclear space of 25 nm, and the outer membrane is studded with ribosomes. The nuclear envelope is visible on light microscopy because of associated chromatin material attached to its inner surface. Karyoplasm is clear-staining, but it contains dispersed chromatin, some granules, and protein. Nuclear *chromatin* appears as irregular, dense, coarsely granular clumps of material both within the nuclear sap and associated with the inner aspect of the nuclear envelope. The chromatin represents regions of condensed or tightly coiled chromosomes in the interphase nucleus.

Nuclei themselves are basically of two types: (1) small, darkly staining "condensed" or hyperchromatic; and (2) larger, paler-staining "vesicular." The nucleolus may be obscured in a nucleus of the condensed type. The nucleolus usually is about 4 μm in diameter, discrete, spherical or ovoid, and lying freely in the karyoplasm or attached to the inner surface of the nuclear envelope. Usually, nucleoli are basophil, larger, and more regular than masses of chromatin; however, the coloration varies because, in addition to RNA and deoxyribonucleic acid (DNA), they contain both basic and acidic proteins. On electron microscopy, the nucleolus contains granular and fibrillar components. Ribosomal RNA is synthesized in the nucleolus, which is prominent and often multiple in protein-secreting cells. Nuclear chromatin, which represents chromosomes in the interphase nucleus, is composed largely of DNA.

Chromosomes, of course, can be seen in cells undergoing mitosis. The process of mitosis will not be discussed here, but examples of cells in the four stages of mitosis are included in the chapter.

Sex chromatin (the *Barr body*) can be seen in some cell types. Human somatic cells contain 46 chromosomes, or 23 pairs: 22 pairs are called *autosomes*; in addition, there are two X chromosomes in the female and one X and one Y chromosome in the male. Occasionally, this number varies, either in multiples or in numbers greater or less but not multiples. In female nuclei, one X chromosome in interphase remains extremely heterochromatic and forms a visible mass called the Barr body. It is about 1 μm in diameter and is found often lying against the inner aspect of the nuclear envelope in a planoconvex form (in epithelial cell nuclei), as a "drumstick" or slender protrusion of the nucleus, or as a small body associated with the nucleolus.

PRIMARY TISSUES

During development in the embryo, there are three primitive cellular layers:
1. *Ectoderm* covers the body surface.
2. *Endoderm* lines the gut tube.
3. *Mesoderm* lies between the other two.
The body develops from these three layers.

In an adult, only four primary tissues are present, each differing in appearance and function from the others. A primary or basic tissue is a group of similar cells specialized in a common function. The four tissues are as follows:
1. *Epithelium.* These are closely apposed cells with little intercellular material;

these cells are arranged in sheets (membranes) covering or lining surfaces or as masses of cells in glands.

2. *Connective tissue.* These cells are usually widely separated by large amounts of intercellular material. This group includes blood, bone, and cartilage.

3. *Muscle.* Muscle consists of elongated cells with fibrillar cytoplasm, relatively closely situated with a little fine vascular connective tissue.

4. *Nervous tissue.* These are groups of cells, often large, with elongated processes usually grouped into bundles or fascicles.

In turn, organs are formed from the primary tissues, often all four being present in an organ.

NOTE ON MAGNIFICATION

In the photomicrographs, only a general indication of magnification is given, but this is adequate for the student's interpretation. Four ranges are used:

1. *Low power* indicates a micrograph taken with approximately a 10 × objective lens or less.

2. *Medium power,* a 25 × objective lens.

3. *High power,* a 40 × objective lens.

4. *Oil immersion,* a 100 × objective lens.

For all ranges, the eyepiece is 10 ×. Thus, as the student uses the microscope, the term "medium power" indicates the area of tissue and the amount of detail he or she can expect to see with a 25 magnification objective lens.

Most material is paraffin-embedded, and the sections are 8 to 10 μm in thickness, except when a "plastic-section" is indicated. A plastic section is of 0.5 to 2 μm thickness and embedded in either methacrylate or epon. While difficult to stain, a plastic section has the advantage of being virtually two-dimensional. A few special preparations are used and so indicated. Details of staining and preparative methods are not given, but the stain used is stated in each case.

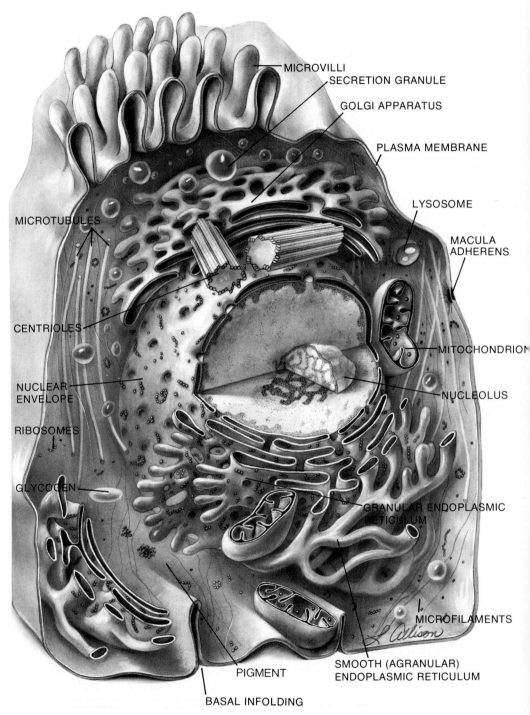

MICROVILLI
SECRETION GRANULE
GOLGI APPARATUS
PLASMA MEMBRANE
LYSOSOME
MACULA ADHERENS
MITOCHONDRION
NUCLEOLUS
GRANULAR ENDOPLASMIC RETICULUM
MICROFILAMENTS
SMOOTH (AGRANULAR) ENDOPLASMIC RETICULUM
PIGMENT
BASAL INFOLDING
GLYCOGEN
RIBOSOMES
NUCLEAR ENVELOPE
CENTRIOLES
MICROTUBULES

Figure 1–1. Schematic diagram of the cell.

Shown are many of the organelles and inclusions as they would be seen on electron microscopy.

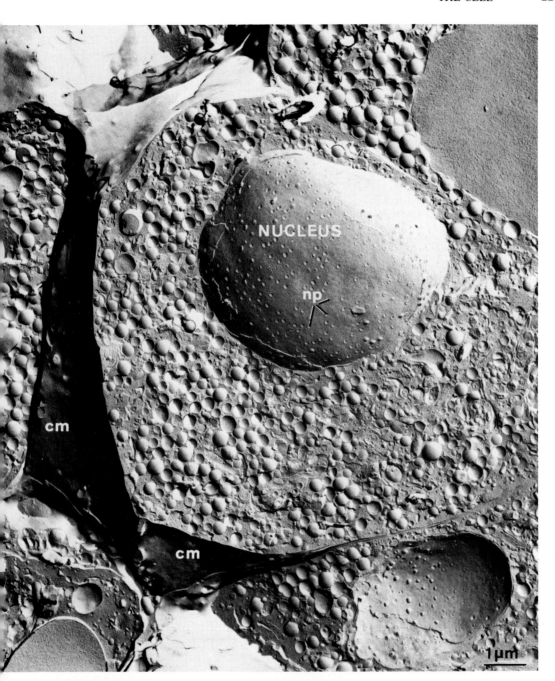

Figure 1–2. Freeze-etch replica from an isolated pancreatic islet.

This technique characteristically reveals face views of membranes. The endocrine cells shown here have been cleaved in such a way that a fracturing plane followed cell membranes (cm) for some distance before breaking through into the interior of the cells, revealing the nucleus with numerous nuclear pores (np) or annuli in the nuclear envelope. Most of the globular cytoplasmic profiles represent secretory granules. (Micrograph courtesy of Dr. L. Orci and reproduced by permission of the Editor, Diabetologia, Springer-Verlag, New York.)

Figure 1–3. Liver. H and E. Low power.

This field shows a portion only of a liver lobule. (See Chapter 11.) At this low magnification, cell boundaries are indistinct; however, liver (parenchymal) cells, which are epithelial, are arranged in irregular cords radiating from a central vein (V) and with vascular or sinusoidal spaces between the cords. Other cell types and structures are present. Note that cytoplasm of the parenchymal cells is abundant, eosinophil, and homogeneous. Nuclei of these cells are generally spheroidal and vesicular in type. Smaller, darker-staining (condensed or hyperchromatic) nuclei of cells associated with the sinusoids also are seen. On the right is a portal area (P) containing several tubes (blood vessels and bile ducts) cut in transverse section. This area appears darker owing to the presence of numerous small cells with dark nuclei, packed closely together.

Figure 1–4. Liver. Plastic section. Toluidine blue. High power.

Anastomosing cords of epithelial (parenchymal) cells are present with vascular, sinusoidal spaces between the cords; these contain erythrocytes that appear as round profiles staining dark blue and are non-nucleated. In the liver cells, cell borders are seen, and the cytoplasm is abundant and shows small dense particles that are mitochondria. Small, spherical, clear spaces represent dissolved lipid. Nuclei (N) are vesicular, some with prominent nucleoli (arrows) and some cells containing two nuclei (arrowheads).

Figure 1–5. Jejunum, villi. Plastic section. H and E. Oil immersion.

Villi are finger-like processes of the lining (mucosa) of the gastrointestinal tract with a core of connective tissue. The simple epithelium on the surfaces of two adjacent villi (C is the connective tissue core of each) is composed of tall columnar cells with densely eosinophil cytoplasm and elongated, ovoid, dark nuclei. At the surface, these cells show a striated or brush border (B) formed by regular, closely packed microvilli. Between these cells are scattered single, flask-shaped cells with basal, irregular nuclei (arrows) and apical cytoplasm filled with pale-staining droplets. These are goblet cells, and the droplets are mucin, the cells secreting mucus.

Figure 1–6. Ductus epididymidis. Plastic section. H and E. Oil immersion.

The tall columnar cells lining the duct show basally located, elongated nuclei and long, apical cytoplasmic (S) processes. These are stereocilia—nonmotile, formed by long, branching microvilli. They are to be distinguished from cilia (see Figure 1–7) by their irregularity in length and diameter and by the lack of basal bodies in apical cytoplasm; that is, they appear as simple, cytoplasmic extensions covered by the cell (plasma) membrane.

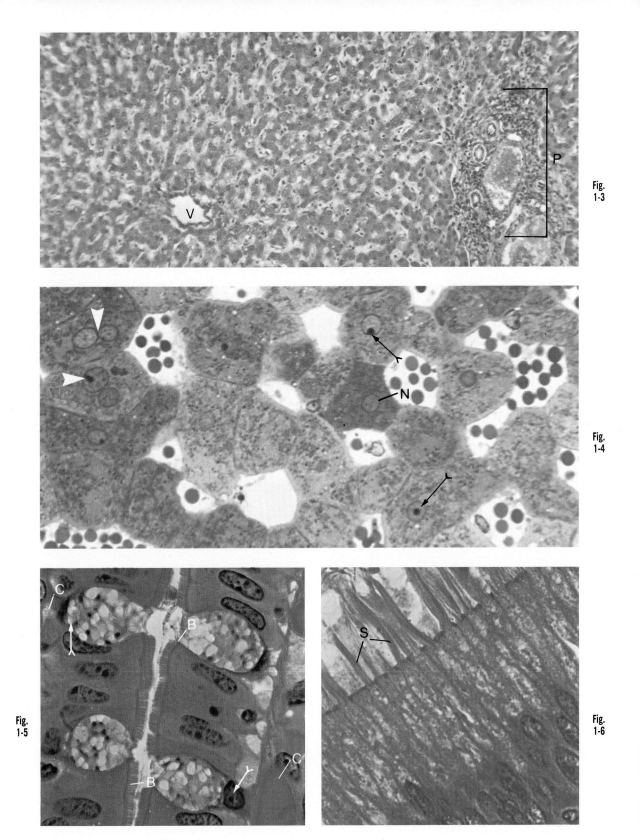

Fig.
1-3

Fig.
1-4

Fig.
1-5

Fig.
1-6

Figure 1–7. Trachea, cilia. Plastic section. H and E. Oil immersion.

At the luminal surface, most cells of the tracheal epithelium show the presence of cilia (C)—long, regular motile processes with basal bodies (B) in apical cytoplasm, giving the appearance of a densely staining (red) line just beneath the apical surface.

Figure 1–8. Pancreas, cytoplasmic basophilia. Plastic section. H and E. Oil immersion.

Cells are arranged in groups or acini around a small central lumen in the exocrine portion of the pancreas. (See Chapter 11.) Each cell is pyramidal in shape with a densely basophil cytoplasm (in the basal portion of the cell) (arrow). This is due to the presence on electron microscopy of an extensive granular endoplasmic reticulum and numerous associated ribosomes. Nuclei are located in basal cytoplasm; they are spheroidal and show prominent nucleoli (N). The apical cytoplasm is filled with eosinophil, closely packed, secretory droplets or granules (D). Also present is a small autonomic ganglion (G). The ganglion cells show large vesicular nuclei with prominent nucleoli, and abundant pale-staining cytoplasm with irregular clumps of basophil material, the Nissl bodies (arrowhead), composed also of granular endoplasmic reticulum.

Figure 1–9. Sensory ganglion, Golgi apparatus. Osmium tetroxide. High power.

The large spheroidal cells are ganglion cells, with large spherical nuclei, of a dorsal root ganglion. In the cytoplasm of these cells is an extensive network of dark (black) small vesicles and tubules. This is the Golgi apparatus appearing as a positive image. In these cells, the Golgi apparatus is scattered throughout the cytoplasm and around the nucleus and is extensive.

Figure 1–10. Duodenal epithelium, Golgi apparatus. Plastic section. H and E. Oil immersion.

The mucosal surface of the duodenum shows a negative image of the Golgi apparatus in a supranuclear position (arrows).

Figure 1–11. Liver, mitochondria. Osmic method. Oil immersion.

These large cells are from amphibian liver. The cytoplasm contains numerous small dark brown bodies, which are mitochondria. Nuclei are vesicular in type with prominent nucleoli.

Figure 1–12. Striated muscle, mitochondria. Plastic section. Toluidine blue. Oil immersion.

The muscle cells (fibers) are cut transversely. The pale (blue)-staining cytoplasm (sarcoplasm) contains myofibrils (not seen), and the dark blue, small spherical profiles are mitochondria. In these cells, mitochondria are elongated in the length of the fiber; thus, here also they are cut transversely and therefore appear small. Nuclei in these cells are peripheral in location and are multiple—the cells (arrows) each contain two nuclei in the plane of section.

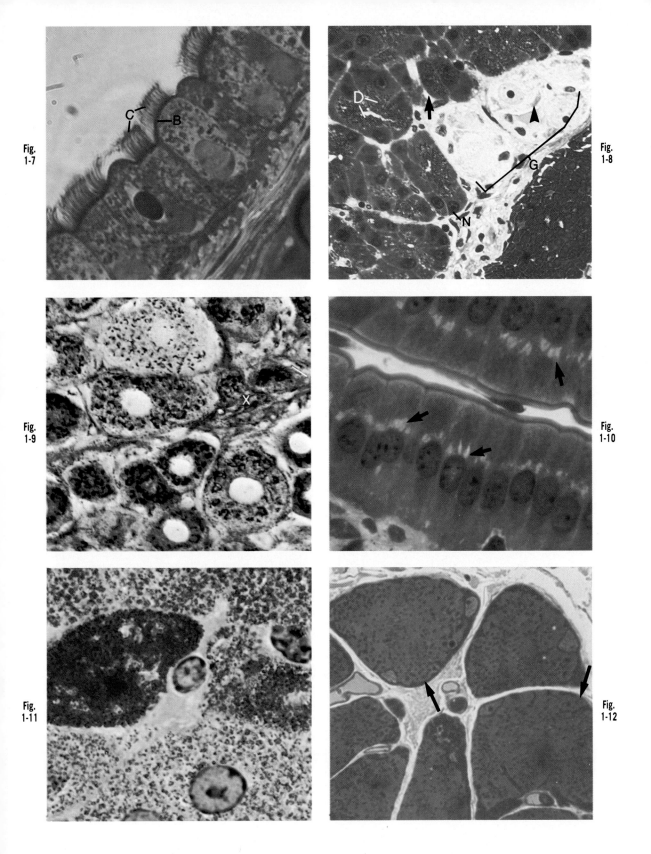

Fig. 1-7

Fig. 1-8

Fig. 1-9

Fig. 1-10

Fig. 1-11

Fig. 1-12

Figure 1–13. Pancreas, granules. Plastic section. Toluidine blue. Oil immersion.

The acini, or berry-like groups of pancreatic (exocrine) cells, are composed of cells with basophil cytoplasm. They contain numerous apical, spherical granules or droplets, here stained black. These droplets contain packets of digestive enzymes, which are later passed into the digestive tract. This is an exocrine (external) secretion. The cells of an islet of Langerhans (bottom left) are arranged in irregular cords and clumps with blood capillaries (C) between the cells. These cells are endocrine (*endos,* within), passing their secretion (hormones) into the blood vascular system. Several cell types are present in the islet, but all contain small dust-like, dark-staining granules. The secretion is mainly insulin and glucagon.

Figure 1–14. Breast, lipid. Sudan IV. High power.

Fat is stained red by this method and is present here in two cell types. The epithelial cells of secretory units (alveoli) (A) contain several small globules of lipid, while in the surrounding connective tissue are fat cells (F), each containing a large single droplet. Lipid normally is removed in preparation, and this is a frozen section. (See also Figures 3–11 and 3–12.)

Figure 1–15. Liver, glycogen. Best's carmine. Medium power.

Parenchymal cells of the liver contain stored glycogen, here seen as irregular, small clumps of red-staining material in the cytoplasm. Other inclusions and organelles are not seen, but nuclei are stained blue and appear vesicular with prominent nucleoli. (See also Figure 1–20.)

Figure 1–16. Epidermis, melanin. H and E. High power.

In the cells of the basal layers of the epidermis of skin are yellowish-brown cytoplasmic pigment granules (arrows). These granules, found characteristically on the apical (surface) side of the nucleus, are composed of melanin, an endogenous pigment formed in melanocytes. This is the pigment of suntanning and is more extensive in negroid races.

Figure 1–17. Ciliary body, melanin. Plastic section. H and E. High power.

The melanin granules are present in the pigmented layer of the ciliary epithelium (arrows), which rests on the stroma of the ciliary body.

Figure 1–18. Lymph node, carbon. H and E. Medium power.

Most cells present in this bronchial lymph node are small lymphocytes and plasma cells, but scattered among them are larger cells. These are macrophages (M) that have phagocytosed carbon, an exogenous pigment present here as black granules.

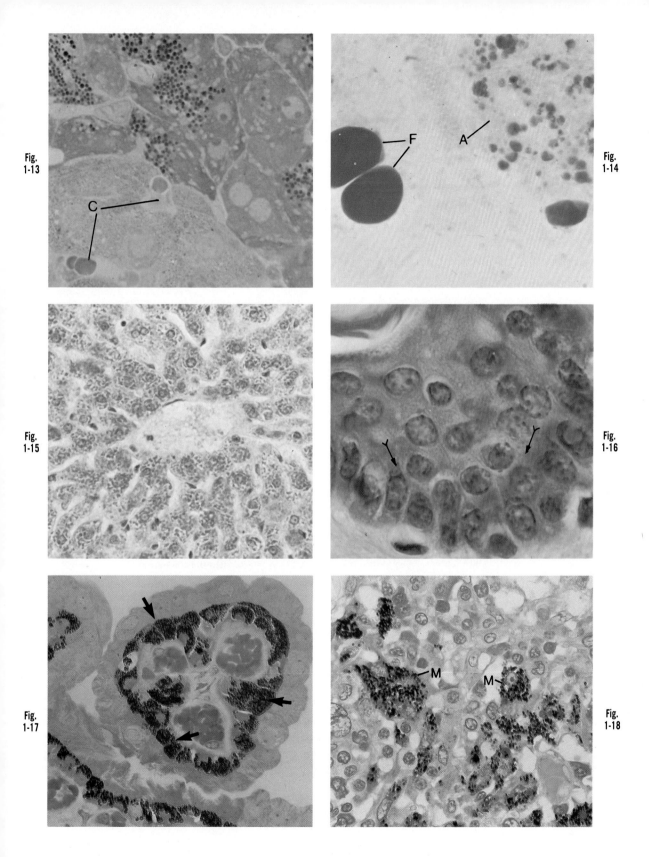

Fig. 1-13

Fig. 1-14

Fig. 1-15

Fig. 1-16

Fig. 1-17

Fig. 1-18

Figure 1–19. Autonomic ganglion, lipofuscin. H and E. High power.

Present in the ganglion cells (G) are discrete, yellowish granules of lipofuscin. These are actually residual bodies and often increase in number with age. Note the large nuclei of the ganglion cells, each showing a nuclear envelope; nuclear sap with fine, speckled chromatin masses; and a prominent nucleolus.

Figure 1–20. Liver, nuclei and glycogen. Plastic section. PAS, toluidine blue. Oil immersion.

Nuclei of parenchymal cells are large, spheroidal, and located centrally in cells. They show a nuclear envelope; irregular chromatin clumps in the nuclear sap; and, in some cells, prominent, large nucleoli (N). Nucleoli may be multiple, and in these liver cells, two nuclei may be present—a condition called polyploidy. In the cytoplasm are irregular masses of pink-staining glycogen. A few small, irregular, hyperchromatic or condensed nuclei (arrows) of cells associated with liver sinusoids also are seen.

Figure 1–21. DNA and RNA. Azure B. Oil immersion.

Both DNA and RNA are basophilic, but with Azure B, DNA stains green and RNA stains purple. DNA is seen only in the nuclei, whereas RNA is present mainly in the cytoplasm but also in the nucleoli. Note that nucleoli may be multiple.

Figure 1–22. Oral smear, Barr body. Aceto-orcein. Oil immersion.

This is a buccal smear, squamous epithelial cells having been scraped gently from the inside of the cheek and smeared onto a microscope slide. The nucleus shows a nuclear envelope, karyoplasm, and nuclear chromatin. Associated with the inner aspect of the nuclear envelope is a small, planoconvex, densely staining body (arrow). This is the Barr body, or sex chromatin, and indicates the presence of two X chromosomes, i.e., female sex. One X chromosome in an interphase nucleus is dispersed, that is, uncoiled. The other X chromosome of a female nucleus remains tightly coiled (i.e., heterochromatic) and is visible as the Barr body.

Figure 1–23. Neutrophil, sex chromatin. Giemsa. Oil immersion.

In this blood smear, many non-nucleated erythrocytes (red blood corpuscles) are present with one nucleated cell. This is a neutrophil, or polymorphonuclear leukocyte, and shows a large, irregularly lobated nucleus. Attached to one lobe of the nucleus by a fine strand of chromatin is a small nuclear appendage (arrow). This "drumstick" probably represents the sex chromosome and is found in only about 3 per cent of neutrophils in female blood.

Figure 1–24. Intestinal glands, mitosis. H and E. High power.

This is a transverse section through the bases of two intestinal glands in the terminal ileum. The tubular glands are lined by simple columnar epithelium. Several "mitotic figures" (cells undergoing mitosis) are seen. For cell division, which is active in the intestinal lining, cells round up, pass toward the lumen, and undergo mitosis to form two daughter cells. The visible stages are a late telophase (T), metaphase plates (M), an anaphase (A), and an early telophase (T_1).

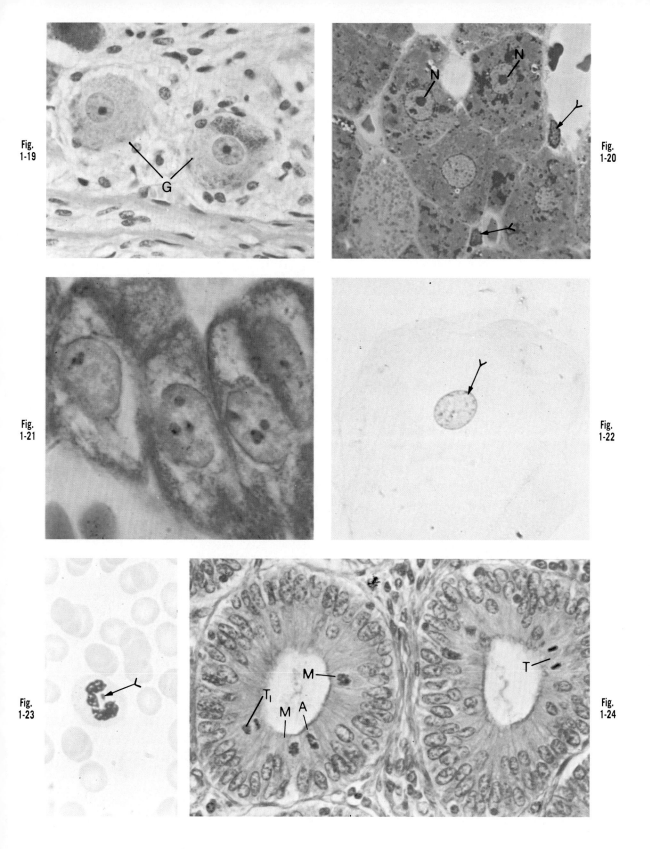

Fig.
1-19

Fig.
1-20

Fig.
1-21

Fig.
1-22

Fig.
1-23

Fig.
1-24

Figure 1–25. Mitosis. Pentachrome. Oil immersion.

This and the following three slides (Figs. 1–26 through 1–28) are of cells in tissue culture and show the stages of mitosis. Interphase nuclei (I) and one early prophase (P) are seen. Here, the cell is "rounding up," i.e., withdrawing its cytoplasmic process, and in the nucleus are irregular, darkly staining threads—these are the chromosomes. The cell at M shows a metaphase plate as seen from one pole of the cell. Chromosomes, or pairs of chromatids, lie at the equator of the cell, and the cell outline is defined clearly; that is, it has withdrawn its processes.

Figure 1–26. Mitosis. Pentachrome. Oil immersion.

The cell at left (P) has rounded up, the nuclear membrane is disappearing, and chromosomes are clearly visible. This is a late prophase. The cell A is somewhat elongated, and two groups of darkly staining daughter chromosomes are passing to opposite poles of the cell in anaphase.

Figure 1–27. Mitosis. Pentachrome. Oil immersion.

Apart from cells in interphase (I), the cell at T is in early telophase. Two daughter nuclei are commencing to re-form, although chromosomes still are visible; the cytoplasm is starting to constrict, the cleavage furrow deepening around the midbody. (The midbody is a mass of microtubules from the mitotic spindle located originally at the equator, now at the site of cytokinesis.)

Figure 1–28. Mitosis. Pentachrome. Oil immersion.

In the center, two daughter cells have nearly separated completely at the cleavage furrow (arrows), and the daughter nuclei are complete. Nuclear envelopes are visible, and chromosomes have dispersed, leaving only a speckling of nuclear chromatin. This is late telophase.

Figure 1–29. Tongue, primary tissues. Plastic section. H and E. High power.

Here, all four primary tissues are seen, each differing in appearance and function from the others. Epithelium (E) is represented by secretory units (acini)—groups of cells containing numerous pink-stained secretory droplets or granules. Connective tissue is present as strands of collagen (C) between acini and around groups of acini, and as fat cells (F). Muscular tissue occurs as striated muscle fibers cut in longitudinal (ML) and transverse (MT) sections, showing cytoplasmic fibrils (myofibrils). These cells have peripherally located nuclei. Nervous tissue is seen as a transverse section of a peripheral nerve (N), a bundle of nerve fibers (nerve cell processes), and supporting tissue. All organs are formed from these four basic tissues, often all four being present in the same organ, as here.

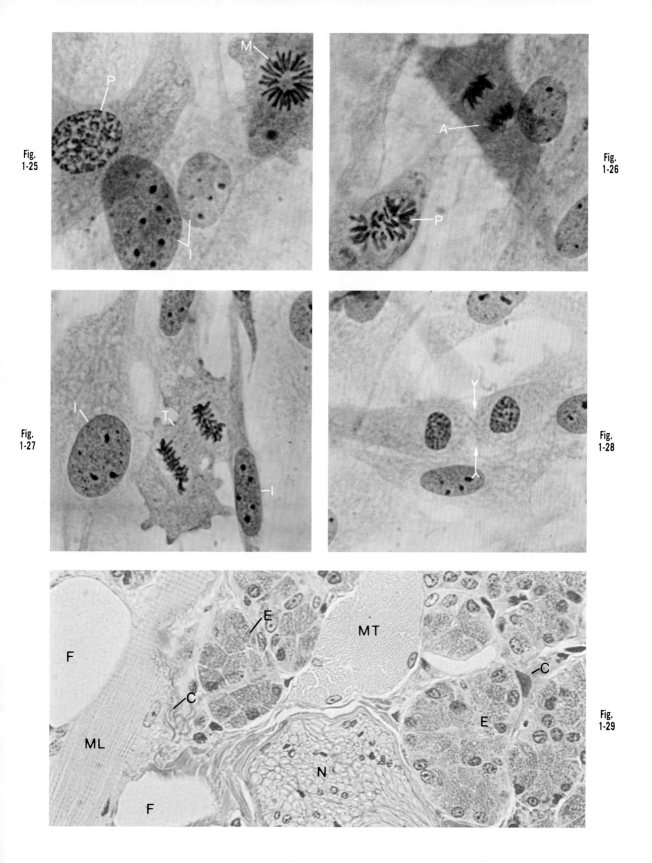

Fig.
1-25

Fig.
1-26

Fig.
1-27

Fig.
1-28

Fig.
1-29

21

TWO

Epithelium

Typically, epithelium consists of closely packed cells with little or no intercellular material between the cells. Epithelial tissues occur as *membranes* and as *glands*.

Membranes are sheets of cells that cover an external surface or line an internal surface; thus, all materials that enter or leave the body either do so through an epithelial membrane or have been secreted, or modified, by epithelial cells. These membranes are involved in one or more of many processes such as protection, absorption, secretion, excretion, digestion, sensation, and contractility. All epithelia rest upon or are surrounded by a basal lamina (please see Chapter 3), and membranes are supported by connective tissue containing blood and lymph vessels and nerves. There are no blood vessels within epithelium itself, and nutrition thus depends upon diffusion of oxygen and metabolites from blood vessels in the underlying connective tissue.

Glands are formed by epithelial cells mainly specialized for secretion, and they develop from epithelial surfaces by downgrowths or ingrowths into underlying connective tissue. In *exocrine* glands, the connection to the surface remains as the duct of the gland, the secretion passing externally to the surface. In *endocrine* glands, the surface connection is lost and the gland secretion (a hormone) passes internally to the vascular system. As with membranes, glands are embedded in and supported by connective tissue containing vessels and nerves.

Characteristically, most epithelia have a capacity for renewal, cell replacement occurring by mitosis. The rate of renewal varies with the location and type of epithelium; for example, the rate is very rapid in the epithelium lining the small intestine (see Figure 1–24).

MEMBRANES

Epithelial cells in membranes are basically of three types only:
1. *Squamous*—cell height is much less than width.
2. *Cuboidal*—height and width are approximately equal.
3. *Columnar*—height exceeds width.
All, however, may be of irregular shape.

Membranes are classified on this basis of cell shape and by their arrangement in one or more layers. *Simple* epithelium consists of cells arranged in a single layer, all cells extending from the basal lamina to the surface. A *pseudostratified* epithelium is one in which all cells contact the basal lamina but not all reach the surface. Thus, while basically it is formed by a single layer of cells, different cell types are present and this gives the appearance of several layers. A *stratified* or *compound* epithelium is composed of several layers of cells, only the deepest being in contact with the basal lamina. By using cell shape, it then is possible to classify further, e.g., simple squamous, simple cuboidal, and simple columnar. Pseudostratified columnar epithelia may be ciliated or nonciliated. In stratified epithelia, it is the shape of the surface layer of cells only that determines the classification of stratified squamous, stratified cuboidal, or stratified columnar. A special type of stratified epithelium is the *transitional epithelium* lining the urinary tract. Examples of varieties of simple squamous epithelium are the lining of vascular and lymphatic vessels and the heart, termed *endothelium*, and that covering serous membranes of the body cavities, called *mesothelium*.

Most epithelial membranes line wet cavities, such as the oral cavity, the ureter, and the intestines, and in these locations they are one component of *mucous membranes*. A mucous membrane, or mucosa, is the moist inner lining of viscera formed by an epithelial membrane supported by a layer of areolar connective tissue (the lamina propria) and separated from it by a basal lamina. In some locations, beneath the lamina propria is a third layer of smooth muscle, the muscularis mucosae. The exception is the epithelium or epidermis on the skin surface, a dry surface; here the stratified squamous epithelium is keratinized, the flat surface cells undergoing a transformation into a tough, resistant, nonliving layer of material called *keratin*.

In all epithelial cells, the shape of the nucleus conforms to that of the cell, being parallel to the long axis of the cell. Thus, the nucleus is spheroidal in cuboidal cells, flattened in squamous cells, and ovoid in columnar cells. In view of the fact that epithelial cell outlines often are difficult to discern (i.e., the plasma membrane may not be seen clearly), nuclear shape often is important in cell identification. Most cells show polarity in respect to organelles, for example, cytoplasmic basophilia and mitochondria basally or mainly infranuclear, a supranuclear Golgi apparatus, and apical secretory material. Also, there are commonly specializations of the cell surface, such as microvilli—which sometimes are so numerous and closely packed as to be visible on light microscopy as a striated or brush border (Fig. 1–5), motile cilia, and nonmotile stereocilia. The lateral cell interfaces may be highly irregular, with "jig-saw" or "zipper" interlocking. Between plasma membranes of adjacent cells is a small amount of cement substance with desmosomes, terminal bars, and junctional complexes. In cells of some stratified epithelia, numerous cell-to-cell contacts are made, these appearing as "intercellular bridges." At basal cell surfaces, invaginations of the plasma membrane may be present, a mechanism for increasing surface area.

Epithelial cells in membranes perform a variety of functions, one of which is secretion. In many locations, the epithelial surface area is insufficient to accommodate the large number of secretory cells required, and glands therefore develop.

GLANDULAR EPITHELIUM

Several criteria are used to classify glands. *Unicellular* glands are seen as goblet, mucus-secreting cells in respiratory and intestinal epithelia, but most glands are *multicellular*. The distinction between exocrine (external secreting) and endocrine (internal or hormone-secreting) glands has already been mentioned. According to the mechanism by which the secretory product is released from the cell, exocrine glands are classified as *merocrine, holocrine,* or *apocrine.* In merocrine glands, secretory droplets or granules are simply extruded from the cell, a process of exocytosis, with no loss of cytoplasm. In holocrine glands, the cells are filled with secretory material and the entire cell is shed and forms the secretion. In apocrine cells, the apical cytoplasm supposedly is discharged and lost with the secretory material.

A further classification involves the nature of the duct system and the shape of the secretory unit. Simple glands have a single duct, whereas in compound glands the ducts branch repeatedly. In most glands, the secretory units may be tubular, either straight or coiled, or acinar (berry- or grape-like). The term *alveolar* (bag-like) is often used synonymously with acinar, although a larger, sack-like secretory unit often is termed *saccular.* In some glands, both acinar (alveolar) and tubular units are present. Additionally, glands are classified on the nature of the secreted material as *serous* (a watery, usually protein- or enzyme-containing fluid) or *mucous* (a sticky, viscid, glycoprotein-containing material). Additionally, *"mixed"* acini are present in some glands. In these, a mucous acinus has at its blind end a few serous cells arranged as a crescent or demilune, these cells passing their secretion to the lumen via slender intercellular channels. Both serous and mucous units may be present in "mixed" glands. Thus, a compound, tubuloalveolar mixed gland is one with repeated branchings of the duct system and both alveolar and tubular secretory units, some being serous and others being mucus-secreting.

Ducts in compound glands are lined by epithelium that varies with the size of the duct and the nature of the gland. In many glands, the duct cells are involved in secretion, or in modifying the secretory product. Most multicellular glands are enclosed in a connective tissue capsule, divided into lobes; the lobes in turn are divided into lobules. Within lobules, the ducts (intralobular) generally are lined by a simple squamous or cuboidal epithelium. Often, one duct (the lobular) leaves each lobule and several join to form interlobular ducts, lying in the connective tissue between lobules and lined usually by a simple high cuboidal or columnar epithelium. In turn, interlobular ducts unite to form a lobar duct, and the lobar ducts join to form a main duct. The larger ducts are lined by stratified epithelia, often with a supporting smooth muscle coat in addition to connective tissue.

Endocrine glands (which will be considered in later chapters) are of two main types according to cell arrangement into groups and hormone storage:

1. Most endocrine cells contain secretory material, and the cells are arranged in anastomosing cords and clumps between blood vessels; such glands are of the "cord and clump" type.

2. In the second type, secretory material is released from cells and stored temporarily in large, usually globular masses surrounded by the secretory cells. These are the "follicle" type.

In some organs, such as the pancreas, both exocrine and endocrine functions are performed.

Figure 2–1. Lip: epithelia. Iron hematoxylin, aniline blue. Medium power.

To the left is a thick, stratified squamous, nonkeratinizing, epithelial membrane (S), the surface cells being squamous, and supported by relatively dense fibroconnective tissue (C). This is a "wet" membrane, and the epithelium together with the supporting connective tissue composes the oral mucous membrane or mucosa. To the right are secretory units, both alveolar (A) and tubular (T), formed by clear-staining mucous cells. Ducts are not apparent, but the duct system is branched in this compound, mucous, tubuloalveolar gland.

Figure 2–2. Mesothelium and endothelium (simple squamous epithelium). Plastic section. Methylene blue, basic fuchsin. Oil immersion.

Shown is the mesothelium (E) *(above)* of the epicardium covering the outer surface of the heart. This is simple squamous in type, although classified as mesothelium, being derived from mesoderm and lining all the serous cavities (pleura, pericardium, and peritoneum). Also seen is endothelium (E_1) lining a blood capillary, simple squamous in type, and both show flattened nuclei and attenuated cytoplasm. The mesothelium is supported by relatively dense connective tissue with collagen fibers (C) and nuclei of fibroblasts (F).

Figure 2–3. Mesothelium. Silver technique. Oil immersion.

This is a flat preparation of the peritoneal lining, where cell outlines are clearly visible and show irregularity. The nuclei of the mesothelial cells (blue) have been counterstained lightly.

Figure 2–4. Kidney, simple epithelia. Plastic section. H and E, PAS. Oil immersion.

These tubules, cut in transverse section, are lined by simple epithelial membranes of several types, each tubule bounded by a basal lamina (here stained dark pink). The epithelial types are simple squamous (S), simple cuboidal (C), and simple columnar (L). Also present are blood capillaries lined by endothelium (E).

Figure 2–5. Seminal vesicle, simple columnar epithelium. Plastic section. H and E. High power.

The lining mucous membrane of the seminal vesicle is composed of loose areolar connective tissue (the lamina propria) (L) and simple columnar epithelium (C), and it is complexly folded. Cell interfaces in the epithelium are seen clearly, nuclei are basal in location, and apical cytoplasm is extensive and pale-staining.

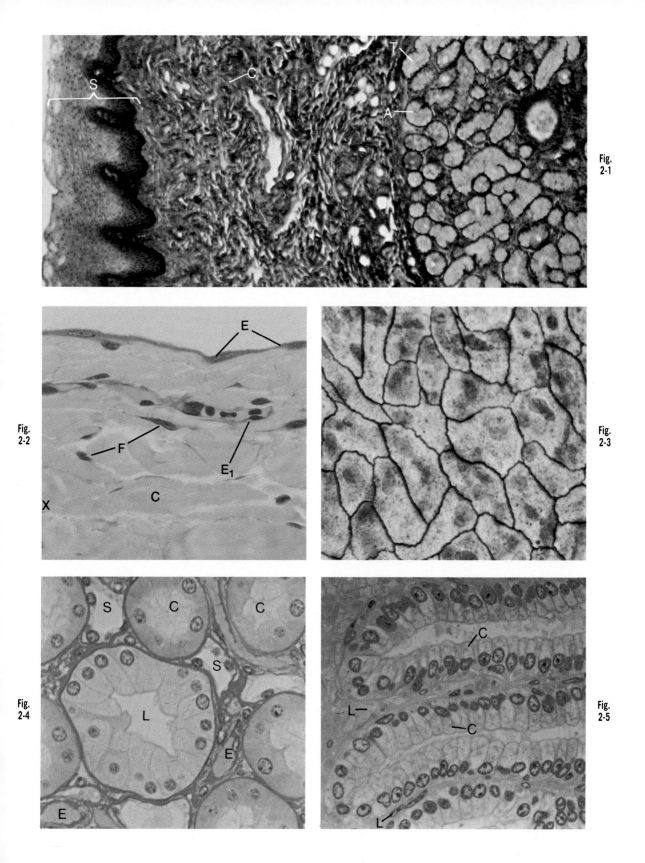

Fig.
2-1

Fig.
2-2

Fig.
2-3

Fig.
2-4

Fig.
2-5

27

Figure 2–6. Vagina, stratified squamous epithelium. Plastic section. H and E. Medium power.

This nonkeratinized epithelium shows a basal layer of cuboidal cells, several layers of polygonal cells that become progressively more squamous, and surface squamous cells. The surface cells desquamate constantly, being replaced by mitosis in the basal layer. There are no glands in the vagina, but the wet mucosal surface is lubricated by mucus from cervical glands. This epithelium is supported by relatively dense connective tissue (the lamina propria) (L), the two forming the vaginal mucosa.

Figure 2–7. Thick skin, epidermis. H and E. Medium power.

Epidermis, the outer covering of skin, is a stratified squamous keratinizing epithelium and is supported by connective tissue of the dermis. The interface between the two is irregular, with pegs and ridges (P) of dermis protruding into epidermis. Several layers or strata are seen in the epidermis—the stratum basale or germinativum (B), a single row; several rows of spiny cells (see Figure 2–8) of the stratum spinosum (S); the granule-containing cells of the stratum granulosum (G); a poorly seen thin, translucent stratum lucidum (L); and, superficially, a thick stratum corneum (C) composed of many layers of clear, dead, scale-like cells lacking nuclei. The duct of a sweat gland (D) is shown.

Figure 2–8. Tongue, intercellular bridges. Plastic section. H and E. Oil immersion.

In both types of stratified squamous epithelia, keratinized and nonkeratinized, cells in the stratum spinosum show "intercellular bridges" (I). There is no cytoplasmic continuity between cells, but each bridge is formed by short cytoplasmic processes of adjacent cells, the two processes meeting at a desmosome, or macula adherens.

Figure 2–9. Stratified columnar epithelium. Plastic section. H and E. High power.

The lobar duct of the sublingual salivary gland lies in dense connective tissue. The epithelium has a basal layer of small cuboidal cells and an apical layer of columnar cells.

Figure 2–10. Transitional epithelium. Plastic section. H and E. High power.

The urinary tract is subject to variations in internal pressure and capacity and is lined by a special type of stratified epithelium (transitional), the appearance of which varies between stratified columnar and stratified squamous. In the relaxed ureter seen here, surface cells are cuboidal; with distention they become squamous.

Figure 2–11. Trachea, pseudostratified, ciliated columnar epithelium. Mallory. Oil immersion.

Several different cell types are present in the epithelium; all contact the basal lamina, but not all reach the lumen. Nuclei appear at different levels. Most of the cells are of the tall columnar type with cilia (C). Also seen are small basal cells (B) and goblet cells (G) with apical, pale-staining cytoplasm distended with mucous secretory material. (See also Figure 1–7.)

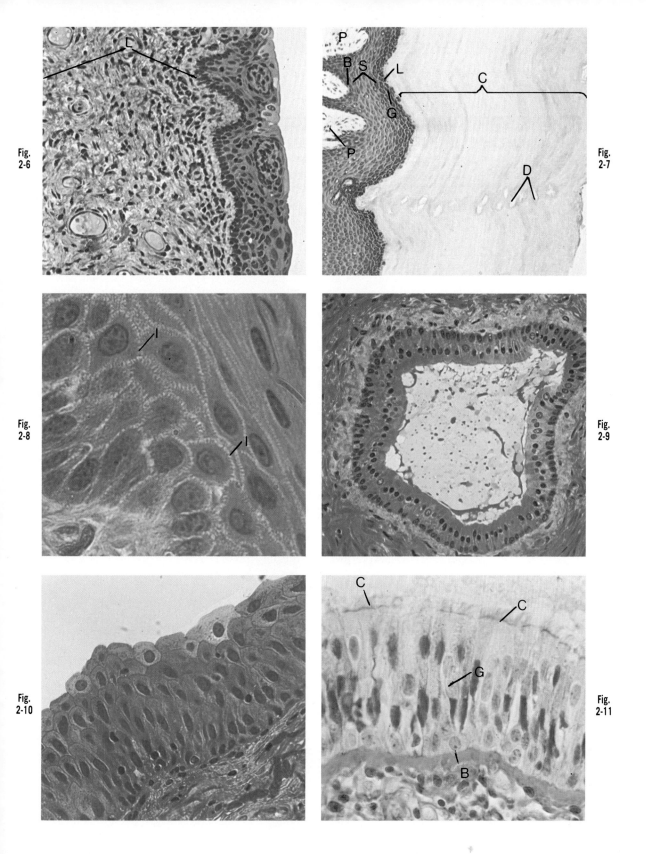

Fig.
2-6

Fig.
2-7

Fig.
2-8

Fig.
2-9

Fig.
2-10

Fig.
2-11

Figure 2–12. Pseudostratified columnar epithelium. Plastic section. H and E. High power.

This epithelium of the ductus epididymidis is formed mainly by tall columnar cells with apical stereocilia (S) and some basal cells (B). Nuclei thus lie at different levels in this pseudostratified epithelium. Terminal bars (T) stain dark pink on cell interfaces near the lumen. (See Figure 1–6.)

Figure 2–13. Goblet cells, jejunum. Plastic section, Mallory trichrome. Oil immersion.

The small intestine is lined by simple columnar epithelium (enterocytes, E) with ovoid nuclei (N) and with a brush border (arrowheads). The dark pink dots on lateral cell interfaces near the lumen represent terminal bars (arrows). Numerous goblet cells (G) are present in the epithelium; these are unicellular glands that secrete a protective lubricating mucus. (Mucus is discharged into the lumen at M.) (See Figure 1–5.)

Figure 2–14. Tongue, mucous and serous acini. Plastic section. H and E. Oil immersion.

Mucous acini (M) have pale-staining cells with "foamy" cytoplasm and dense, irregular nuclei at their bases, seemingly compressed against the basal lamina. Serous acini (S) are seen as clusters of cells with basally located, spherical, vesicular nuclei and apical cytoplasm filled with discrete, eosinophil secretory droplets or granules. Also present are striated muscle fibers (F) and a small peripheral nerve (N).

Figure 2–15. Mixed acini, submandibular gland. Plastic section. Masson. Oil immersion.

A branching mucous acinus (M) shows serous crescents or "demilunes" (S). The mucous cells are pale-staining with condensed basal nuclei. The serous cells of the crescents contain pink-staining discrete cytoplasmic droplets or granules and pass their secretion into the lumen of the acinus by slender intercellular canals between mucous cells.

Figure 2–16. Simple tubular glands, colon. H and E. Medium power.

Simple tubular glands (crypts) pass from the surface (arrows) into the underlying connective tissue (lamina propria) (L) and are lined by a simple columnar epithelium with numerous pale-staining goblet cells (G). Underlying the lamina propria is a thin muscularis mucosae (M) of smooth muscle.

Figure 2–17. Myoepithelial cells. Masson trichrome. High power.

These are the ducts of labial mucous glands, lined by pale-staining, simple cuboidal epithelium (C). Thin slips of dark pink cytoplasmic processes (arrows), some containing nuclei (arrowheads), lie within the basal laminae of the ducts and are seen particularly well in ducts cut obliquely (top center and left). These are processes of myoepithelial (basket) cells that have an octopus-like shape, are contractile, are of epithelial and not mesodermal origin, and surround the acini and smaller ducts of many glands.

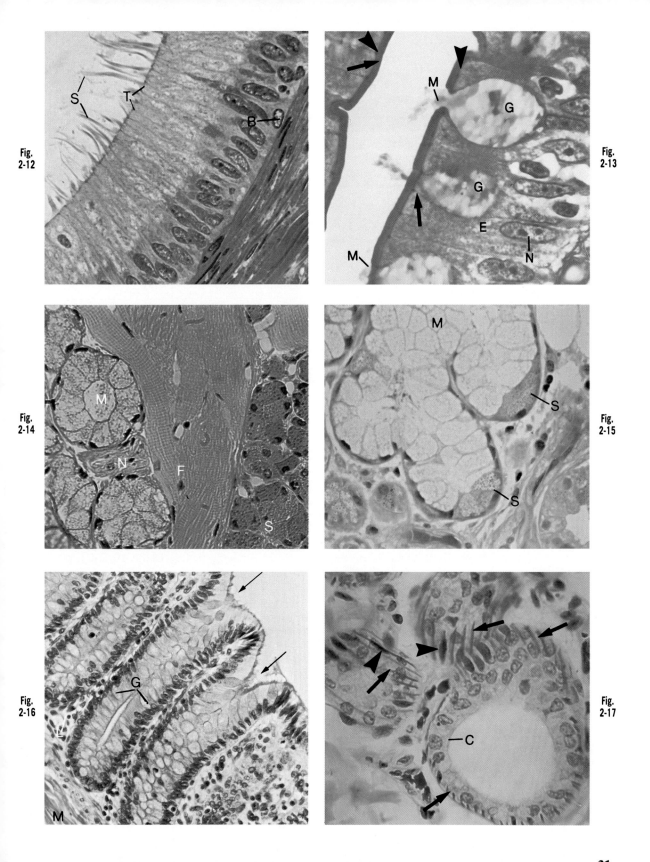

Fig. 2-12

Fig. 2-13

Fig. 2-14

Fig. 2-15

Fig. 2-16

Fig. 2-17

Figure 2–18. Submandibular gland. Hematoxylin, phloxine, safranin. Low power.

This gland is classified as a compound, tubuloalveolar, mixed gland. This implies that the duct system is branched (compound), that there are both tubular and alveolar types of secretory units (tubuloalveolar), and that both serous- and mucous-secreting cells are present (mixed). In fact, some acini are serous and some are mucous, and mixed acini also are present. The gland is divided into lobes, each lobe subdivided into lobules, with fine connective tissue around lobules and denser connective tissue (yellow) between lobes. Details of alveoli and ducts cannot be seen. Parts of several lobes are seen, each composed of several lobules, one lobule being outlined by the interrupted line. Ducts are labeled as intralobular (1), lobular (i.e., the main duct leaving a lobule) (2), interlobular (3), and lobar (4). Lumen diameter increases from intralobular to lobar, and the lining epithelium increases in height. Thus, it is simple cuboidal in type in intralobular ducts and stratified columnar in the lobar duct. As ducts increase in size, they are associated with increasingly denser connective tissue.

Figure 2–19. Endocrine gland, cord and clump type. Plastic section. H and E. High power.

Blood vessels (V), mainly capillaries, lie around and between groups of epithelial cells arranged in short, anastomosing cords. These are cells of the suprarenal medulla, and they have large vesicular nuclei and finely granular cytoplasm. The arrangement of cells and blood vessels is such that each medullary cell is believed to be related on one surface to a capillary and on one other to a venule. These cells contain epinephrine and norepinephrine and also are called *chromaffin* cells because their granular content is oxidized by potasssium bichromate (the chromaffin reaction), their granules becoming brown. (See also Figure 1–13.)

Figure 2–20. Endocrine gland, follicle type. Plastic section. H and E. High power.

Whereas secretory material of cord- and clump-like endocrine glands is stored within the secretory cells (i.e., it is intracellular), in the follicle type the secretion is released from the cells and stored in follicles. In the thyroid gland, seen here, secretory material stains pink and is present in follicles (vesicles) of various sizes, each follicle having a "wall" of low, cuboidal, secretory cells (T). Between follicles is a little connective tissue containing numerous blood capillaries (C). The pink-staining material in the follicles is called *colloid*, and, when required, it passes back through the cells lining the follicle and into neighboring capillaries.

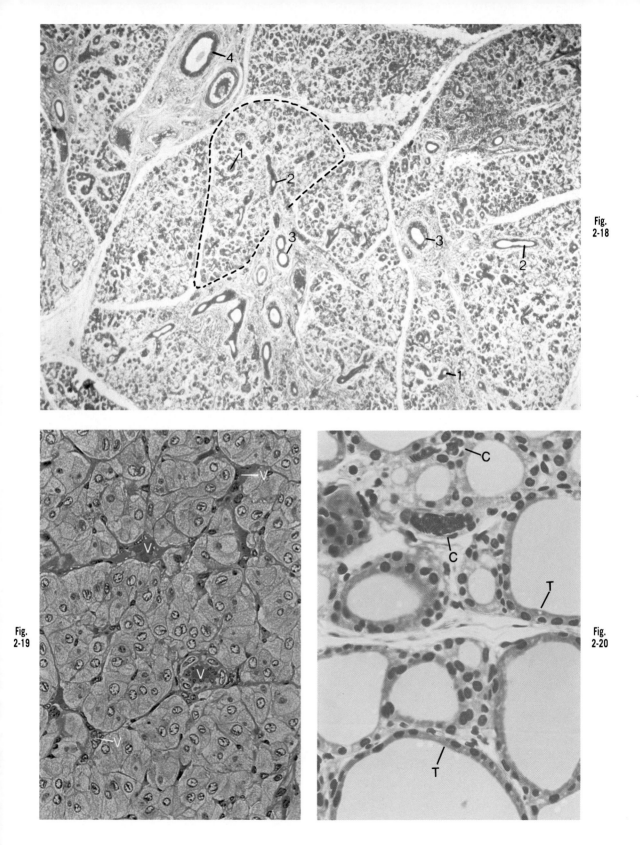

Fig.
2-18

Fig.
2-19

Fig.
2-20

33

THREE

Connective Tissue Proper

Mesenchyme, derived from mesoderm, the third germ layer, gives rise to the connective, or supporting, tissues of the body. These include the connective tissue proper, cartilage, bone, and blood.

Connective tissues differ from epithelia in the presence of abundant intercellular material or matrix. Matrix is composed of fibers and an amorphous ground substance. In connective tissues, the proportions of cells and intercellular substance show considerable variation and form the basis of classification, which is inexact since various types are linked by transitional forms. In any type of connective tissue, therefore, there are three elements to consider: (1) amorphous ground substance, (2) fibers, and (3) cells.

AMORPHOUS GROUND SUBSTANCE

This material, semifluid to solid in consistency, occupies the spaces between the cells and fibers of connective tissue. It provides a medium through which tissue fluid, containing nutrients and waste products, can diffuse between cells and the blood vascular system. It contains glycosaminoglycans, glycoproteins, carbohydrates, lipids, and water. Usually, two kinds are recognized: *ground substance,* which is soft, and *cement substance,* which is firmer. The material exists as sols and gels and, having the same refractive index as water, is invisible in fresh preparations. It is not a conspicuous feature of routine sections, since much of it is extracted by the usual fixatives. It does stain metachromatically (purple) with toluidine blue because of a content of glycosaminoglycans.

Basal laminae, or basement membranes, are layers of condensed intercellular material present at the boundaries between epithelium and connective tissue and around muscles, nerves, capillaries, and fat cells. They vary in thickness and are rich in proteoglycans. They stain intensely with the periodic acid–Schiff (PAS) reaction and with silver techniques, but are poorly demonstrated in hematoxylin and eosin (H and E) preparations. Basal laminae are synthesized by the related cells and probably play an important role in the diffusion of oxygen and metabolites. In addition, they serve as limiting and supporting membranes around epithelia and other cell types.

FIBERS

Fibers are the chief factor responsible for strength and support of tissues. Three types of formed fiber exist, and they are distinguished by their appearance and chemical reactions. All are complex proteins, and are comparatively insoluble in neutral solvents. Thus, they exist as fibers in the fluid internal environment of the body.

Collagenous Fibers. Collagenous or white fibers are formed extracellularly from tropocollagen molecules that are only 280 nanometers (nm) long and 1.4 nm in diameter. These molecules are lined up in parallel rows to form a microfibril or unit fiber of collagen, visible by electron microscopy as a thread with characteristic cross-banding, 4.5 to 100 nm in diameter and of indefinite length. In turn, bundles of microfibrils form a collagen fibril, 0.3 to 0.5 micron, or micrometer (μm), in diameter and visible with the light microscope. The fibrils do not branch or unite, and groups of fibrils are held together by cementing substance to form fibers, varying in diameter from 1 to 12 μm. The fibers show a longitudinal striation and may appear to branch and reunite owing to an interchange of fibrils between fibers. They are acidophil and stain pink or red with H and E, red with van Gieson's stain, blue with Mallory's stain, and blue or green with Masson's trichrome stain.

Reticular Fibers. Reticular fibers are of small diameter (0.2 to 1 μm) and typically branch to form a network or reticulum around, for example, small blood vessels, muscle and nerve fibers, fat cells, and underlying epithelia. They can be stained specifically with the PAS technique and with silver (hence, they often are termed "argyrophil"). They are composed of unit fibers of collagen, having an identical periodicity or cross-banding. Their staining properties, which are different from those of collagen fibers, probably are due to their high content of hexoses.

Elastic Fibers. Elastic fibers occur both as individual fine fibers and as extensive broad sheets or laminae. The fibers are thick, highly refractile, and occur either as cylinders or as flat ribbons that range in diameter from less than 1 μm to 4 μm or more. They are formed from the union of a globular protein, elastin, with microfibrils of glycoprotein. On electron microscopy, elastic fibers show a central amorphous material with peripheral microfibrils 13 nm in diameter. In fresh material, elastic fibers are visible as highly refractile, homogeneous, shining threads. In fixed material, they stain lightly with eosin but are best demonstrated by special stains that contain orcein or resorcin fuchsin. With the latter, they appear as a network of long, delicate, anastomosing fibers.

CELLS

The cells of connective tissue proper may be grouped according to the frequency of their appearance. The two most common cells are fibroblasts and macrophages (or histiocytes). Less common are undifferentiated mesenchymal cells, fat cells, mast cells, and lymphoid cells. Eosinophil cells, plasma cells, and pigment cells generally are seen rarely.

Fibroblasts. Fibroblasts are the most characteristic cells and are associated with the production of collagenous, reticular, and elastic fibers. They are fusiform or stellate cells with long cytoplasmic processes. After fixation, however, little cytoplasmic detail can be recognized, and the principal feature is an elongated, ovoid nucleus with fine chromatin granules and one or more large nucleoli.

Macrophages. Macrophages, or tissue *histiocytes,* belong to the macrophage (reticuloendothelial) system, a collective term applied to a widespread system of highly phagocytic cells. The cells possess no morphological characteristics that distinguish them with certainty from other cells. Generally they are ovoid or irregular in shape, with plentiful cytoplasm and an oval or reniform nucleus that is smaller and more densely staining than that of a fibroblast. They are identified by their ability to engulf nontoxic colloidal dyes and particulate matter.

Mesenchymal Cells. Undifferentiated mesenchymal cells are thought to persist in adult connective tissue. They are difficult to distinguish from fibroblasts, but in general are smaller and often are located along the walls of blood vessels, particularly capillaries, where they are referred to as *perivascular cells.*

Fat Cells. Fat cells are large, ovoid or spherical, with a thin rim of cytoplasm and a flattened or compressed nucleus at the periphery. A large lipid inclusion occupies the majority of the cytoplasm. In fresh or formalin-fixed tissue, the lipid inclusion can be stained with osmic acid or with one of the Sudan dyes, but in most preparations the lipid is extracted, leaving only the delicate protoplasmic envelope.

Mast Cells. Mast cells are large and frequently are associated with blood vessels. They contain numerous prominent cytoplasmic granules that stain metachromatically with basic aniline dyes such as azure A and toluidine blue. Mast cell granules, which also can be visualized by supravital staining with neutral red, contain both heparin and histamine.

Lymphoid and Plasma Cells. Lymphocytes and plasma cells also occur within connective tissue and play an important role in the defense mechanism. Lymphocytes are small cells with little visible cytoplasm and a spherical, deeply stained nucleus. Plasma cells, spherical or ovoid in shape, have a spherical nucleus that usually is eccentrically situated and exhibits coarse chromatin granules. The chromatin often is clumped at the margin of the nucleus in a cartwheel pattern.

Eosinophil Cells. Eosinophil granulocytes possess reniform or bilobed nuclei and a cytoplasm that contains spherical granules which are highly refractile and stain with acid dyes. Other white blood cells that may be found in connective tissue are neutrophil granulocytes, but generally these escape into connective tissue from capillaries only in regions of inflammation. They may be recognized by the multilobation of the nucleus.

Pigment Cells. Pigment cells are rarely seen in connective tissue. Some pigment cells, the melanocytes, have irregular cytoplasmic processes that contain small pigment granules, the melanosomes. In addition to melanocytes, the connective tissue dermis of the skin may contain melanophores—macrophages that have phagocytosed melanosomes from disintegrating melanocytes.

CLASSIFICATION OF CONNECTIVE TISSUES

The major subdivision in the classification of connective tissues is determined by the concentration of fibers. Connective tissues that show an abundance of compactly arranged fibers are referred to as *dense* connective tissues. In *loose* connective tissues, there are fewer fibers and relatively more cells. Loose connective tissues may be further subdivided into those that are present only in the embryo (*mesenchyme* and *mucous* connective tissue) and those that are found in the adult. The latter include loose *areolar* connective tissue, *adipose* tissue, and *reticular* tissue.

Loose Connective Tissue

Mesenchyme. Mesenchyme is the unspecialized connective tissue of early embryonic life. It is composed of mesenchymal cells and of a ground substance that is fluid in the earliest stages but later contains fine fibrils.

Mucous Connective Tissue. This is a transient tissue that appears during the normal development and differentiation of the connective tissues. Component cells are large and stellate fibroblasts. The ground substance is soft and contains a delicate meshwork of fine collagenous fibers.

Areolar Tissue. Loose (areolar) connective tissue is formed by direct differentiation of mesenchyme. It forms the *stroma,* or framework, of organs and is the embedding medium of many structures, including blood vessels and nerves. All the structural elements—cells, fibers, and ground substance—are present within it. In some sites, it forms the supporting framework for the epithelium of mucous membranes, and here it is referred to as the *lamina propria.* In such sites, the connective tissue usually is very cellular and may contain large numbers of lymphoid cells.

Adipose Tissue. Fat cells are scattered in loose connective tissue, but when they form large aggregations and are the principal cell type, the tissue is designated adipose tissue. The closely packed fat cells form lobules, separated by fibrous septa.

Reticular Tissue. A primitive type of connective tissue, reticular tissue is characterized by the presence of a network of reticular fibers associated with primitive reticular cells, not unlike mesenchymal cells in appearance. Reticular tissue forms the framework of lymphoid organs, bone marrow, and liver.

Dense Connective Tissue

Dense connective tissues show a close packing of fibers. In areas where tensions are exerted in all directions, the fibers are without regular orientation and the tissues are termed *irregularly arranged.* In structures subject to tensions principally in one direction, the fibers show an orderly parallel arrangement and are designated *regularly arranged.* In most regions collagenous fibers are the main component, as in fascia, fibrous capsules, tendons and ligaments, but in a few ligaments, elastic fibers predominate.

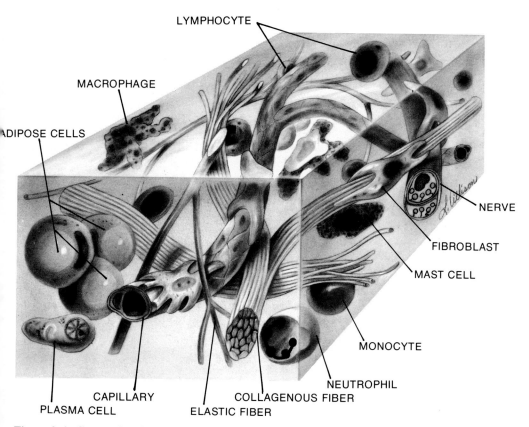

Figure 3–1. Connective tissue.

This is a diagrammatic representation of subcutaneous, loose areolar connective tissue. The characteristic cell and fiber types are shown.

Figure 3–2. Kidney: basal laminae. Plastic section. PAS and hematoxylin. High power.

The red-staining material that surrounds each cross section of the kidney tubules and blood capillaries is a basal lamina, or basement membrane. It is a complete thin layer intimately related to the epithelial cells of the tubules or to the endothelium of the capillaries.

Figure 3–3. Connective tissue of lip: fibers. Iron hematoxylin, aniline blue. High power.

Two fiber types, collagenous and elastic, are demonstrated. Collagenous fibers (blue) generally are coarse and show a faint longitudinal striation owing to their component fibrils. Elastic fibers (black) are less numerous and more delicate than collagenous fibers and appear homogeneous. Fat cells (arrows) occur between the fibers.

Figure 3–4. Liver: reticular fibers. Wilder's silver method. High power.

The section shows the central vein of a liver lobule with radiating columns of liver cells. The black-staining reticular fibers are concentrated around the central vein and extend between the columns of liver cells in relation to blood vascular spaces (sinusoids). The fibers are of small diameter and form a delicate network.

Figure 3–5. Lymph node: reticular fibers. Plastic section. Silver. High power.

Delicate reticular fibers (brown-black) are present within the capsule (top) and in relation to a concentration of lymphocytes (center). The space beneath the capsule, the subcapsular sinus, also contains numerous lymphocytes. The cells generally exhibit a dense, spherical nucleus and a thin rim of cytoplasm.

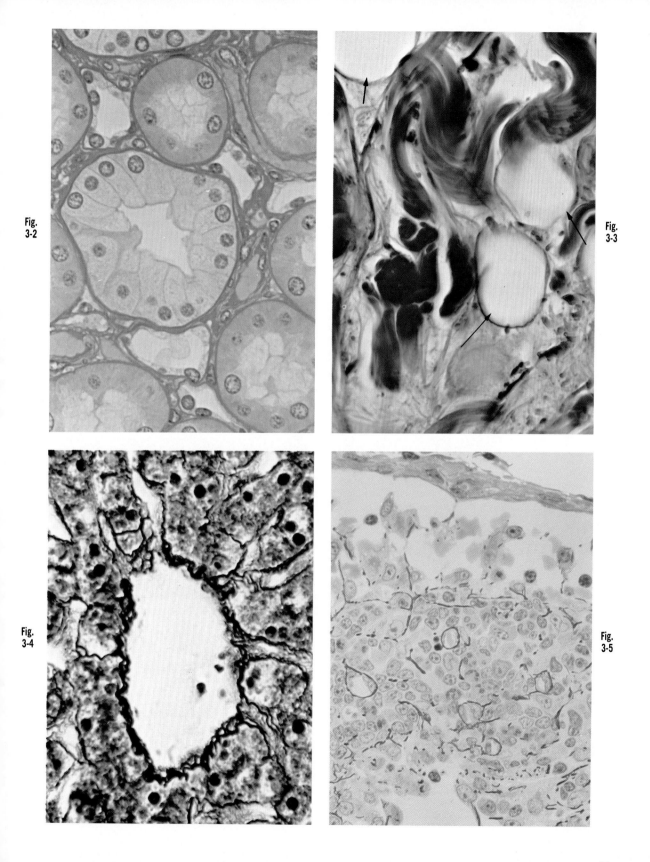

Fig.
3-2

Fig.
3-3

Fig.
3-4

Fig.
3-5

Figure 3–6. Areolar connective tissue: elastic fibers. Verhoeff's elastic stain. Medium power.

This is a "spread" preparation, not a section, of mesentery. Elastic fibers (dark brown-black) are thin, homogeneous threads that branch and anastomose to form a loose network. Most appear straight (under tension), but some are curled into loose spirals (relaxed).

Figure 3–7. Vein: elastic fibers. Weigert's stain. Medium power.

Elastic fibers, stained brown, are concentrated in relation to the lumen of the vein (above) as a convoluted, complete internal elastic lamina, and appear as individual fibers, often sectioned transversely or obliquely, in the underlying coats of the venous wall.

Figure 3–8. Dense connective tissue: fibroblasts. H and E. High power.

Coarse collagenous fibers are sectioned longitudinally and exhibit a faint longitudinal striation. A few cells, mostly fibroblasts (arrows), lie within the matrix between fibers. Generally, they appear fusiform in shape and show a pale nucleus, with a distinct nucleolus, and little cytoplasm. A macrophage (M) exhibits a distinct cell outline and a dense, spherical nucleus.

Figure 3–9. Lymph node: macrophages and reticular cells. H and E. High power.

The section shows a portion of the subcapsular sinus, which is bridged by reticular cells that are interconnected by delicate cytoplasmic processes. Also present are macrophages that show accumulations of carbon particles within their cytoplasm. This particulate matter has been ingested by the cells from the surrounding lymph.

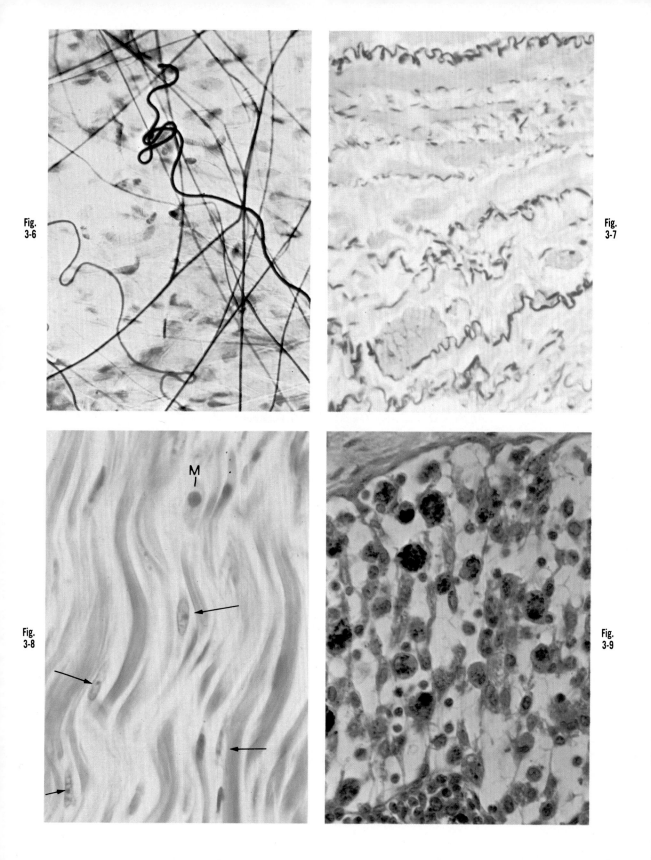

Fig.
3-6

Fig.
3-7

Fig.
3-8

Fig.
3-9

M

Figure 3–10. Mesenchyme. Plastic section. H and E. High power.

The tissue is composed of irregularly spindle-shaped cells with processes that extend into a relatively homogeneous ground substance devoid of formed fibers. The cells show a spherical or ovoid nucleus with a distinct nucleolus. Two cells (arrows) are in the process of mitosis. The tissue is vascular, and portions of three small blood vessels (C), lined by a delicate endothelium, are present.

Figure 3–11. Fat cells. Plastic section. Toluidine blue. High power.

Three fat cells are present. The cell to the right contains a single large droplet of fat surrounded by a thin rim of cytoplasm that contains a distinct oval nucleus. Because this tissue was fixed in osmic acid, the fat has been preserved. This section also shows a transverse section of a small nerve (N) and a mast cell (M), from which some granules have escaped into the surrounding tissue.

Figure 3–12. Fat cells. Osmic acid. Medium power.

Fat cells, in which the content of fat has been preserved, appear closely opposed in this section of adipose tissue. No details of the protoplasmic envelope can be discerned.

Figure 3–13. Mast cells. Plastic section. Toluidine blue. High power.

In this section of tongue, mast cells lie within the connective tissue between skeletal muscle fibers (M). They are ovoid in shape and show large numbers of granules that stain metachromatically (dark purple). The cells show nuclei, although commonly nuclei are masked by the crowded granules. Also present are collagenous fibers and a fibroblast (F).

Figure 3–14. Plasma cells. Plastic section. H and E. High power.

In this section of the mucosa of the gastrointestinal tract, the epithelium is of the tall columnar type (upper left) and the loose areolar tissue of the lamina propria (lower right) is very cellular and contains numerous plasma cells. The cells generally are ovoid in shape, with a densely staining nucleus that is eccentrically placed. Clumping of chromatin at the margin of the nucleus is apparent in most cells, and some show a negative Golgi image (arrows).

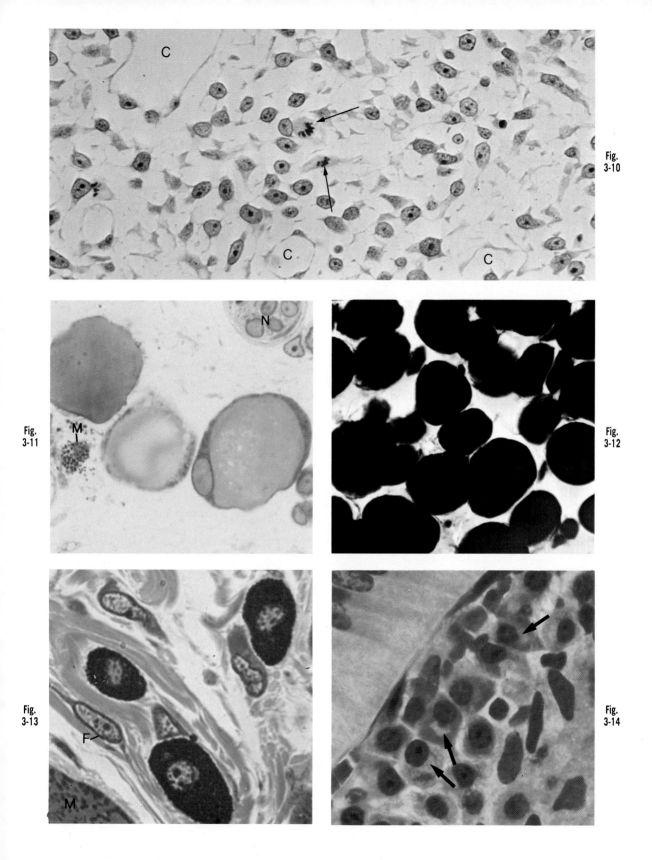

Figure 3–15. Mucous connective tissue. H and E. Medium power.

Component cells are large, stellate fibroblasts with spherical or ovoid nuclei. Delicate collagenous fibers (pink) form a loose network within the ground substance and show no definite spatial organization.

Figure 3–16. Fetal hypodermis: differentiation of loose (areolar) connective tissue. H and E. Medium power.

Early during fetal life, the hypodermis is composed of mesenchyme. As development proceeds, differentiation into loose connective tissue occurs. In this section fibroblasts constitute the principal cell type. They appear fusiform in shape; since they generally have been sectioned on the side, their nuclei appear slender and densely stained. The tissue is vascular and shows numerous small blood vessels, sectioned transversely.

Figure 3–17. Loose areolar connective tissue. Spread preparation. H and E, orcein. High power.

Elastic fibers (black) are slender and form a branching three-dimensional network. The large, ovoid, darkly staining cells are mast cells, the nuclei of which are masked by large numbers of cytoplasmic granules.

Figure 3–18. Adipose tissue. Mallory's stain. Medium power.

A portion of a lobule of adipose tissue is shown, and a fibrous septum, composed principally of collagenous fibers, is present at the top left. In this preparation, only the delicate protoplasmic envelope (blue) of each fat cell is seen. Occasional nuclei (red) may be seen within the thin rim of cytoplasm. Blood capillaries (arrows), containing red blood cells, indicate the rich vascularity of this tissue.

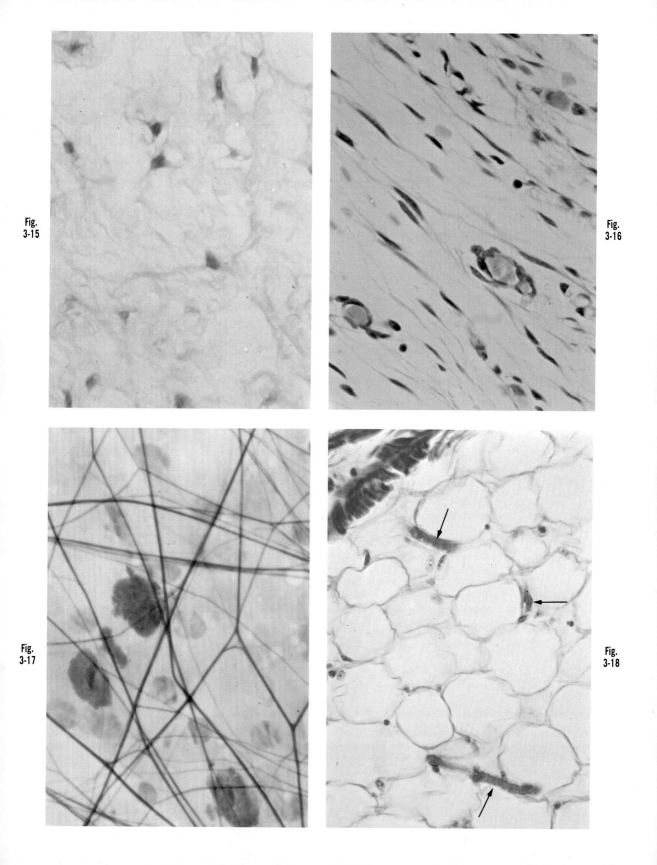

Fig.
3-15

Fig.
3-16

Fig.
3-17

Fig.
3-18

Figure 3–19. Adipose tissue. Plastic section. H and E. High power.

A thin rim of cytoplasm (red) surrounds the large fat globule, which has been dissolved in preparation. Occasional nuclei (blue), with distinct nucleoli, may be seen within the thin rim of cytoplasm.

Figure 3–20. Brown adipose tissue. Plastic section. H and E. Medium power.

Portions of two lobules of brown adipose tissue are shown, separated by loose connective tissue containing small blood vessels (bottom center). The fat cells contain numerous lipid droplets that do not coalesce. Thus, brown adipose tissue is referred to as *multilocular*, in contrast to *unilocular* white adipose tissue.

Figure 3–21. Reticular tissue. Mallory's stain. Medium power.

In this section of the medulla of a lymph node, the majority of the field is occupied by reticular tissue. Reticular cells, interconnected by delicate cytoplasmic processes, form a network that delineates irregular medullary sinuses. The cells are supported by reticular fibers, not stained specifically in this preparation. At the periphery, there are concentrations of small lymphocytes that form medullary cords.

Figure 3–22. Tendon. H and E. Medium power.

Tendon, here sectioned longitudinally, is an example of dense regular connective tissue in which the principal fibrous component is collagen. Each collagenous fiber (pink), or primary tendon bundle, possesses a longitudinal striation, since it is composed of a large number of fibrils. The fibers tend to follow a wavy course. Fibroblasts are aligned in rows between the collagenous fibers. Their cytoplasm is indistinct, and only the elongated nuclei are seen. The collagen fibers are grouped into fascicles, each bounded by a more cellular connective tissue, the peritendineum (arrows).

Figure 3–23. Tendon. Plastic section. H and E. High power.

Portions of two fascicles, sectioned longitudinally, are shown. In the right-hand fascicle, collagen fibers are separated by fibroblast nuclei that appear ovoid. No associated cytoplasm is visible. In the left-hand fascicle, fibroblast nuclei are sectioned on the side and appear dense and elongated. A portion of the cellular peritendineum, containing small blood vessels, occupies the center of the field.

Figure 3–24. Tendon. Transverse plastic section. H and E. High power.

The fibroblasts, or *tendon cells*, appear stellate in shape with delicate cytoplasmic processes extending between the large collagenous fibers. Blood capillaries lie within a connective tissue septum (bottom).

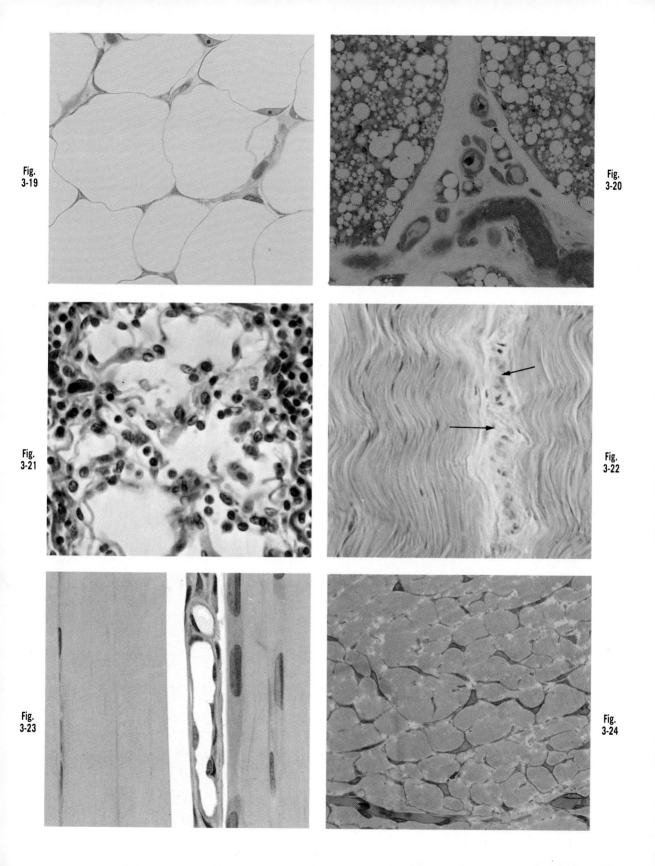

CHAPTER
FOUR

Specialized Connective Tissue: Cartilage and Bone

Cartilage and bone, the skeletal tissues, are specialized connective tissues and, like all connective tissues, are composed of three elements: (1) *cells*, (2) *fibers,* and (3) *ground substance*, the latter two constituting the intercellular substance or matrix. Skeletal tissues differ from the connective tissues proper in the rigidity of their matrices.

CARTILAGE

Cartilage, like other connective tissues, develops from mesenchyme. Mesenchymal cells round up and become closely packed, and collagenous fibers are deposited within the ground substance. The cells, now termed *chondroblasts*, elaborate further ground substance and the fibers become masked. As the cells differentiate further and gradually become more separated as a result of the elaboration of matrix around them, they acquire the characteristics of mature cartilage cells, or *chondrocytes*. The cells occupy small cavities or lacunae within the matrix. The ground substance is gel-like and consists principally of proteoglycans, which have a protein core with covalently bound chondroitin sulfate and keratan sulfate side chains. Ground substance is markedly basophil and stains metachromatically with toluidine blue. It also gives a positive reaction with periodic acid-Schiff (PAS) staining.

Cartilage increases in size by two methods:

1. *Interstitial growth*, which occurs in relatively young cartilage that is malleable enough to allow internal expansion.

2. *Appositional growth*, a process in which new layers of cartilage are added

to the surface from activity within the inner layer of perichondrium, the fibrous envelope surrounding cartilage.

Mature cartilage is a nonvascular tissue and is classified on the basis of differences in type and amount of fibers present within the matrix:

1. *Hyaline cartilage* is the fundamental and most common type. Its matrix contains collagenous fibers that are not visible in ordinary preparations.

2. *Elastic cartilage*, fundamentally similar to hyaline cartilage, has a preponderance of elastic fibers that frequently concentrate in the walls of the lacunae that surround chondrocytes.

3. *Fibrocartilage*, which never occurs alone but merges gradually into neighboring hyaline cartilage or with dense fibrous tissue, contains massed, coarse collagenous fibers within its matrix. The fibers run parallel to the direction of the principal stress on the structure of which the fibrocartilage is a part, and chondrocytes typically are aligned in rows between the collagenous bundles, with little matrix around the cells.

BONE

Composition. Bone (or osseous tissue) is a rigid form of connective tissue that constitutes most of the adult skeleton. The matrix contains an inorganic component, principally calcium phosphate, that accounts for approximately two thirds of the weight of bone. Macroscopically, bone is either spongy (*cancellous*) or compact (*dense*). The differences between the two types depend on the relative amount of solid matter and the size and number of spaces in each. They both contain the same histological elements: bone cells (osteoprogenitor cells, osteoblasts, osteocytes, and osteoclasts) and matrix. The osteocytes lie principally within small cavities or lacunae in the matrix, which consists of collagenous (osteocollagenous) fibers arranged in bundles with a cementing substance between that contains the inorganic salts. Characteristically, the matrix is arranged in layers or lamellae and is permeated by fine canaliculi linking adjacent lacunae and occupied in part by fine cytoplasmic processes of the osteocytes. The outer surface of bone is covered by a fibrous sheath (the periosteum), and a delicate layer of connective tissue (endosteum) lines the marrow cavity and extends as a lining into the canalicular system of compact bone.

Preparation. Because of its mineral content, special preparations are needed to examine bone: Two of the most common are *ground sections* and *decalcified sections*.

Ground sections are prepared from bone that is allowed to dry and is then cut into thin slices with a saw. The slices then are ground to sufficient thinness with fine grinding stones. The architecture of dense bone is well displayed, but unfortunately the relationship of bone to soft tissues is destroyed. The preparations may be treated with India ink to highlight the spaces that formerly were occupied by organic matter. In such material, the canaliculi, lacunae, and Haversian canals (occupied by blood vessels) appear black.

In decalcified sections, the cellular and organic components are retained, and the mineral content is removed by treating the tissue with demineralizing solutions such as chelating agents or acids. After decalcification, bone can be embedded and sectioned in the normal manner. These preparations retain the relationships between bone and related soft tissues, but cells tend to be shrunken and details of the matrix are blurred owing to swelling of osteocollagenous fibers caused by the reagents used.

Growth and Development. Bone has certain unique qualities that must be borne in mind when consideration is given to the methods by which a bone develops and increases in size. Briefly, these are:

1. The presence of a canalicular system, tiny canals which allow for the exchange of metabolites between the blood stream and the bone cells.

2. The presence of an internal vascular system located within Haversian and Volkmann's canals.

3. The presence of an inorganic component within the matrix that prevents expansion within the interior. Consequently, bone can grow only by the appositional mechanism.

4. The nonstatic nature of bone architecture—bone is destroyed locally and re-formed repeatedly. There is thus a continuous process of reconstruction.

Bone development is of two types, *intramembranous* and *endochondral* (or *intracartilaginous*). The actual process of bone deposition is the same in both cases.

In intramembranous ossification, bone develops directly on or within membrane (i.e., a condensed sheet of mesenchyme). Osteoblasts differentiate within primitive loose connective tissue, thin bars of dense intercellular substance appear between them, and minerals are deposited in an orderly fashion. Some osteoblasts are engulfed in the matrix and become osteocytes; others proliferate and form a layer on the surface of the new island of bone. These cells continue to elaborate and mineralize bone matrix. As growth continues at several foci of bone formation, initially the bone consists of spicules and trabeculae, and it is spongy in type. Later, some of this spongy bone is replaced by compact bone as the areas between trabeculae are filled with concentric lamellar bone.

Endochondral ossification occurs in those bones in which, after the laying down of bone matrix, continued growth in length is necessary. The early cartilage model, surrounded initially by a perichondrium, increases in size by both interstitial and appositional growth. Bone formation is initiated within a band-shaped area of perichondrium surrounding the diaphysis, and simultaneously there is calcification of the cartilaginous matrix within the center of the diaphysis. The area is invaded by blood vessels from the bony collar and is replaced by bone. It constitutes the primary ossification center. Later, secondary centers of ossification, the epiphyseal centers, develop toward the ends of the cartilage model. Continued longitudinal growth of the model occurs in the cartilage between the primary and secondary centers. As a result of this and of extension of the primary ossification center, definite zones of activity become established within the cartilage. Passing toward the primary ossification center, the following zones can be recognized:

1. *Quiescent or reserve zone.* This zone, composed of primitive hyaline cartilage, shows growth in all directions.

2. *Zone of proliferation.* This is an active zone showing numerous mitoses. The daughter cells resulting from the mitotic activity align themselves in distinct rows or columns parallel to the long axis of the bone.

3. *Maturation zone*. Cells lying in continuity with the columns of the previous zone enlarge owing to accumulation of glycogen in their cytoplasm. Mitoses no longer occur.

4. *Zone of calcification*. The matrix surrounding the enlarged cells becomes calcified and stains deeply basophil owing to the deposition of minerals.

5. *Zone of retrogression*. The cartilage cells die and undergo dissolution, as does the matrix between cells. Vascular primary marrow extends into the spaces resulting from the destruction of cells and matrix.

6. *Zone of ossification*. Osteoblasts that accompany the vascular tissue deposit bone matrix on the surface of the remnants of calcified cartilage.

7. *Zone of resorption*. As ossification extends toward the ends of the cartilage, resorption of bone occurs in the center of the diaphysis to extend the marrow cavity.

Eventually, with the spread of ossification, there is replacement of cartilage by bone except in two regions. Cartilage remains over the free ends as articular cartilage and as a plate, the epiphyseal plate or disc, between the primary and secondary ossification centers. When growth ceases, the epiphyseal plate is replaced by bone. Later, as a result of extensive remodeling, the initial spongy bone is mostly replaced by compact bone.

JOINTS

Two principal types of joints are distinguished:

1. *Synarthroses*, those that are immovable or only slightly movable.

2. *Diarthroses*, or synovial joints, freely movable joints with a joint cavity interposed between the participating bones.

In synarthroses, the union may occur by dense fibrous tissue (syndesmoses) or by cartilage (synchondroses). In diarthroses, the articular cartilage usually is hyaline in type, but often the matrix contains abundant collagenous fibers. Its deepest layer is calcified and firmly adherent to the bone it covers. The bones of the joint are united by a joint capsule of dense fibrous tissue continuous with the periosteum of the bones. Often it is thickened in regions to form the ligaments of the joint. Its inner layer, the synovial membrane, lines the joint cavity, except over articular cartilages. This synovial membrane is thin and vascular, containing large caliber capillaries and, more deeply, concentrations of fat cells. At its surface are one to three layers of synovial cells, the majority of which resemble macrophages and are phagocytic, with fewer cells that have the appearance of fibroblasts. It is the synovial membrane that produces the synovial fluid which acts as a lubricant and contributes to the nutrition of the articular cartilage.

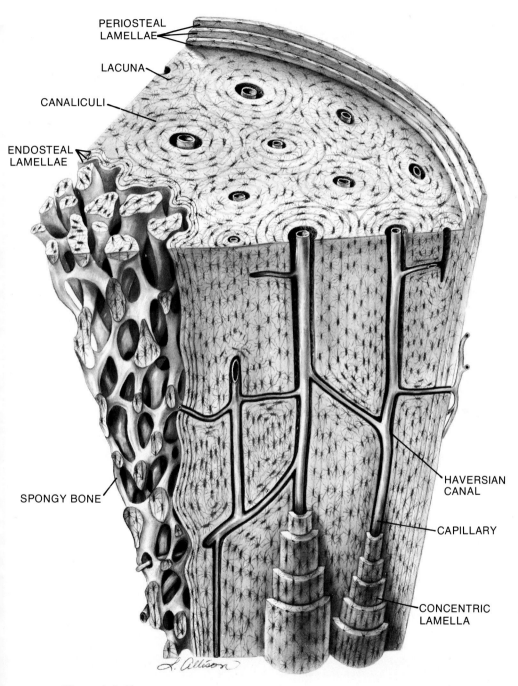

Figure 4–1. Bone.

This is a diagrammatic representation of a small portion of compact bone.

Figure 4–2. Embryonic hyaline cartilage. Mallory's stain. Medium power.

Chondrocytes, with spherical nuclei (red) and a vacuolated cytoplasm, are closely packed and generally uniform in size. They are separated by little intercellular substance (pale blue). At the periphery of the cartilage mass, the surrounding mesenchyme is concentrated as the perichondrium (left and right). Component cells here are elongated and are associated with concentrations of collagenous fibers (dark blue). The perichondrium merges gradually into the cartilage on one side and into the surrounding mesenchyme on the other.

Figure 4–3. Hyaline cartilage. H and E. Medium power.

The chondrocytes that lie centrally within mature hyaline cartilage are large and tend to be arranged in groups or cell "nests" (arrows). Each group represents the offspring of a single parent chondrocyte (interstitial growth). Peripherally the cells are smaller and individually arranged. All chondrocytes occupy lacunae within the matrix, which appears homogeneous and stains blue-gray. Collagenous fibers within the matrix are not readily apparent. The perichondrium (left) is composed of fibroblasts, with dense, elongated nuclei, and of elastic and collagenous fibers (pink). Next to the cartilage, the perichondrium appears more cellular and merges into cartilage. This appearance indicates that cells of the inner zone of perichondrium may transform into cartilage cells and surround themselves with intercellular substance (appositional growth).

Figure 4–4. Hyaline cartilage. Plastic section. Alcian blue. High power.

This section shows a narrow band of hyaline cartilage surfaced by perichondrium (lower left). Lacunae within the matrix, occupied by chondrocytes, are not readily apparent, since the chondrocytes completely fill and conform to the shape of the lacunae. The cells show a finely granular cytoplasm that contains discrete vacuoles, which represent the sites of fat droplets, lost during preparation. The matrix surrounding chondrocytes is rich in proteoglycans and stains intensely (territorial matrix or the cartilage capsules).

Figure 4–5. Elastic cartilage. Verhoeff's elastic stain. Medium power.

Within the matrix, there are extensive networks of specifically stained elastic fibers. Generally, the fibers are large and densely packed within the interior of the cartilage. Chondrocytes also are large within the interior and tend to be smaller toward the perichondrium (left and right).

Figure 4–6. Elastic cartilage. Weigert's stain. High power.

The arrangement of elastic fibers (purple) within the matrix is clearly apparent. They are concentrated in the matrix immediately in relation to the lacunae. Chondrocytes tend to be large and arranged in small cell nests centrally, but are smaller and individually aligned toward the periphery (left).

Figure 4–7. Fibrocartilage. H and E. Medium power.

Fibrocartilage is composed principally of bundles of dense collagenous fibers (pink) that are regularly arranged. Between the bundles are chondrocytes that lie in lacunae within small regions of hyaline cartilaginous matrix (pale blue–purple). The chondrocytes typically occur in short rows between the collagenous bundles.

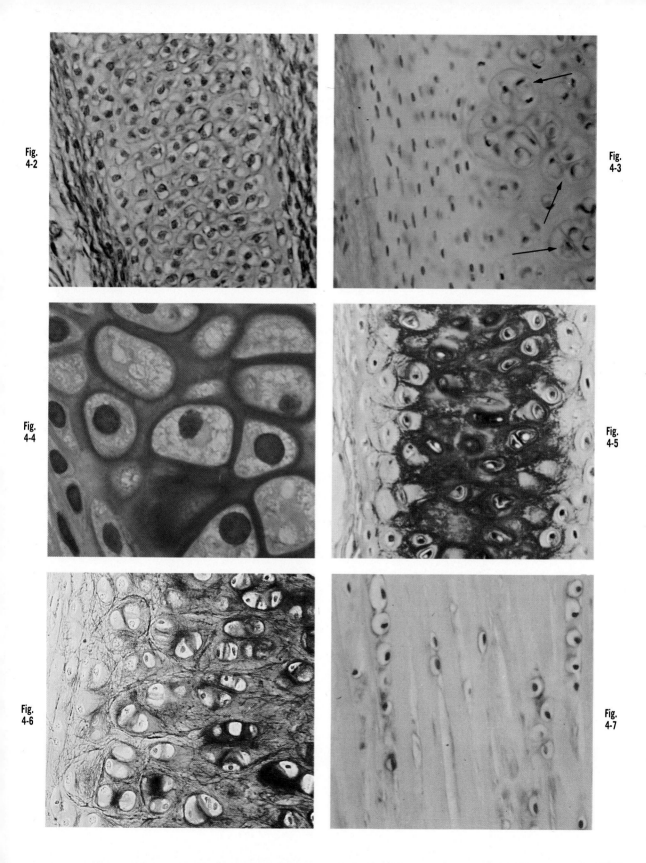

Fig.
4-2

Fig.
4-3

Fig.
4-4

Fig.
4-5

Fig.
4-6

Fig.
4-7

Figure 4–8. Spongy (cancellous) bone. Decalcified section. H and E. Low power.

In a decalcified section such as this, details of the matrix are not apparent. It appears homogeneous (pink), and the small dark areas within it are lacunae occupied by osteocytes. The spicules of bone are separated by bone marrow.

Figure 4–9. Compact (dense) bone. Ground section. Medium power.

In compact bone, the arrangement of lamellae is determined by the distribution of blood vessels, which lie in channels within the matrix. Volkmann's canals enter the bone and communicate with Haversian canals that run in the longitudinal axis of the bone. Each Haversian canal is surrounded by a number of concentric lamellae. The lamellae, the cells, and the central canal constitute the Haversian system. Here, several Haversian systems are sectioned transversely. Each Haversian canal is surrounded by lamellae, and lacunae, which in life contain osteocytes, occur between the lamellae. At the lower right (arrows), there is a small group of interstitial lamellae. These represent the remnants of Haversian systems that were partially destroyed during internal reconstruction of the bone.

Figure 4–10. Compact (dense) bone. Ground section. High power.

The central portion of one Haversian system or osteon in transverse section is shown. The Haversian canal (center) is surrounded by concentric lamellae, with lacunae (black) between the lamellae. In life, the lacunae contain osteocytes. Fine canaliculi radiate from them to interconnect all lacunae with the central canal, thus permitting nutrition of all osteocytes by vessels in the canal.

Figure 4–11. Compact bone. Ground longitudinal section. High power.

Portions of two Haversian systems are separated by an artefactual gap, representing a Haversian canal. Although lamellae, lacunae, and canaliculi are well defined, the concentric nature of the lamellae is not apparent in longitudinal sections.

Figure 4–12. Osteoblasts and osteoclasts. Azan. High power.

Two spicules of bone (blue), developing in mesenchyme, are shown. Numerous osteoblasts, cuboidal or pyramidal in shape, form an almost continuous row in relation to the surface of the bony trabeculae. They have large nuclei and a markedly basophil cytoplasm. Three large osteoclasts (arrows) also occur in relation to the developing bone. These are multinucleated giant cells with a granular cytoplasm.

Figure 4–13. Sharpey's fibers. H and E. Medium power.

At lower right is bone (B) with osteocytes (dark blue) in lacunae. The bone surface is covered by periosteum (P). Above are two bundles of collagenous (tendon) fibers (T), which penetrate the periosteum (arrowheads) to enter bone matrix as Sharpey's fibers, thus anchoring the tendon firmly to bone. Around the tendon and between the two bundles is adipose tissue (a). (See Figure 11–17.)

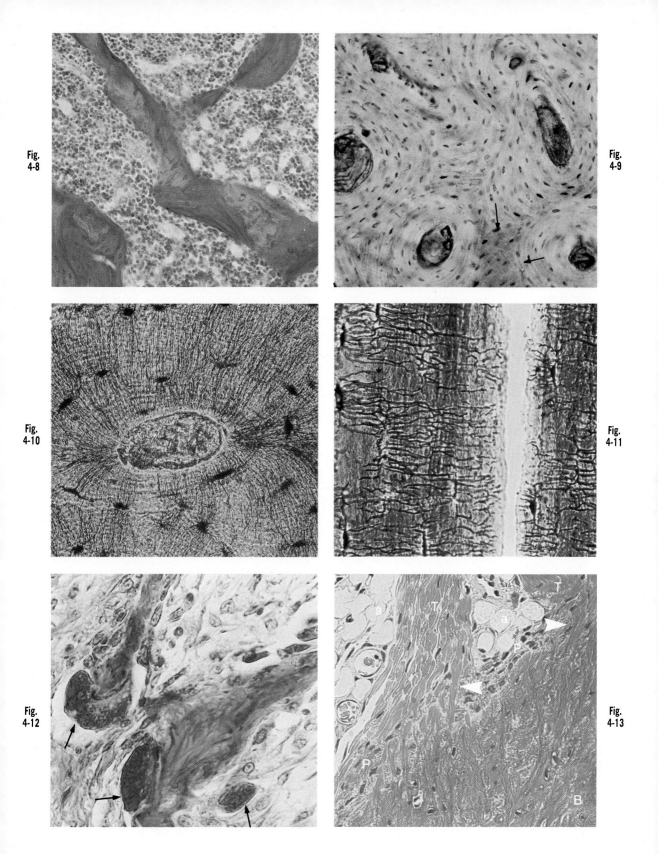

Fig.
4-8

Fig.
4-9

Fig.
4-10

Fig.
4-11

Fig.
4-12

Fig.
4-13

Figure 4–14. Intramembranous bone formation. Azan. Medium power.

One bar or trabecula of bone occupies the center of the field. Within the bone matrix (deep blue), a few osteocytes, each within a lacuna, are present. The bone is surrounded by a continuous layer of osteoblasts, which generally appear cuboidal in shape, with large nuclei and a basophil cytoplasm. The surrounding mesenchyme contains numerous blood vessels. Through the activity of osteoblasts, the bone increases in thickness. Successive layers of matrix are added by apposition, and osteoblasts, which initially lie on the surface, become included within the matrix as osteocytes.

Figure 4–15. Intramembranous bone formation: late. Decalcified section. H and E. Low power.

This section of the developing calvarium shows two plates of bone separated by a marrow cavity or diplöe (D). The dense concentrations of osteoblasts on the outer surface of one plate and on the inner surface of the other (arrows) indicate active addition of bone matrix at these sites.

Figure 4–16. Endochondral bone formation: finger. Mallory-Azan. Low power.

The three phalanges of a finger are shown. The process of endochondral bone formation is seen best in the intermediate phalanx. The cartilage model (pale gray) is surrounded by perichondrium (dark blue), later to become periosteum, except over the joint surfaces. Around the center of the diaphysis, a periosteal bony collar (dark purple) has formed. Centrally within the diaphysis, a primary center of ossification (O) is present. In the proximal phalanx, the process of ossification is more advanced (arrow). The section shown here is tangential and passes obliquely through the bony collar (dark purple), demonstrating the spongy nature of the bone at this stage.

Figure 4–17. Endochondral bone formation. Plastic section. H and E. Low power.

The periosteal bony collar (arrows) is limited to one extremity of the diaphysis, but the primary marrow cavity (O) is extensive. To the left of this, the cartilage model shows definite zones of activity and the establishment of cartilage columns and calcification of the matrix (dark blue). Details of the zones are depicted in Figures 4–19 through 4–21.

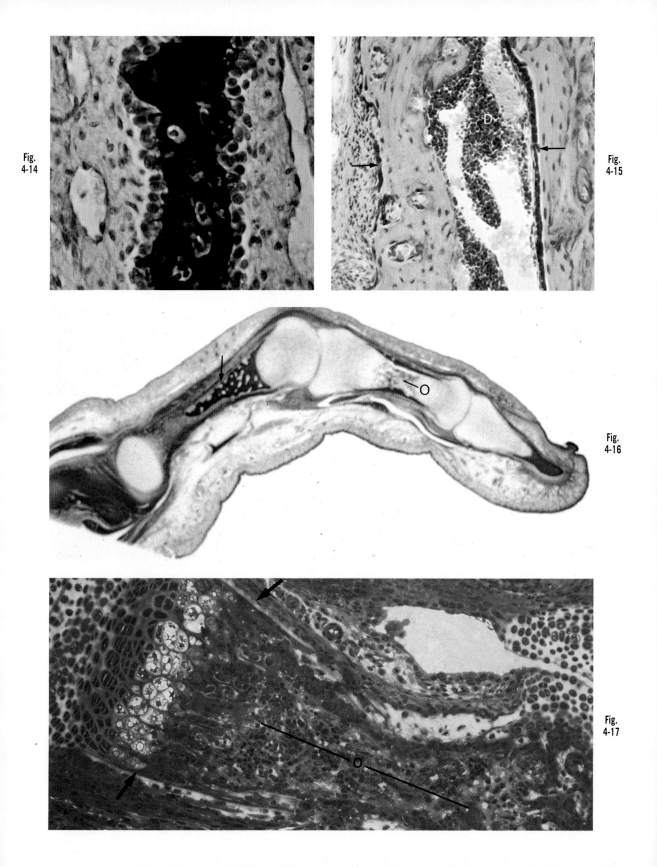

Fig.
4-14

Fig.
4-15

Fig.
4-16

Fig.
4-17

Figure 4–18. Endochondral bone formation. Mallory-Azan. Low power.

A more advanced stage of ossification than that shown in Figure 4–16. The periosteum (P) covers the developing bone, and a wide periosteal collar of spongy bone (dark blue) encloses the diaphysis. In the primary ossification center (right center), which appears red owing to the marked vascularity, cells of the original periosteal bud have opened up wide cavities, the primary marrow spaces. In the epiphysis (left), there is a reserve or quiescent zone of hyaline cartilage, and, toward the diaphysis, the cartilage cells become larger and the region appears pale. A joint cavity (arrow) is present beyond the epiphysis.

Figure 4–19. Endochondral bone formation. Plastic section. H and E. Medium power.

Details of the zones of activity within the cartilaginous epiphysis are shown. The quiescent or reserve zone (top right) gives way to a zone of proliferation where cartilage cells are aligned in distinct rows. Below this zone, there is maturation of cells and calcification of the matrix (dark blue) surrounding the cells. The zone of retrogression occupies the lower left part of the field. A small portion of the periosteal bony collar appears to the right (arrow).

Figure 4–20. Endochondral bone formation. Plastic section. H and E. High power.

Above, the cartilage cells of the epiphysis are aligned in rows in the zone of proliferation. Below, the cells are large and vesicular as a result of the accumulation of glycogen within their cytoplasm; this is the maturation zone.

Figure 4–21. Endochondral bone formation. Plastic section. H and E. High power.

Above, the zone of proliferation gives way to the maturation zone. Below this, there is the zone of calcification, where the matrix appears deeply basophil, and the narrow zone of retrogression, where cartilage cells die and undergo dissolution (arrow). The lower left part of the field shows the ossification zone. Here, bone matrix (pink) is being deposited upon the surface of the remnants of calcified cartilage matrix by osteoblasts (O).

Figure 4–22. Endochondral bone formation. Decalcified section. H and E. Medium power.

A portion of a trabecula in the ossification zone is shown. Bone matrix (pink) has been deposited upon the calcified cartilage matrix (purple). A few osteocytes within lacunae are present within the bone matrix. The presence of an osteoclast (arrow) indicates that bone resorption also is occurring here to enlarge the primary marrow spaces that surround the trabecula.

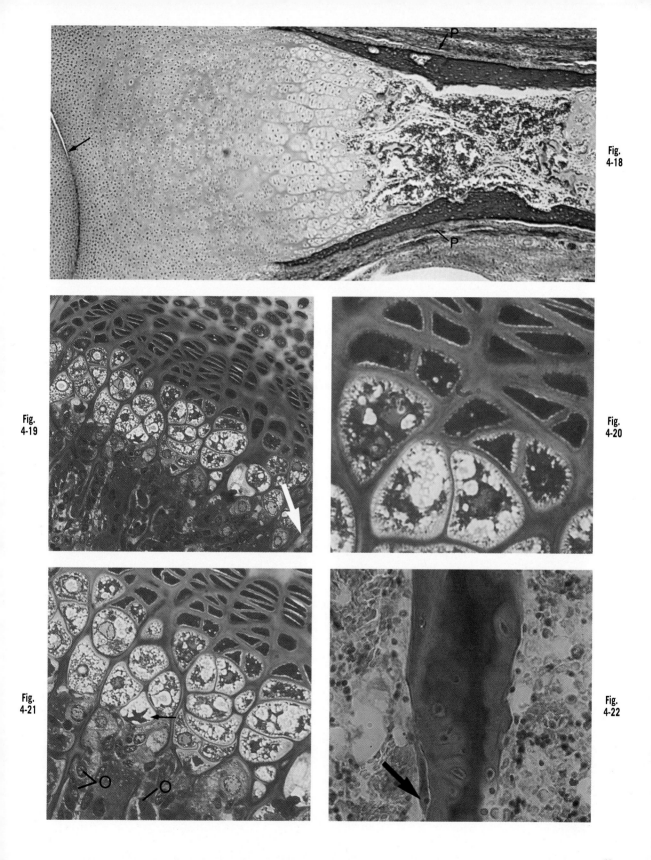

Fig.
4-18

Fig.
4-19

Fig.
4-20

Fig.
4-21

Fig.
4-22

63

Figure 4–23. Secondary ossification center. Azan. Low power.

A secondary center of ossification (C) has appeared in the head of a developing femur. Below is the diaphysis, with a periosteal collar of bone (dark blue) and a marrow cavity containing a few spicules of spongy bone. Above right, small bony trabeculae are present within the secondary ossification center. This center is surrounded by hyaline cartilage of the original cartilage model. The epiphyseal disc (arrows) appears as a pale band between the epiphysis and the shaft. Above left, the greater trochanter is composed solely of hyaline cartilage; a secondary ossification center has yet to appear within it.

Figure 4–24. Epiphyseal disc. Azan. Medium power.

The secondary ossification center (C) exhibits more extensive ossification than the one shown in Figure 4–23. Ossification has spread peripherally, and cartilage remains only as articular cartilage over the free surface (not shown) and as a plate, the epiphyseal disc (D), between the epiphysis and the diaphysis. The formation of cartilage columns (arrows), the calcification of cartilage, and the deposition of bone continue here as earlier in the shaft. Below is the marrow cavity (M) of the diaphysis.

Figure 4–25. Primitive Haversian systems. Mallory-Azan. High power.

This is a transverse section through spongy bone which is in the process of being transformed into compact bone. Longitudinal cavities, sectioned transversely, appear as pale, rounded areas surrounded by bone. The spongy bone matrix (blue) contains numerous osteocytes within lacunae and shows no obvious lamellar pattern. Each large cavity contains a blood vessel centrally, embedded within a primitive connective tissue. Peripherally, osteoblasts (arrows) form an irregular row of cells directly in relationship to the bone matrix. As this layer elaborates additional bone matrix and becomes incorporated within it, a further layer of osteoblasts will differentiate from the primitive connective tissue. In this way, there is a rhythmical deposition of concentric lamellae to form a primitive Haversian system.

Figure 4–26. Diarthrosis: knee joint. Van Gieson. Low power.

In this section, the distal end of the femur (F) and the proximal end of the tibia (T) are shown. The epiphyses of both these bones are cartilaginous at this stage, and there is no distinction between articular cartilage and the main mass of each epiphysis. The joint space between the epiphyses is limited by the joint capsule (arrows). No details of the capsule are apparent at this magnification, but the inner layer is becoming specialized as the synovial membrane, which lines the joint cavity, except over articular surfaces.

Figure 4–27. Diarthrosis: articular cartilage. H and E. High power.

This is a section through the synovial joint between two of the small bones (ossicles) of the middle ear. The participating bones (B) are covered with articular (hyaline) cartilage (C). Near the joint surface, the nuclei of chondrocytes appear flattened and more densely stained than those within the interior of the cartilage. The interface between articular cartilage and the underlying bone (arrows) is irregular.

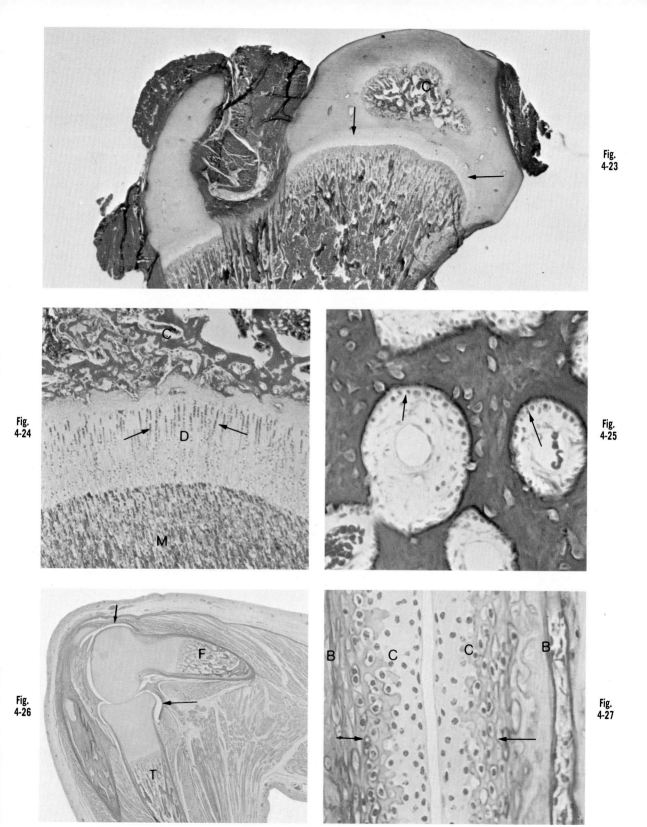

Fig.
4-23

Fig.
4-24

Fig.
4-25

Fig.
4-26

Fig.
4-27

65

Specialized Connective Tissue: Blood

COMPOSITION

Blood is a specialized and somewhat atypical form of connective tissue. It consists of *formed elements* (principally cells) and of a fluid intercellular substance, the blood *plasma.* Fibers appear in the plasma as fibrin, but only when blood is exposed to air and clots. Blood cells are of two main types: red *(erythrocytes)* and white *(leukocytes).* Other formed elements are blood platelets.

Erythrocytes are highly differentiated cells that functionally are specialized for the transport of oxygen. In mammals, they have lost their nuclei and cell organelles during development. Each is a biconcave disc and averages about 7.6 microns, or micrometers (μm), in diameter. In human blood, there are approximately 5 million erythrocytes per cubic millimeter. The cells are extremely elastic and flexible, properties that allow them to pass along small blood vessels whose diameter often is less than theirs.

Leukocytes, or white blood corpuscles, are complete cells with nuclei and the usual cell organelles. There are approximately 5000 to 9000 leukocytes per cubic millimeter in normal human blood. Leukocytes are of two main types, agranular and granular. *Agranular leukocytes,* which possess a cytoplasm that generally appears homogeneous and nuclei that are spherical to reniform in shape, include *lymphocytes,* small cells with scanty cytoplasm; and *monocytes,* slightly larger cells containing greater amounts of cytoplasm. *Granulocytes* (granular leukocytes) are of three types: *neutrophil, basophil,* and *eosinophil,* and are distinguished by the affinity of their cytoplasmic granules for neutral, basic, and acidic stains, respectively. It must be appreciated that leukocytes in the living state or in routine histological sections appear quite different from the same cells seen in dried smears. In the latter, the cells flatten and appear larger than in life, and many structural details are altered or destroyed.

Blood platelets are small protoplasmic discs varying in diameter from 2 to 4 μm. Their number varies considerably but usually the range is 200,000 to 350,000 per cubic millimeter. They function in hemostasis; for instance, they adhere to injured regions of blood vessels and participate in the clotting mechanism.

Plasma, the liquid intercellular substance, constitutes 55 per cent of the blood and transports all nutritive materials. When blood clots, one of the globulins of plasma (fibrinogen) precipitates as a network of fine filaments. The contraction of clotted blood or plasma expresses a clear, yellowish fluid, *serum.*

Formed elements of blood are short-lived and continuously are being destroyed and replaced by a process called *hemopoiesis* (or *hematopoiesis*), which occurs in the hemopoietic tissues. The formed elements are divided into two groups according to the sites of their development in the adult: (1) lymphocytes and monocytes are developed chiefly in the lymphoid tissues; and (2) erythrocytes, granulocytes, and platelets normally are produced within the bone marrow (myeloid tissue). The latter group consists of a framework or *stroma,* blood vessels, and free cells lying within the meshwork of the stroma. The stroma is a loose latticework of reticular fibers in close association with primitive and phagocytic reticular cells. Cells lying free within the stroma represent all stages in the maturation of erythrocytes and granulocytes. The stroma of lymphoid tissue is similar to that of myeloid tissue, and the sinuses present within it are lined by littoral cells of the reticuloendothelial system. The meshes of the stroma contain the free cells, principally lymphocytes.

DEVELOPMENT OF FORMED ELEMENTS

All formed elements of blood develop in all probability from a common ancestor, the *hemocytoblast.*

Erythrocytes. In the development of an erythrocyte, the hemocytoblast gives rise via an intermediary, the proerythroblast, to the basophil erythroblast, which has a dense nucleus and an intensely basophil cytoplasm. This cell divides repeatedly and eventually produces the polychromatophil erythroblast, the cytoplasm of which stains either lilac or gray owing to the presence within the basophil cytoplasm of pink-staining hemoglobin. After numerous divisions, the polychromatophil erythroblast gives rise to the normoblast. This cell has a small, dense nucleus and a cytoplasm that is acidophil owing to the increased concentration of hemoglobin within it. There is no further mitotic activity. The nucleus of the normoblast is extruded from the cell, which now is termed a *reticulocyte.* This cell eventually loses its reticular structure to become an erythrocyte.

Leukocytes. Granular leukocytes develop from hemocytoblasts via the promyelocyte, a cell with a cytoplasm that generally is basophil but is characterized by the presence of scattered, azurophil granules. Promyelocytes proliferate and differentiate into myelocytes, which contain specific granules. These granules have the size, shape, and staining characteristics that allow them to be recognized as neutrophils, basophils, or eosinophils. As the specific granules appear, the primary, azurophil granules are lost. After numerous divisions, the myelocytes in turn give rise to metamyelocytes, which are incapable of further division. These cells are juvenile forms of granular leukocytes and have a characteristic granular content.

Their nuclei, at first horseshoe-shaped, indent further and the cells are termed *band forms*. Later, the nuclei acquire their typical lobation and the mature granulocytes enter the blood stream.

Platelets. In the formation of platelets, the hemocytoblast gives rise to the megakaryocyte, a multinucleated giant cell, when the nucleus undergoes numerous mitotic divisions without cytoplasmic division. After its formation, the megakaryocyte extends cytoplasmic processes that become pinched off and released as platelets into the blood vessels of the bone marrow.

Figure 5–1. Development of myeloid elements.

The double line in the illustration separates the cells that are found in the bone marrow from the mature cells (below the line) seen normally in peripheral blood. (Courtesy of J. H. Cutts.)

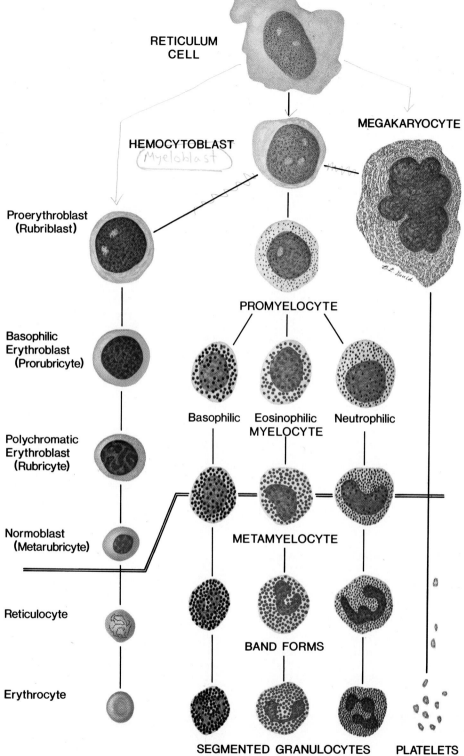

RETICULUM CELL

HEMOCYTOBLAST
(Myeloblast)

MEGAKARYOCYTE

Proerythroblast
(Rubriblast)

Basophilic
Erythroblast
(Prorubricyte)

Polychromatic
Erythroblast
(Rubricyte)

Normoblast
(Metarubricyte)

Reticulocyte

Erythrocyte

PROMYELOCYTE

Basophilic   Eosinophilic   Neutrophilic
MYELOCYTE

METAMYELOCYTE

BAND FORMS

SEGMENTED GRANULOCYTES   PLATELETS

Fig.
5-1

71

Figure 5–2. Peripheral blood. Plastic section. H and E. High power.

In this section, blood within the lumen of a vein is shown. A portion of the endothelial lining of the vein (arrows) appears below, and the lumen contains numerous erythrocytes, some sectioned on the flat, others on the side. Many appear grouped in columns or irregular rows, a phenomenon termed *rouleaux* formation. Also shown are two granulocytes (G).

Figures 5–3 to 5–9. Peripheral blood smears. Wright's stain. Oil immersion.

Figure 5–3. Erythrocytes and a neutrophil granular leukocyte.

The erythrocytes possess no nuclei, and their cytoplasm stains more densely pink at the periphery, an indication of their biconcave disc shape. The neutrophil possesses a lobed nucleus, and the individual lobes are joined by filaments. The neutrophil also shows a small appendage (arrow) attached to one lobe, the "drumstick," or Barr body. The abundant cytoplasm contains numerous fine granules.

Figure 5–4. Eosinophil (left) and neutrophil (right) granular leukocytes.

The eosinophil shows a bilobed nucleus and a cytoplasm crowded with large, eosinophil granules.

Figure 5–5. Eosinophil granular leukocyte.

The nucleus is partially obscured by the large cytoplasmic granules that are uniform in size.

Figure 5–6. Basophil granular leukocyte.

The cytoplasm contains coarse basophil granules that are variable in size.

Figure 5–7. Small lymphocyte.

The cell is a little larger than erythrocytes and has a large, dense nucleus and a thin rim of basophil cytoplasm. (See Figure 5–15.)

Figures 5–8 and 5–9. Monocytes and platelets.

Monocytes possess an indented or irregularly ovoid nucleus in which the chromatin is less dense than that of lymphocytes. The cytoplasm is finely granular. Platelets (arrows) are small, irregular protoplasmic fragments. In Figure 5–9, the peripheral dense staining of erythrocytes is well shown.

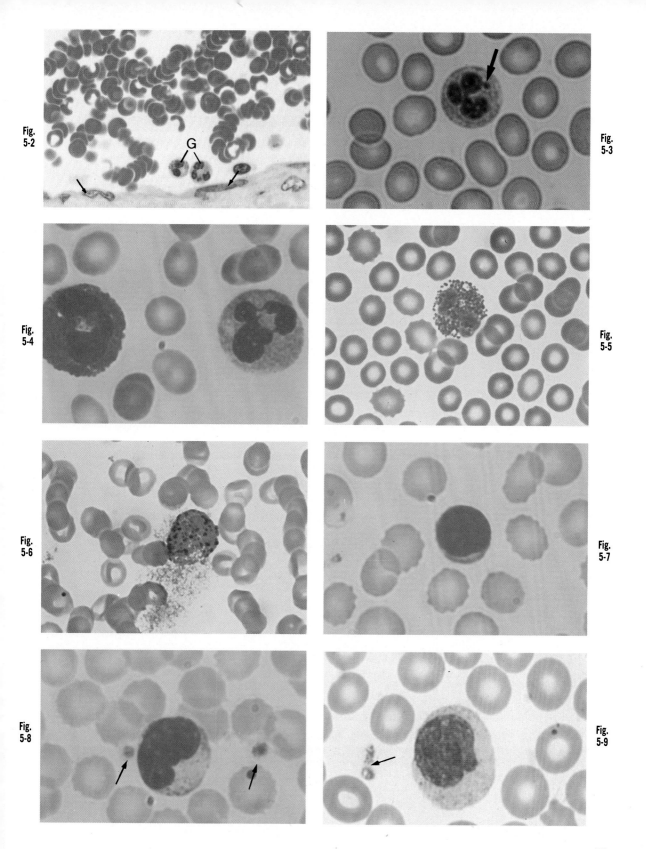

Fig.
5-2

G

Fig.
5-3

Fig.
5-4

Fig.
5-5

Fig.
5-6

Fig.
5-7

Fig.
5-8

Fig.
5-9

Figure 5–10. Bone marrow section: hemopoiesis. Plastic section. H and E. High power.

The bone marrow, or myeloid tissue, consists of a stroma (not stained specifically here), blood vessels, and free cells. The free cells represent all stages in the maturation of red and white blood cells. Individual cell types generally cannot be recognized. The large cell in the center, with a large lobed nucleus, is a megakaryocyte. The large, clear areas within the stroma are fat cells (arrows).

Figure 5–11. Embryonic liver: hemopoiesis. Plastic section. Paragon. High power.

Blood cells are formed in different sites at different stages during development, and in the fetus they appear successively in the yolk sac, mesenchyme, liver, spleen, and lymph nodes. Blood formation commences in the liver at about 6 weeks and gradually diminishes during the middle of fetal life. This section demonstrates active hemopoiesis within the liver. Hepatic cells are large and contain large vesicular nuclei. The cells are arranged in plates that radiate out from the central vein (V). Between the plates of liver cells are numerous hemopoietic elements (arrows), principally of the red cell series. A large megakaryocyte (M), with a complex lobed nucleus and finely granular cytoplasm, also is present. With the development of bone marrow (during the third fetal month), hemopoiesis wanes in the liver.

Figure 5–12. Bone marrow smear. Wright's stain. High power.

Erythrocytes are pale yellow, anucleate, and homogeneous. The nucleated cells are immature elements, principally of the white cell series.

Figures 5–13 to 5–15 are bone marrow smears illustrating erythrocyte formation. Wright's stain. Oil immersion.

Figure 5–13. Reticular cell (left) and hemocytoblast (right).

The reticular cell shows a large, pale nucleus and a faintly basophil, granular cytoplasm. The hemocytoblast possesses a large, ovoid nucleus with a fine pattern of chromatin material; a large, pale nucleolus; and a basophil cytoplasm.

Figure 5–14. Basophil erythroblast (B), polychromatophil erythroblast (P), and normoblast (N).

The basophil erythroblast is smaller than the hemocytoblast (Fig. 5–13), and its nucleus possesses coarser chromatin granules. The cytoplasm is markedly basophil. The polychromatophil erythroblast, smaller than the basophil erythroblast, shows coarse clumping of nuclear chromatin and a cytoplasm that is gray in color owing to the presence of hemoglobin within the basophil cytoplasm. The normoblast, no larger than surrounding erythrocytes, contains a small, dense nucleus and a thin rim of pale cytoplasm, which later in development will be acidophil as a result of the accumulation of hemoglobin.

Figure 5–15. Polychromatophil erythroblasts.

The four polychromatophil erythroblasts exhibit large nuclei, with coarse chromatin clumps, and a polychromatophil cytoplasm owing to the presence of hemoglobin within the basophil cytoplasm. Also present are a juvenile (band) neutrophil (N) and a small lymphocyte (L).

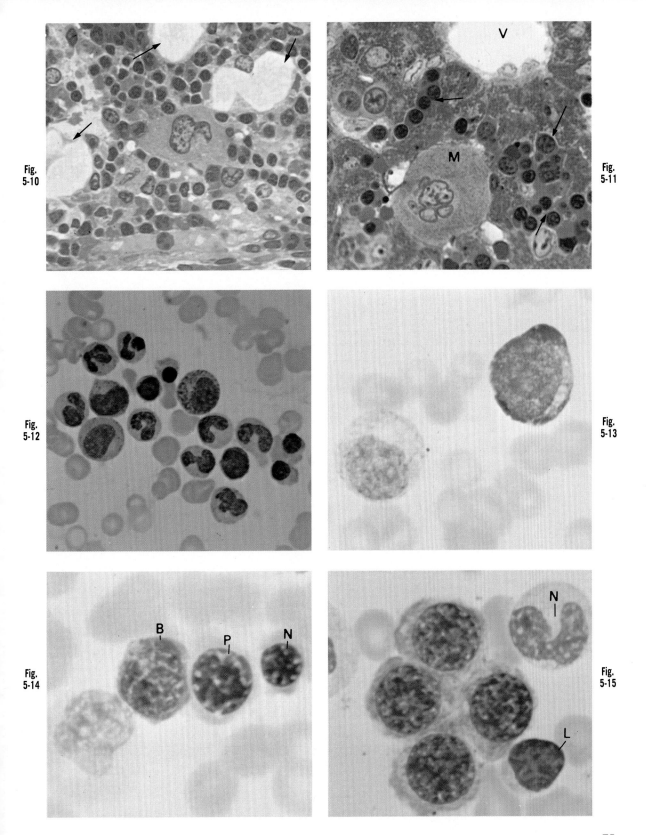

Fig.
5-10

Fig.
5-11

Fig.
5-12

Fig.
5-13

Fig.
5-14

Fig.
5-15

Figures 5–16 to 5–20. Bone marrow smears illustrating white cell formation. Wright's stain. Oil immersion.

Figure 5–16. Promyelocyte.

The large cell, a promyelocyte, exhibits an ovoid nucleus with coarse chromatin strands and two nucleoli (arrows). The cytoplasm is basophil and contains a few nonspecific granules (pink). The other cell is a mature neutrophil granular leukocyte.

Figure 5–17. Neutrophil myelocyte (left) and band neutrophil (right).

The neutrophil myelocyte, somewhat smaller than a promyelocyte (Fig. 5–16), shows more compact nuclear chromatin and fine cytoplasmic granules. The band neutrophil contains an irregular lobed nucleus and fine, specific cytoplasmic granules.

Figure 5–18. Eosinophil (E) and neutrophil (N) myelocytes.

The late eosinophil myelocyte shows an indented nucleus and large eosinophil granules. The early neutrophil myelocyte possesses a condensed ovoid nucleus and fine neutrophil granules. Also present are three neutrophil metamyelocytes with fine, specific granules and reniform nuclei.

Figure 5–19. Basophil myelocyte.

The outline of the nucleus appears indefinite, and the cytoplasm contains specific basophil granules.

Figure 5–20. Bone marrow smear.

Present in this field are eosinophil myelocytes (E), neutrophil metamyelocytes (M), band neutrophils (B), and a mature neutrophil granular leukocyte (N).

Figure 5–21. Bone marrow smear: megakaryocyte. Wright's stain. Medium power.

This giant cell, which occupies the majority of the field, has a large, irregular nucleus and a finely granular cytoplasm that exhibits a patchy basophilia.

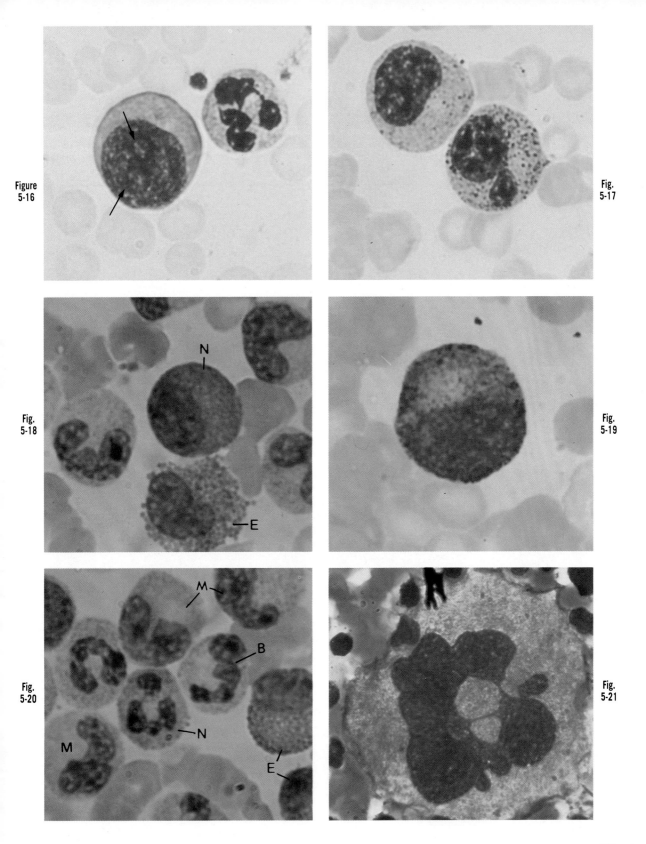

Figure
5-16

Fig.
5-17

Fig.
5-18

N

E

Fig.
5-19

Fig.
5-20

M

B

M

N

E

Fig.
5-21

CHAPTER
SIX

Muscle

Muscle cells are specialized for contraction, producing movement of the body as a whole and of the many parts with respect to one another. All types of muscle cells are elongated in the axis of contraction and thus usually are termed *muscle fibers*. Muscle fibers must not be confused with *connective tissue fibers* (which are extracellular) or with *nerve fibers* (which are cell processes).

Muscle tissue consists of (1) muscle fibers, occasionally occurring as single elements, but usually arranged in bundles or fasciculi; (2) fibroconnective supporting tissue with fibroblasts, collagenous fibers, and some elastic fibers; and (3) a rich capillary network to provide oxygen and nutrients and to eliminate toxic waste materials. Nerve fibers also run in the connective tissue.

CLASSIFICATION

There are three types of muscle, classified both on a structural and on a functional basis. Functionally, muscle is either *voluntary* (under the control of the will) or *involuntary*. Structurally, it is either *striated* (cross-striped) or *smooth* (unstriped). On this basis, there are three types:

1. Smooth involuntary muscle, present in the walls of hollow viscera and blood vessels.

2. Striated voluntary or skeletal muscle, forming the flesh of the limbs and body wall and attached to bones and fascia.

3. Striated involuntary or cardiac muscle, located in the heart and adjacent major blood vessels.

STRUCTURE

A special terminology is used with respect to muscle (*sarcos* = muscle). The protoplasm is referred to as *sarcoplasm;* mitochondria as *sarcosomes;* endoplasmic reticulum as *sarcoplasmic reticulum;* and the plasma membrane complex of plasmalemma, with its basal lamina and associated collagen microfibrils, as *sarcolemma.*

Contained in muscle cells are *myofibrils,* the contractile elements that run in the long axis of the cells and are responsible for the longitudinal striation seen in all muscle fibers. Each myofibril is a bundle of smaller myofilaments, invisible by light microscopy and composed of the contractile proteins of actin and myosin. In the two types of striated muscle, the orientation of the myofilaments is regular, giving a cross-striation to the myofibrils with alternating light (isotropic or I band) and dark (anisotropic or A band) bands. The I band is bisected by a thin dark Z line, the A band by a light or less dense H band. At the center of the H band, a thin dark M band or middle stripe may be visible. These bands are not visible in a cross section and, in longitudinal section, while they are distinct in relaxed muscle, they are not so in contracted muscle. The segment of a myofibril between adjacent Z lines is called a *sarcomere;* this is not merely a structural unit but the basic contractile unit. In contraction, the muscle fiber becomes shorter and thicker and the sarcomeres progressively shorter. The ends of the A bands move toward Z lines, eventually eliminating the I bands; that is, A and I bands become indistinguishable, but the length of the A band in contraction remains constant. In smooth muscle, the arrangement of myofilaments is not so regular, and no cross-banding is visible.

CONTRACTION

Contraction of muscle involves a process termed the "sliding filament mechanism." As stated already, myofilaments are linear units and are of two types, thin (actin-containing) and thick (myosin-containing). The thick filaments lie in the center of the sarcomere occupying the A band. The thin filaments at one end are attached to a Z line and extend through the I band into the A band to the edge of the H band. At the extremities of the A band, they intermesh with the thick filaments. The H band is simply the center portion of the A band that is free of thin filaments. This is the situation in a relaxed, noncontracted fiber. Thus, in transverse section, the I band contains only thin filaments, the extremities of the A band contain both thick and thin, and the H band contains only thick filaments. During contraction, the thin filaments slide past the thick filaments so that their free ends extend further toward the M band, i.e., toward the center of the sarcomere. This draws adjacent Z lines closer together, with decrease in width of the I band and the H band. In full contraction, the ends of the thick filaments approach Z lines, the H band is obliterated by approximation of the free ends of thin filaments from both extremities of the sarcomere; thus, throughout the length of the sarcomere, both thick and thin filaments are present. Each sarcomere thus is shortened. On relaxation, the two sets of filaments slide back past each other to their original, relaxed position of partial overlap.

Smooth muscle fibers in general contract slowly, but they can sustain contraction for long periods. Striated muscle fibers can contact rapidly and powerfully, but they become fatigued relatively quickly. Cardiac muscle contracts rhythmically, constantly, and automatically.

SIZE AND ARRANGEMENT

In general, smooth muscle fibers are small, fusiform in shape, about 20 to 200 microns, or micrometers (μm), in length and about 6 μm in diameter, with a single, central, elongated nucleus. Striated muscle fibers are larger, with a diameter of 10 to 60 μm and a length of 1 to 4 mm, and with numerous ovoid nuclei located peripherally in the fiber. A cardiac muscle fiber is actually a linear unit of several cells joined end to end at specialized junctional zones called intercalated discs, each cell being about 100 μm long and 15 μm in diameter. The cell may branch at its ends to meet another cell, or cells, at intercalated discs, giving an overall but false impression of a synctium or network. Nuclei are elongated and centrally located in the fiber.

In all three types, there is associated fibroconnective tissue carrying blood vessels and nerves, and providing a "harness" or attachment for the muscle fibers. Smooth muscle, while found in some locations as single cells, usually is arranged in sheets. In striated muscle, a named "muscle" of gross anatomy is enveloped in substantial connective tissue, the epimysium, within which are bundles or fascicles of fibers surrounded by less dense connective tissue, the perimysium. Around individual fibers is fine reticular connective tissue, the endomysium. At the ends of the muscle, connective tissue blends with tendon, periosteum, raphe, or dermis. In cardiac muscle, there is only delicate endomysium around muscle fibers.

INNERVATION OF SKELETAL MUSCLE

Skeletal muscle fibers have associated nerve terminals, the motor neuron cell body lying in the anterior horn of the gray matter. At its termination, the axon may branch to supply 1 to about 100 muscle fibers, and each point of contact between a muscle fiber and a terminal branch of a nerve shows a complex dilatation of the nerve. These are called *motor end-plates*, or *myoneural junctions*. Here, the terminal nerve fiber loses its myelin sheath and forms a plate-like mass or a series of branches with terminal swellings. The muscle fiber at the point of contact is swollen with a local mass of sarcoplasm (the soleplasm) with numerous sarcosomes and nuclei.

Sensory (proprioceptive) endings also are found in muscle tissue. Neuromuscular spindles are small groups of slender muscle fibers (intrafusal fibers) enclosed in a connective tissue capsule. Afferent sensory nerves contact the intrafusal fibers and are stimulated by their contraction. Neurotendinous endings are located in tendons near muscle-tendon junctions, with sensory nerve endings terminating between bundles of tendon (collagen) fibers. These nerve endings are stimulated by tension or stretching of the tendon that occurs during muscle contraction.

Figure 6–1. Teased skeletal (striated) muscle fibers. Iron hematoxylin. Oil immersion.

Shown are parts of two skeletal muscle fibers teased from a mass of muscle; i.e., the entire thickness of the fibers is seen, and they are not sectioned. The fibers are cylindrical, of considerable length, and multinucleated, the nuclei (N) located peripherally in the fibers. Some fibers are not in sharp focus, owing to the thickness of the preparation. In the cytoplasm, an obvious cross-striation of alternating light (isotropic—I) and dark (anisotropic—A) bands is present with a light central H band in the A band. The bands appear to cross the full thickness of the fibers, which are in a relaxed state.

Figure 6–2. Tongue, striated muscle. Plastic section. Methylene blue, basic fuchsin. Medium power.

Muscle fibers are cut mainly transversely, with one fiber in longitudinal section (left), with A and I bands shown. In transverse section, the muscle fibers are packed closely and show darkly staining myofibrils with small areas of clear sarcoplasm between. Nuclei are peripheral (arrows). Between the muscle fibers is fine connective tissue (endomysium), with nuclei of fibroblasts (arrowheads) and some capillary blood vessels (asterisks). A small peripheral nerve (N) is seen in transverse section.

Figure 6–3. Tongue, striated muscle. Plastic section. Toluidine blue, safranin. Oil immersion.

Each fiber, cut in transverse section, is delineated clearly by the sarcolemma. Nuclei are peripheral—one fiber shows two nuclei (N), and some nuclei show prominent nucleoli (O). The sarcoplasm contains many sarcosomes (black dots) between the myofibrils. Between muscle fibers is supporting connective tissue, collagen staining pink, with numerous blood capillaries (B), also sectioned transversely, and containing erythrocytes in their lumens. Also present is a small peripheral nerve (T) with two myelinated nerve fibers (black). (See Figure 1–12.)

Figure 6–4. Striated muscle. Plastic section. H and E. Oil immersion.

These fibers are cut longitudinally to show Z, A, I, and H bands. A sarcomere (S)—the unit between adjacent Z bands—is indicated.

Figure 6–5. Diaphragm, striated muscle. Plastic section. Toluidine blue. Oil immersion.

Note that in this figure, which is similar to Figure 6–4, the A, I, and Z bands are seen clearly. The longitudinal pale streaks (arrows) are clear sarcoplasm between myofibrils, and the bands do not pass across this sarcoplasm; i.e., banding is confined to the myofibrils.

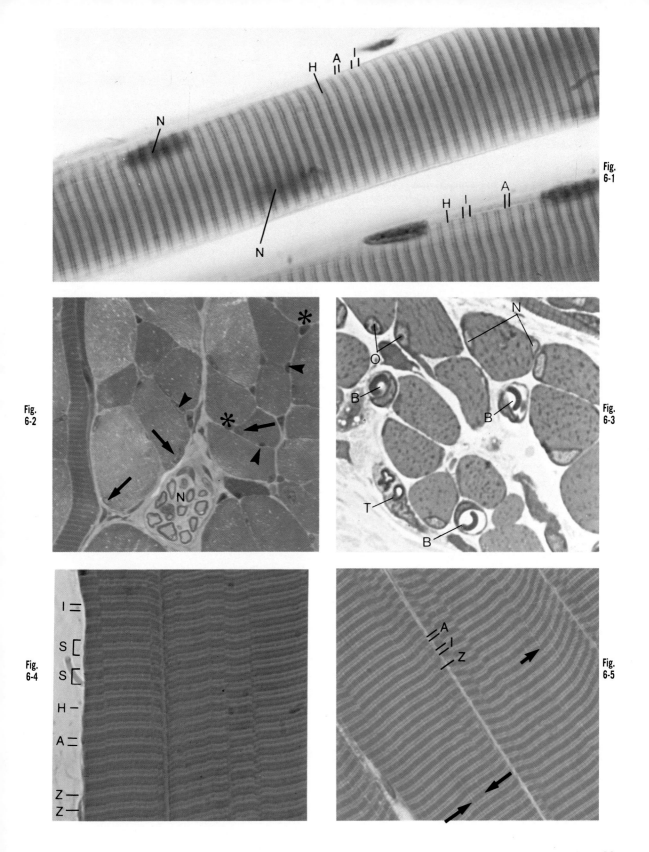

Figure 6–6. Muscle, tendon. Plastic section. Masson's trichrome. Oil immersion.

The muscle fibers (top) in longitudinal section show A, I, Z, and H bands with thin slips of clear cytoplasm between myofibrils. Thin endomysium envelops the fibers; the fibroblast nuclei of endomysium are shown by arrows. The tendon (below) stains pink with nuclei of fibroblasts (tenocytes) (N) between collagen bundles. At its extremity, the muscle fiber shows "ridges" passing from which there are slips of connective tissue (endomysium, blue-staining) (arrowheads). These are attached to the sarcolemma at one end (right) and at the other blend with the tendon (left).

Figure 6–7. Muscle, tendon. Plastic section. H and E. High power.

In transverse section, the muscle fibers are below, the tendon above. Nuclei of fibroblasts (tenocytes) of the tendon lie between collagen bundles (dark pink). A few fibroblasts of endomysium are seen between muscle fibers (arrow), while nuclei of muscle cells are located peripherally (N).

Figure 6–8. Muscle, capillaries. Phosphotungstic acid. Medium power.

In this preparation, the arterial supply to a muscle has been injected with colored (red) gelatin to demonstrate the rich capillary plexus. The muscle fibers have been stained lightly with phosphotungstic acid and are sectioned longitudinally. Note the capillaries run longitudinally (L) between muscle fibers, with numerous cross-connections. A small arteriole supplies the plexus (arrow). The coiling of capillaries probably is due to contraction of the muscle.

Figure 6–9. Neuromuscular junction. Gold chloride. Medium power.

Several striated muscle fibers are present with a small nerve (N) with several terminal branches, some terminating in myoneural (neuromuscular) junctions or motor end-plates (J). The motor end-plate is disc-shaped and plexiform; the nerve terminals are dilated and associated intimately with a muscle fiber.

Figure 6–10. Neuromuscular spindle. Plastic section. H and E. Medium power.

Bundles of striated muscle (extrafusal) fibers (E) are seen at left and right, in transverse section. Centrally located is a muscle spindle (S) with seven intrafusal fibers (I), smaller than the extrafusal fibers, with a connective tissue capsule. Afferent nerve fibers (not seen) contact the intrafusal fibers. A small artery (A) is also present.

Figure 6–11. Striated muscle, endomysium. Gridley's reticulin. Medium power.

Striated muscle fibers of the tongue are seen in transverse and longitudinal section, arranged in bundles. Those in longitudinal section show transverse striations, and nuclei are peripheral and multiple (arrowheads). Each fiber is surrounded by fine reticular fibers (brown) of the endomysium, this network containing numerous blood capillaries. (See Figure 6–8.)

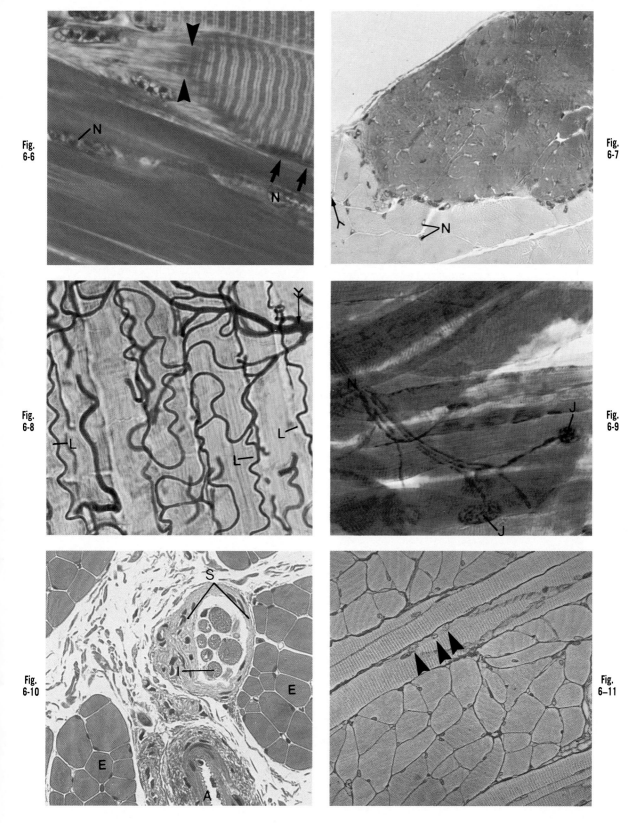

Figure 6–12. Cardiac muscle. Plastic section. Weigert. Medium power.

The muscle is cut longitudinally and shows a pseudosyncytial arrangement with branching of the fibers or trabeculae and capillary blood vessels (C) between the trabeculae. Nuclei (N) are located centrally in the muscle fibers with sarcoplasm free of myofibrils at their poles. Intercalated discs (arrowheads) cross the fibers either transversely (left) or in a zig-zag manner (right).

Figure 6–13. Cardiac muscle. Plastic section. Methylene blue, basic fuchsin. Medium power.

Muscle fibers, cut transversely, show variation in size and shape. Nuclei (N) are located centrally, and sarcoplasm (pale-staining) appears reticular between the irregular, darker-staining myofibrils. Numerous capillaries (C), also cut transversely, are seen.

Figure 6–14. Cardiac muscle. Plastic section. H and E. Medium power.

Muscle fibers, cut transversely, show darkly staining central nuclei (N); pink-staining, irregular myofibrils; and pale-staining sarcoplasm between the myofibrils. Numerous capillaries (C) lying in endomysium are seen between the fibers.

Figure 6–15. Cardiac muscle. Plastic section. H and E. Oil immersion.

This is a higher magnification to show variation in diameter of cardiac muscle fibers in transverse section, central nuclei (N), and abundant sarcoplasm with myofibrils (dark pink) and pale-staining sarcoplasm between the myofibrils. A capillary (C) also is present in the field.

Figure 6–16. Cardiac muscle. Plastic section. Azocarmine and thionin. Oil immersion.

Here, in longitudinal section, a nucleus (N) is elongated, centrally located in a fiber, and shows several nucleoli. In the sarcoplasm, A and I bands are seen clearly. Intercalated discs (I) are present, located at Z bands, and often cross fibers in a stepwise fashion (arrows). Note also the "branching" of muscle fibers (arrowheads) with cross beams or trabeculae.

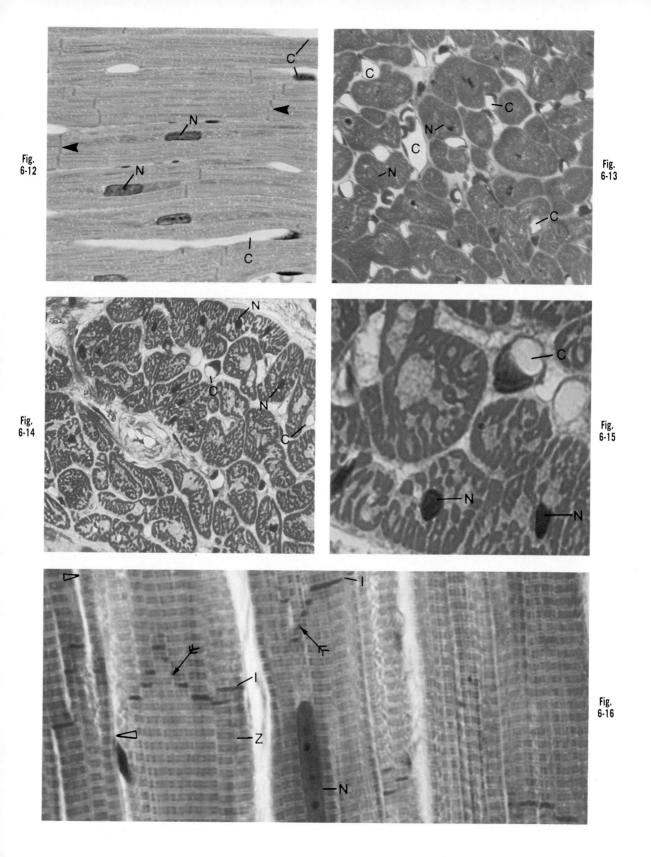

Fig. 6-12

Fig. 6-13

Fig. 6-14

Fig. 6-15

Fig. 6-16

Figure 6–17. Smooth muscle (of duodenum). Plastic section. H and E. Medium power.

The muscularis or muscle coat of the intestine is arranged in two layers, inner circular and outer longitudinal. In this longitudinal section of the gut, the inner layer is cut transversely (left) and the outer layer longitudinally (right), with connective tissue between the layers containing blood vessels (V) and a small nerve (N), the latter part of the intermyenteric plexus. In transverse section, nuclei are round profiles seen in the centers of some fibers. In longitudinal section, they are elongated and appear "folded" (arrow), an indication that the cells were fixed in contraction. Cytoplasm appears homogeneous.

Figure 6–18. Uterine cervix. Van Gieson. Medium power.

In this picture, similar to Figure 6–17, the cytoplasm of smooth muscle stains yellow, the nuclei black, and the collagen (extracellular) fibrils and fibers bright red. A few fibroblast nuclei are seen between collagen fibrils. Note the thin, slender collagen fibrils (reticular fibers) between individual smooth muscle cells.

Figure 6–19. Gallbladder. Plastic section. H and E, PAS. Oil immersion.

Smooth muscle cells are cut both longitudinally (L) and transversely (T). Note elongated nuclei located centrally in cells cut longitudinally; in cells cut transversely, nuclei appear to vary in size. This results from the section cutting either the central portion or the extremity of a nucleus, and many cells show absence of a nucleus where the section was outside the nuclear area, i.e., at either end of a cell. The slender, pink-magenta fibrils between the closely packed muscle cells are reticular (PAS-positive) fibers. Larger collagen fibrils are seen between groups of muscle cells (arrow).

Figure 6–20. Duodenum. Plastic section. H and E. Oil immersion.

In this transverse section, smooth muscle fibers of the inner circular layer of the muscularis are cut longitudinally (left), those of the outer longitudinal layer transversely (right). (Compare with Figure 6–17.) The fibers are elongated and spindle-shaped, wider centrally where the nucleus is located, and tapering at each end. Close packing is achieved by not having nuclear areas of adjacent cells close to each other; i.e., the cells are staggered.

Figure 6–21. Bladder. Plastic section. Toluidine blue. Oil immersion.

Smooth muscle cells are sectioned transversely. Nuclei are seen in some cells and vary in size; these facts indicate that the cells are elongated. Note the close packing of the cells and the presence of small dark bodies both at the surface sarcolemma and within sarcoplasm. These are attachment plaques and dense bodies, regions for the attachment of myofilaments.

Figure 6–22. Esophagus. H and E. Medium power.

The muscularis of the middle esophagus seen here is composed of a mixture of smooth (M) and striated (T) muscle fibers in both the inner circular layer (cut transversely, above) and the outer longitudinal layer (cut longitudinally, below). Note the difference in size of the two types.

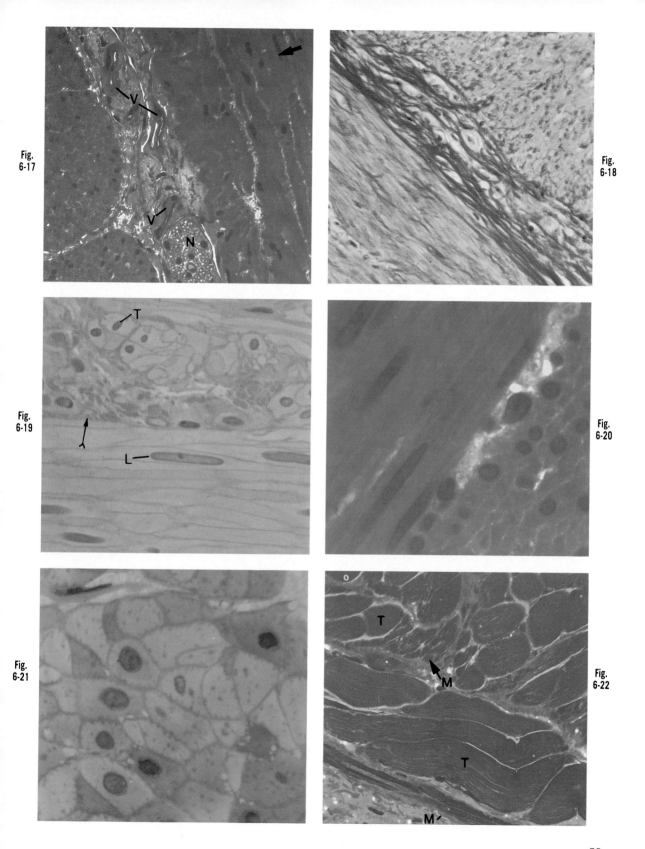

Fig.
6-17

Fig.
6-18

Fig.
6-19

Fig.
6-20

Fig.
6-21

Fig.
6-22

SEVEN

Nervous Tissue

GENERAL ARRANGEMENT

Nervous tissue is distributed widely in the body. The peripheral nervous system (PNS) collects stimuli from the environment, and passes them as nervous impulses to a large central reception and correlation center, the central nervous system (CNS). The CNS, in turn, initiates further impulses and passes them on via the PNS to effector organs to institute appropriate responses. These functions are performed by highly specialized cells called *neurons*. Together with their supporting or *neuroglial* cells and associated extracellular material, the neurons form this integrated communications network. The CNS, consisting of the brain and spinal cord, is protected by bone of the cranium and vertebral column and by a covering of meninges. The basic structural unit of the nervous system is the neuron, in which two properties of protoplasm are developed highly. These are *irritability,* the capacity to respond to physical and chemical stimuli by initiation of an impulse, and *conductivity,* the transmission of this wave of excitation. Thus, neurons are excitable and react to stimuli, often by stimulating or inhibiting other neurons with which they are in contact at specialized regions called *synapses.*

NEURON

Each neuron consists of a cell body (also called the *perikaryon* or *soma*) containing the nucleus and one or (usually) more cell processes. These processes are of two types:

1. *Dendrites* conduct toward the soma, usually are branching and multiple, and together with the soma form the main area for receipt of impulses at synapses.

2. The *axon* conducts away from the soma, is single, and usually is more slender than the dendrite.

The perikarya of nerve cells usually are large, varying in size from 4 to 135 microns, or micrometers (μm), in diameter, and varying in shape depending on the number of cell processes. Nuclei characteristically are large (up to 20 μm), euchromatic, spherical, centrally located and with prominent nucleoli. Sex chromatin (Barr body) may be seen in the neuron of the female as a *nucleolar satellite.* The cytoplasm contains patches of basophil material called *Nissl bodies,* which are formed by stacks of granular endoplasmic reticulum and associated ribosomes and polysomes. Numerous mitochondria and an extensive perinuclear Golgi apparatus also are prominent; best demonstrated by silver techniques are *neurofibrils,* formed by neurofilaments (microfilaments of 10 nm, the intermediate type) and neurotubules (microtubules). Other organelles, such as lysosomes, and inclusions (pigment granules or residual bodies) may be present. Most of the nerve cell bodies lie in or near the CNS collected into groups, called nuclei in the CNS and ganglia in the PNS. In the CNS, neurons are supported by neuroglial cells, mainly of the type called *oligodendroglia,* whereas neurons of ganglia in the PNS have a "capsule" of small satellite cells.

Types of Neurons

Neurons of several types are recognized:

1. Most neurons are *multipolar* with several, branching dendrites and an axon, plus a soma that is polygonal and varies in shape from stellate to pyramidal to globular.

2. A neuron with a single process is *unipolar;* this process later branches to form axon and dendrites. Unipolar neurons are rare in vertebrates.

3. *Bipolar* neurons are also uncommon. These have a single axon and a single dendrite at opposite poles of a spindle-shaped soma. They are found in the retina, cochlear and vestibular ganglia, and olfactory epithelium.

4. In craniospinal ganglia, neurons originally are bipolar in type, but during development, the two processes migrate toward each other and fuse to form a single process. At some distance from the soma, this process branches into axon and dendrite; these neurons are *pseudounipolar.*

Additionally, several different types of multipolar neurons are recognized by shape and location, and, of these, two are important:

1. *Golgi type I neurons* have an extensive dendritic tree and a long axon that enters white matter to terminate in another area of the CNS or to contribute to a peripheral nerve to end in tissue such as muscle or skin. Examples are the *motor (anterior horn) neurons* of the spinal cord, *Purkinje cells* of the cerebellum, and *pyramidal cells* of the cerebral cortex.

2. In contrast, *Golgi type II* neurons have short axons that do not leave the general area of their perikarya, running only a short distance. Examples are the interneurons (internuncial neurons), numerous in cerebral and cerebellar cortices. These connect or lie between other neurons in a pathway.

Nerve Cell Processes

Most neurons have several dendrites and these branch repeatedly, thus increasing the cell surface for impulse reception and making it possible for a large number of axons from other nerve cells to terminate on one neuron. Dendrites contain organelles similar to those found in the perikaryon, with the exception of the Golgi apparatus. They usually are covered by small projections called *dendritic spines or gemmules,* which represent sites of synaptic contact.

Neurons have only a single axon, a cylindrical process that varies in length and diameter with the type of neuron, some being as long as 100 cm. The axon originates from the perikaryon or at the root of a major dendrite, with an adjacent clear area in the perikaryon (the axon hillock). It is distinguished from the dendrites by the absence of Nissl bodies and by having a regular arrangement of neurofibrils in the hillock and root; also, the axon is usually more slender and of more uniform diameter. Terminally, an axon usually branches into a few telodendria, terminating on other neurons, muscle, or glands.

Any long process of a neuron is called a *"fiber,"* a useful term because often the distinction between axons and dendrites is not clear and, also, these nerve cell processes often have additional coats. Nerve fibers may be *myelinated* or *unmyelinated,* the former with a sheath of myelin. Myelin is actually a "jelly-roll" of the plasma membrane of supporting (surrounding) cells, these being oligodendroglia within the CNS and neurolemma (Schwann) cells in the PNS. Individual cells, oligodendrocyte or neurolemma, "wrap" segments of a nerve cell process with junctions between segments, these being the nodes of Ranvier; in other words, an internode or segment between two nodes is wrapped in myelin of a single supporting cell. Myelin acts as an insulator and myelinated fibers conduct more rapidly than unmyelinated fibers.

Within the CNS, nerve fibers run in bundles, these being called *tracts.* In the PNS, bundles of nerve fibers constitute a peripheral nerve. In a nerve, each nerve fiber is surrounded by delicate connnective tissue, the *endoneurium;* bundles of fibers by stronger connective tissue, the *perineurium;* and a main nerve trunk composed of several bundles enveloped in relatively thick connective tissue, the *epineurium.*

THE SYNAPSE

A synapse, the site of transneuronal transmission of a nerve impulse, is a specialized membranous contact between the axon of one neuron and a dendrite (axodendritic synapse) or perikaryon (axosomatic) of another neuron, occasionally between dendrites (dendrodendritic) or between axons (axoaxonic). Functionally, both excitatory and inhibitory synapses occur. Histologically, the presynaptic element usually is a small terminal bulb or bouton of an axon that closely contacts the postsynaptic element, either a dendritic spine, the surface of a dendrite, or the perikaryon, the two elements separated by a slender interval called the synaptic cleft. By synapses, neurons are connected into chains for impulse transmission.

SUPPORTING CELLS

Some supporting cells of nervous tissue already have been mentioned, e.g., capsule or satellite cells of peripheral ganglia and Schwann cells. In the CNS there are other elements. These include *ependymal cells* lining the cavities of the brain and spinal cord, and three types of neuroglial cells—*astrocytes, oligodendroglia,* and *microglia*—the supporting elements of the CNS.

Astrocytes are star-shaped cells with pale nuclei and many processes related closely to blood vessels. Two varieties of astrocytes are present: *protoplasmic* astrocytes have relatively thick processes that branch repeatedly and are found in gray matter (related to nerve cells). *Fibrous* astrocytes have slender and fewer processes and are found in white matter (related to nerve fibers).

Oligodendroglia are smaller, have a denser nucleus and few processes, and form myelin sheaths of nerve fibers in white matter and are the satellite cells of neurons in gray matter.

Microglia, the third type of neuroglial cell, is the smallest. It has a dense nucleus, usually of irregular shape, and is phagocytic. These cells may be derived from several sources.

MENINGES

Additionally, the CNS is protected by several protective layers—the meninges. Externally is the *dura mater* of dense connective tissue containing major blood vessels; then the *arachnoid,* a delicate fibrous network with a trabecular space beneath it—the subarachnoid space, filled with cerebrospinal fluid; and internally a delicate, vascular layer, the *pia mater,* in contact with the brain (and spinal cord) surface. *Cerebrospinal fluid* is secreted by the choroid plexus, a collection of tufts of small arteries and capillaries of the pia mater that invaginate into the ventricular cavities, covered by a simple cuboidal epithelium.

FUNCTIONAL DIVISIONS OF THE NERVOUS SYSTEM

Functionally, the nervous sytem is divided into *somatic* and *autonomic* divisions. The somatic part is concerned with all structures derived from embryological somites, i.e., muscles, bones, and skin. The autonomic nervous system (ANS) innervates smooth and cardiac muscles and all viscera.

SPECIAL STAINS

To demonstrate all the features of nervous tissue, special staining techniques are required. No single stain will demonstrate nerve cells and their processes and all the supporting elements. Several methods are encompassed in this chapter, each stain demonstrating only a few specific features.

Peripheral receptors detecting special senses and the eye and ear are covered mainly in Chapter 17.

Figure 7–1. Composite diagram of a neuron of the central nervous system.

Top left: As seen by light microscopy, a large vesicular nucleus; prominent nucleolus (with nucleolar satellite above); and, in the cytoplasm, Nissl bodies (dots) and neurofibril bundles extending into the dendrites and axon (top right). The axon becomes myelinated, and below it is a small nucleus of an oligodendrocyte. *Center:* This oligodendrocyte is shown forming myelin sheaths for several nerve fibers, with a node of Ranvier. *Bottom:* The neuron, as seen by electron microscopy, demonstrates the perikaryon, its processes, and types of synapse. The large vesicular nucleus (N), with nucleolus (Nu) and nucleolar satellite (NS) containing the heterochromatic X chromosome, occupies much of the soma. In the cytoplasm, Nissl bodies (Ni) of granular endoplasmic reticulum and ribosomes are prominent, with Golgi apparatus (G), smooth endoplasmic reticulum (Ser), lysosomes (L), mitochondria (M), and bundles of microtubules (neurotubules) (T) and neurofilaments (F). Six dendrites (D) are shown with dendritic spines (DS), and the axon (A, top right) leaves at the axon hillock (AH). In the bracket at top, the relation of the neuronal surface to synapses (S) and glial processes (P) is shown. Types of synapse seen are axodendritic (1), axosomatic (2), and axoaxonic (3). The dendrodendritic type is not seen. At right, in the bracket, is a typical (asymmetrical) synapse with the direction of conduction arrowed.

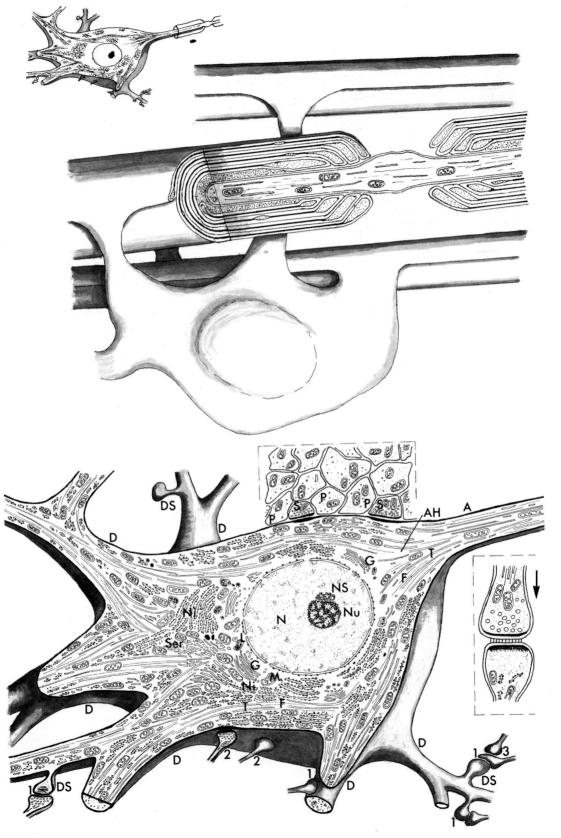

Figure 7–2. Pyramidal neuron of rat cerebral cortex.

This electron micrograph shows most of the features illustrated in Figure 7–1. In the perikaryon is the nucleus (N) with its nucleolus (nl), cytoplasm with Nissl bodies (B), elements of the Golgi apparatus (G), mitochondria (m), free ribosomes (r), lysosomes (L), and microtubules (t). Microtubules are more prominent in the cell processes of which the root of an axon (A, lower right) and apical (D1) and basal (D2) dendrites are seen. An axon terminal (At) forms a synapse with the neuron, and a capillary (C) also is seen. Approx. × 7000. (Reproduced with permission from Peters, A., Palay, S. L., and Webster, H. de F.: *The Fine Structure of the Nervous System.* Philadelphia, W. B. Saunders Company, 1976.)

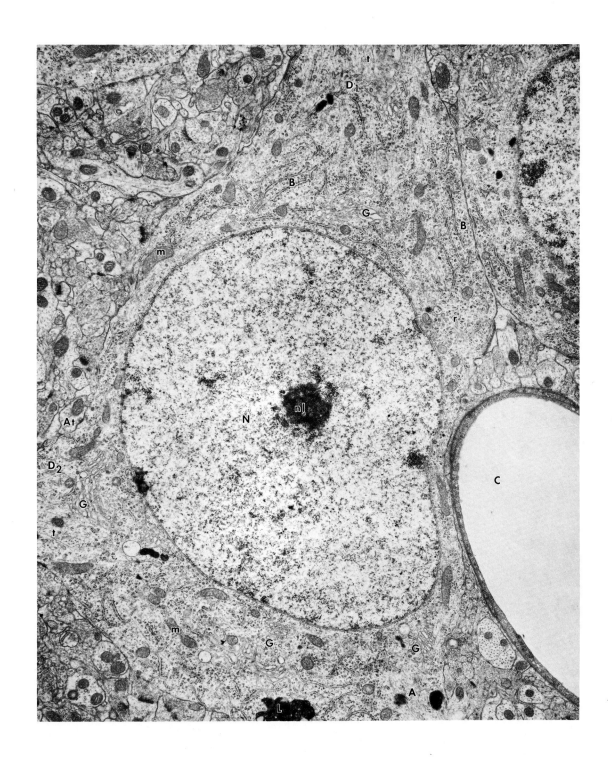

Figure 7–3. Anterior horn (multipolar, motor) neuron. Plastic section. Methylene blue, basic fuchsin. High power.

Nerve cell bodies (perikarya, soma) of motor neurons of the spinal cord are seen. They are large, and one (bottom) shows a typical, large vesicular nucleus with a prominent nucleolus (the "owl's-eye" appearance). Perikarya show clumps of blue-purple staining material, the Nissl bodies, that extend into dendrites. The central cell shows a branching dendrite (D) and an axon (A) devoid of Nissl substance and arising from the soma at the axon hillock (AH). Smaller nuclei present are mainly of oligodendrocytes with numerous capillaries (arrows).

Figure 7–4. Anterior horn, multipolar cell. Plastic section. Silver stain. High power.

This staining method demonstrates the shape of the perikaryon, which is multipolar with the roots of three large dendrites, and the presence in both soma and cell processes of neurofibrils, appearing here as dark strands and clumps. Clear cytoplasmic areas probably represent Nissl bodies (unstained). The central large nucleus is stained black. The neuropil around the motor neuron shows cell processes of other neurons, small dark nuclei of neuroglia, and capillaries.

Figure 7–5. Pyramidal cell. Silver impregnation. Medium power.

In this preparation, only the cell outline is seen. It shows two pyramidal cell bodies, long branching dendrites (D), and the root of one axon (A). Note on the dendritic branches the presence of small spines, the sites of synaptic contact (arrows).

Figure 7–6. Pseudounipolar cell. H and E. Oil immersion.

Although most ganglion cells of autonomic ganglia are multipolar, a few pseudounipolar cells may be present, as here. Note the single process (arrow) leaving the perikaryon, the large vesicular nucleus with prominent nucleolus, and the granular, basophil cytoplasm. Small nuclei of supporting cells, here resembling fibroblasts, surround the ganglion cells.

Figure 7–7. Multipolar cell. H and E. High power.

This is a smear preparation, not a section, and shows an anterior horn cell of the spinal cord. The nucleus is pale and spherical, and has a large, dense nucleolus. The cytoplasm is fibrillar, and the cell has numerous processes. Small dense nuclei around the nerve cell are composed mainly of oligodendrocytes.

Figure 7–8. Sympathetic (autonomic) ganglion cells. H and E. Medium power.

These multipolar cells are interspersed between nerve fibers, and several contain in their cytoplasm yellowish-brown pigment granules (lipochrome, an endogenous pigment). The amount of pigment appears to increase with age.

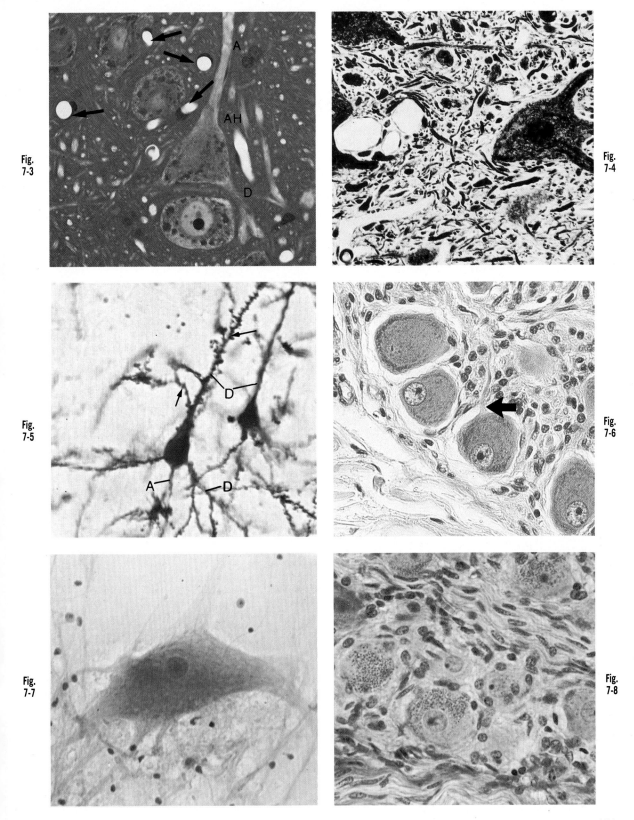

Fig.
7-3

Fig.
7-4

Fig.
7-5

Fig.
7-6

Fig.
7-7

Fig.
7-8

Figure 7–9. Astrocytes, fibrous. Silver preparation. Medium power.

This section is of white matter of the brain and shows two capillary blood vessels (C) with numerous fibrous astrocytes (A). These cells, also called spider cells, are small with numerous long, slender processes, some of which contact the walls of the blood vessels as perivascular feet.

Figure 7–10. Astrocytes, protoplasmic. Protargol. Medium power.

Blood vessels (C) are present in the gray matter of the brain. Closely adjacent to them are protoplasmic astrocytes (P), also called *mossy cells*. They differ from fibrous astrocytes not only in location but also in their having more numerous processes that show many branches. As in the case of fibrous astrocytes, some of the processes contact blood vessels as perivascular feet.

Figure 7–11. Microglia. Silver preparation. High power.

Microglia, the smallest neuroglial cells, are phagocytic and may be derived from several sources. They show small nuclei (arrows) with two or more short cytoplasmic processes. A blood vessel also is seen (C); microglial cells often are found near blood vessels throughout the gray and white matter.

Figure 7–12. Neuroglia, ependyma. Methylene blue, basic fuchsin. High power.

Most of the field shows the substance of the thalamus (diencephalon) adjacent to the third ventricle (right). In the area are numerous capillary vessels (V) with many small nuclei of neuroglial cells in the neuropil, some showing thin cytoplasmic rims. The larger, vesicular, ovoid nuclei probably are of astrocytes; the darker, smaller, more irregular ones are of oligodendrocytes. Lining the third ventricle is ependyma (arrows) (see also Figure 7–13), the remnants of the embryonic neuroepithelium that lines the entire ventricular system of the central nervous system. Ependyma appears as a simple cuboidal epithelium, here with apical cilia.

Figure 7–13. Ependyma, spinal cord. Plastic section. Methylene blue, basic fuchsin. High power.

The central canal (C) of the spinal cord is seen, lined by ependyma, here appearing as a simple low columnar epithelium. The free (apical or luminal) border of the cells appears irregular owing to the presence of microvilli, and a few cells show cilia (arrows). This is usual in the adult, although in the embryo most, if not all, the cells are ciliated. (Compare with Figure 7–12.)

Figure 7–14. Choroid plexus. Plastic section. Toluidine blue. Oil Immersion.

The choroid plexuses of the brain secrete cerebrospinal fluid and are formed by the ventricular lining (ependyma) protruding into the ventricular spaces and associated with blood capillaries of the pia mater. Here, the epithelium is cuboidal with central vesicular nuclei. Cytoplasm contains numerous mitochondria (blue-staining dots and short rods) and has an apical brush or striated border (B) composed of bulbous microvilli. Beneath the epithelium are numerous thin-walled capillary blood vessels containing erythrocytes stained black (arrows).

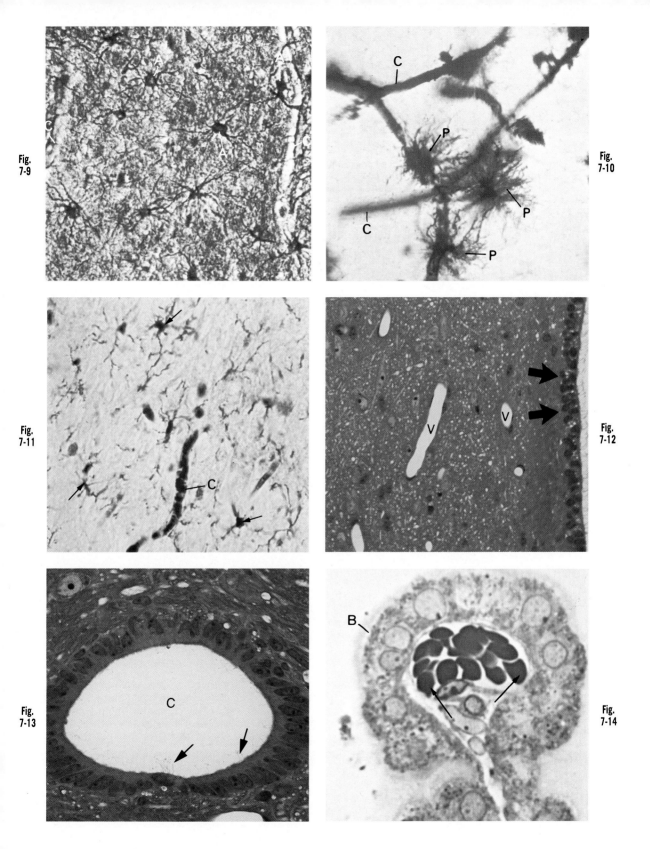

Figure 7–15. Peripheral nerve, transverse section. H and E. Low power.

The nerve fibers are arranged in bundles or fascicles (F), each surrounded by a pink-staining collagenous sheath—the perineurium (P). Finer connective tissue of the endoneurium extends around and between individual nerve fibers. Fascicles of nerve fibers are held together by stronger connective tissue of the epineurium (E). Blood vessels pass to the nerve in its connective tissue.

Figure 7–16. Peripheral (sciatic) nerve. Hematoxylin, aniline blue. Medium power.

Part of one fascicle of the nerve is seen with its perineurium (P) and surrounding epineurium (E). Collagen stains blue. Note fine strands of collagen of endoneurium between nerve fibers, here cut transversely, and in relation to a blood vessel (V). Each nerve fiber shows a dark central core, the axon, with a pale-staining cylinder of myelin around it.

Figure 7–17. Small peripheral nerve of tongue in transverse section. Methylene blue, basic fuchsin. High power.

A nerve fascicle (center) and portions of two others are seen, each enveloped in perineurium (P) and lying in striated muscle cut longitudinally and transversely (t). In each nerve bundle, myelinated axons are cut transversely and show a central, unstained axon surrounded by pink-staining myelin. Nuclei within the fascicle are of Schwann cells (arrowheads) and endoneurium (e).

Figure 7–18. Spinal nerve, transverse section. Methylene blue.

Here, only myelin is seen (stained blue) surrounding unstained nerve fibers. Fibers are of similar size, and the ring shape of the blue-staining myelin indicates that it has the form of a tubular cylinder around nerve axons. The myelinated fibers are collected into fascicles.

Figure 7–19. Nerve, transverse section. Plastic section. Toluidine blue. Medium power.

Parts of two fascicles are seen, each enveloped in perineurium (P) (light blue). Note the blood vessels (V) in connective tissue between the fascicles. Myelin is stained dark blue and appears as a ring around each unstained nerve fiber. Schwann or neurolemma cells are seen clearly in relation to some of the nerve fibers (arrows). Note the variation in size of both the nerve fibers and the thickness of the myelin. (See also Figure 7–20.)

Figure 7–20. Nerve, transverse section. Plastic section. Toluidine blue. Oil immersion.

Portions of two fascicles are seen, surrounded by perineurium (P). Myelinated nerve fibers vary in size and the myelin, stained dark blue, varies in thickness. Some show a clear relation to Schwann cells; i.e., the myelinated axon is "enclosed" within a Schwann cell, and in a few a Schwann cell nucleus (N) is seen. Endoneural nuclei (e) also are seen.

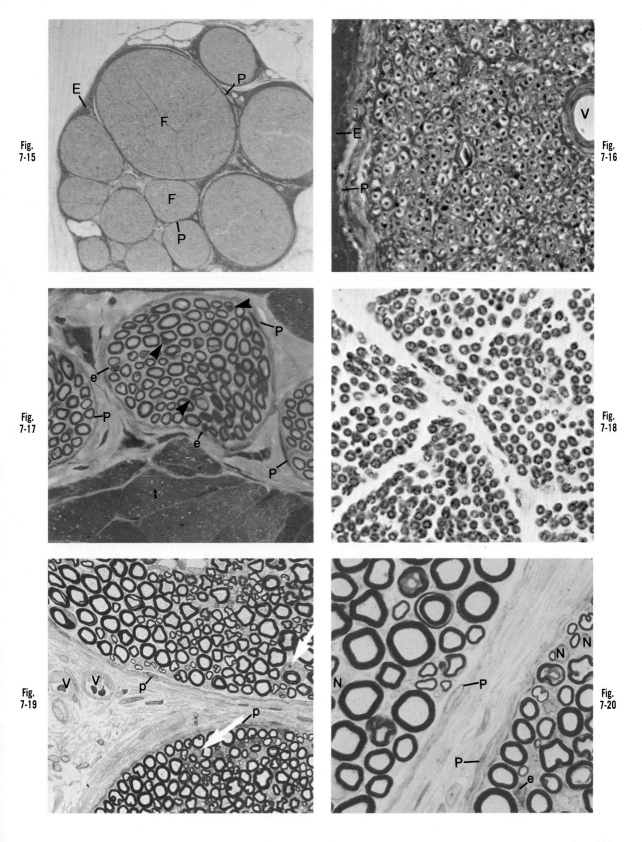

Fig.
7-15

Fig.
7-16

Fig.
7-17

Fig.
7-18

Fig.
7-19

Fig.
7-20

Figure 7–21. Teased nerve. Iron hematoxylin. High power.

A single myelinated nerve fiber is seen, surrounded by strands of endoneurium (e) (pale blue). The nerve fiber shows the neurokeratin network and a node of Ranvier (arrows).

Figure 7–22. Node of Ranvier, spinal nerve, longitudinal section. Iron hematoxylin, phosphotungstic acid. Oil immersion.

In this longitudinal section, only a few myelinated nerve fibers are seen, two of which show axons (A) traversing nodes of Ranvier (arrows), the axons ensheathed in myelin (M). A nucleus (N) of the endoneurium also is present in the field.

Figure 7–23. Dorsal root (sensory) ganglion. Plastic section. H and E. Medium power.

Part of a spinal dorsal root ganglion is seen, with nerve cell bodies in groups, mainly at the periphery of the ganglion, and bundles of nerve fibers (arrows) between the groups. Small, dark nuclei of satellite cells surround the nerve cell bodies.

Figure 7–24. Dorsal (spinal) root ganglion. Silver, aniline blue. Low power.

A portion of the ganglion shows groups of pseudounipolar nerve cell bodies with pale-staining nuclei, the cell bodies mainly located in the cortical (peripheral) zone *(top, left)*. The perikarya vary in size, the smaller with unmyelinated fibers, the larger with myelinated fibers. The fibers (darkly stained) are gathered into groups, mainly in the medullary (central) zone of the ganglion *(right).* (See also Figure 7–23.)

Figure 7–25. Sensory ganglion cells. Plastic section. Methylene blue, basic fuchsin. High power.

Several perikarya of sensory, pseudounipolar neurons are seen, and they vary in size. Some show a large vesicular nucleus with prominent nucleolus—the "owl's eye" appearance. Blue-staining Nissl bodies are prominent in the cytoplasm of the cells. Around the ganglion cells are small satellite cells (arrowheads) with nerve processes in small groups (arrows) between the cells.

Figure 7–26. Dorsal root ganglion, pseudounipolar cell. Plastic section. Toluidine blue. Oil immersion.

This perikaryon of a pseudounipolar cell of a sensory ganglion shows a globular shape with a large, centrally located, spherical nucleus. The cytoplasm is occupied largely by blue-staining Nissl bodies. At the top, the single cell process leaves the soma at an area devoid of Nissl substance (arrowhead), called the axon hillock. Around the soma are small satellite or supporting cells (arrows). (See also Figure 7–6.)

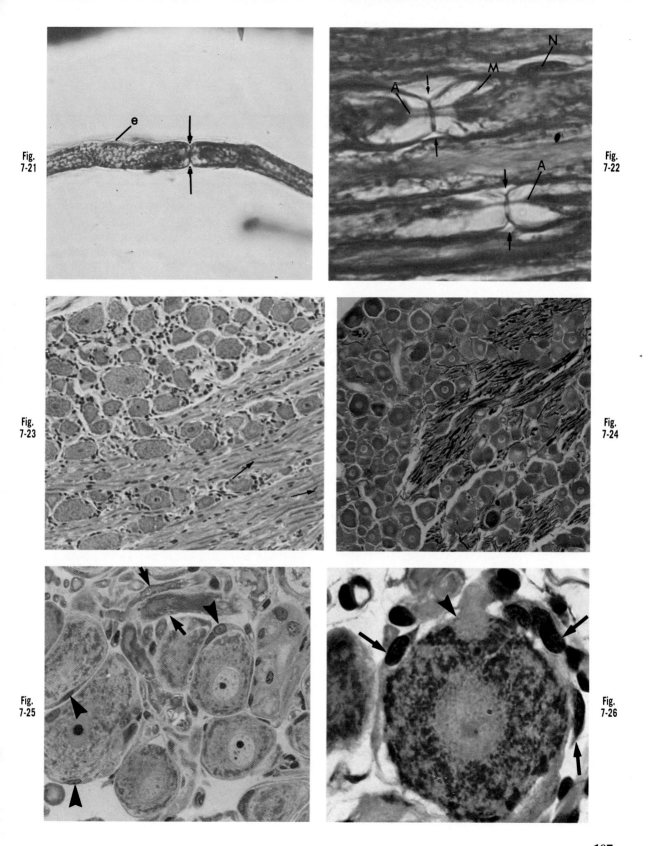

Fig.
7-21

Fig.
7-22

Fig.
7-23

Fig.
7-24

Fig.
7-25

Fig.
7-26

Figure 7–27. Autonomic ganglion. Plastic section. Methylene blue, basic fuchsin. High power.

This small peripheral ganglion from the tongue has a thin capsule (C) of connective tissue and contains large nerve cell bodies, some with large vesicular nuclei and prominent nucleoli and with Nissl bodies in the cytoplasm. A few small capsule cells (arrowheads) lie around the perikarya; these nerve cells are multipolar. To the left is an associated small nerve (N), and the whole lies between striated muscle fibers. Note the mast cell (M) also.

Figure 7–28. Ganglion cell, sympathetic ganglion. H and E. Oil immersion.

This large cell shows granular cytoplasm and a large vesicular nucleus with a prominent nucleolus. Surrounding it are small nuclei of satellite cells (arrows); these cells form a "capsule" around the ganglion cell. (See Figure 7–8.)

Figure 7–29. Spinal cord and canal, transverse section. H and E. Low power.

This low-power view shows muscle fibers (M) around bone (B) of the vertebra. In the vertebral canal lies the spinal cord (S), showing anterior (ventral) motor roots (V) and posterior (dorsal) sensory roots (D). On the latter is located the dorsal root ganglion (G). No detail of structure is seen in the spinal cord. (See Figures 7–30 and 7–31.)

Figure 7–30. Spinal cord, transverse section. Weigert's stain. Low power.

White matter, i.e., nerve fibers in tracts, stains dark gray and lies peripherally. Central gray matter (that is, where nerve cells are located) stains lighter and is in the form of an "H." The spinal cord is divided into right and left halves by the anterior median fissure (F) and the posterior median septum (arrow). The gray matter is divided into large anterior and smaller posterior (P) horns. Large motor neurons lie in the anterior horns (A).

Figure 7–31. Spinal cord, anterior horn. Silver, aniline blue. High power.

The large, multipolar cell in the gray matter (G) is a motor neuron of the anterior horn. The soma shows a large central vesicular nucleus, and the cytoplasm and cell processes contain faintly stained neurofibrils. (See also Figure 7–4.) The axon (cut short, A) is at bottom. Small nerve fibers in the neuropil around this cell are stained black. The long process (top left) is a dendrite (D) with synapses on it and the cell bodies (arrowheads). To the right is white matter (W), with axons stained black (dots) surrounded by clear, unstained myelin (arrows).

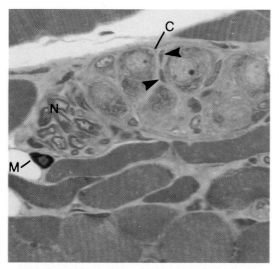

Fig.
7-27

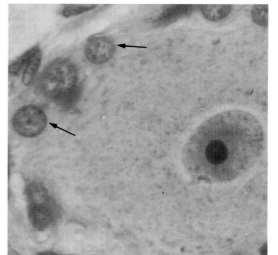

Fig.
7-28

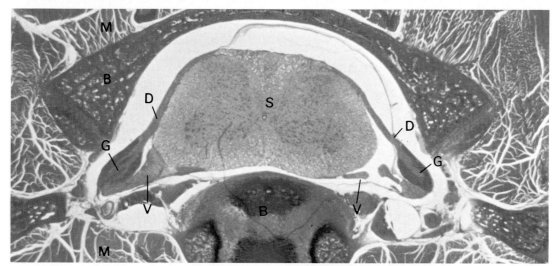

Fig.
7-29

Fig.
7-30

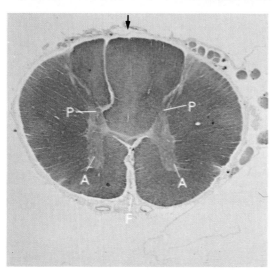

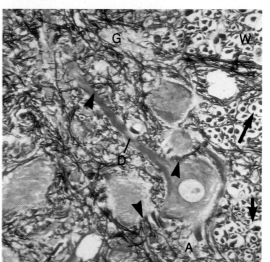

Fig.
7-31

Figure 7–32. Cerebellum. Plastic section. H and E. Medium power.

Part of one folium of the cerebellar cortex is seen with peripheral gray matter (G) and central white matter (W). In the cortex are three layers: (1) the outer, thick, molecular layer (M) with few, scattered, small nerve cell bodies; (2) a single layer of large, spaced Purkinje cells (P); and (3) an inner granular layer (L) of small, closely packed cells.

Figure 7–33. Cerebellum, Purkinje cell. Plastic section. Methylene blue, basic fuchsin. High power.

The flask-shaped perikaryon of the Purkinje cell contains a large vesicular nucleus with a prominent nucleolus. The cytoplasm shows blue-staining Nissl bodies. The single large branching dendrite (D) passes upward into the molecular layer (M) with a few small granule cells (G) below. Also seen in the molecular layer are nuclei of neuroglia (n).

Figure 7–34. Purkinje cells. Golgi. High power.

Only surface features are seen in this preparation. Purkinje cells have large, flask-shaped cell bodies with a single large dendrite (D) entering the molecular layer. This dendrite branches into a flat, fan-shaped network with numerous spines or gemmules. The single axon (A) leaves the base of the cell, passes through the granular layer, and either terminates in a deep central nucleus of the cerebellum or travels to another part of the cerebellar cortex.

Figure 7–35. Cerebral cortex. H and E. Low power.

White matter lies deeply (right) with gray matter superficially (left). Six layers are recognized in the cortex, and, while not clear here, obvious layering is seen. Large pyramidal cells (P) lie in layers 3 and 5.

Figure 7–36. Cerebral cortex, pyramidal cells. Golgi. Low power.

This illustrates layer 3 of the cerebral cortex with large pyramidal cells. (See also Figure 7–5.) These cells show several large branching dendrites and a single basal axon. By this method, only the cell surface is seen.

Figure 7–37. Neurovascular bundle. Plastic section. H and E. High Power.

Peripheral nerves of all sizes often are associated closely with arteries and veins in so-called "neurovascular bundles," even small nerves as illustrated here. The small nerve (N) here lies adjacent to and runs with a small arteriole (A) and a small venule (V), lying in connective tissue (collagen is pink). (See also Chapter 8.) This association is useful in identifying small peripheral nerves, which not always are identified easily; i.e., if a companion artery and vein (or arteriole and venule) can be seen, an accompanying nerve probably is present also.

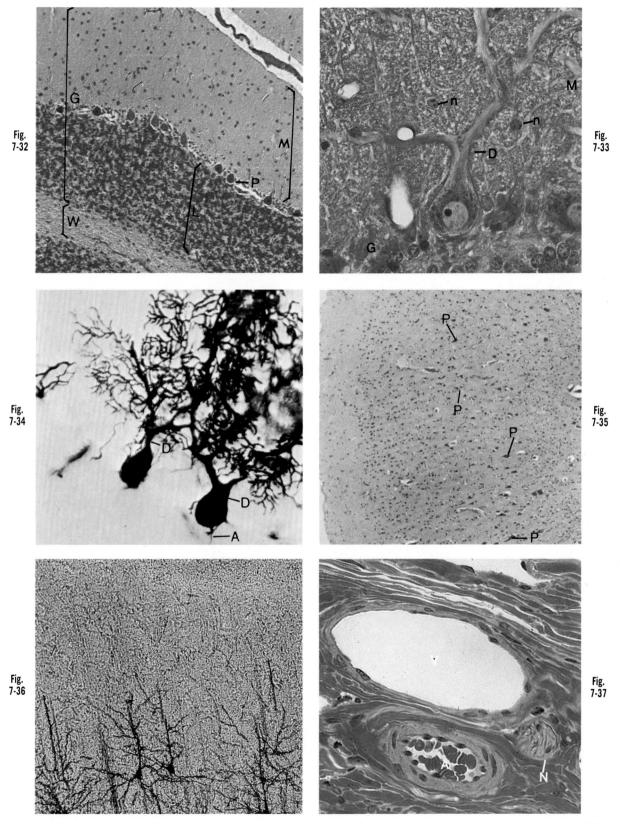

Fig.
7-32

Fig.
7-33

Fig.
7-34

Fig.
7-35

Fig.
7-36

Fig.
7-37

CHAPTER
EIGHT

The Circulatory System

The circulatory system consists of the *blood vascular system* and the *lymph vascular system.* The heart, the arteries, the capillaries, and the veins make up the blood vascular system, which distributes nutritive materials, oxygen, and hormones to the tissues and removes the cellular products of metabolism. The lymph vascular system commences in the tissues as blind tubules and consists of lymph capillaries and variously sized lymphatic vessels that return lymph from tissue spaces to the blood stream via the large veins in the neck. Lymphatic nodes are interposed along the course of lymphatic vessels and add lymphocytes to the lymph passing through them.

Frequently, nerve fascicles lie in company with arteries and veins as they course through the various tissues. These complexes are the so-called neurovascular bundles.

BLOOD VASCULAR SYSTEM

Capillaries. The blood vascular system has a continuous lining that consists of a single layer of endothelial cells. These cells generally have simple intercellular boundaries, which are formed by a close apposition of adjacent cell membranes with little intervening intercellular substance, but occasionally they show delicate interdigitations. In the capillaries, where the interchange of elements between the blood and other tissues occurs, the endothelial cells form the major component of the wall. They are separated from the supporting bed of connective tissue by a basal lamina. Recent electron microscopic studies form the basis of a classification of capillaries into three major types, continuous (Type I, or nonfenestrated), fenestrated (Type II), and sinusoidal (or discontinuous). Capillaries have an average diameter of about 8 microns, or micrometers (μm), and form a meshwork, the closeness of which is determined by the intensity of metabolism in each region. Arterial (pre-) and venous (post-) capillaries are vessels intermediate between arteries and capillaries, and capillaries and veins respectively.

Larger Vessels. All larger blood vessels exhibit a common plan of organization, and each specific type of vessel merely shows adaptations for particular purposes. Each vessel contains three concentric coats. The inner coat, or *tunica intima,* is composed of the endothelial cell layer exposed to the blood, a delicate subendothelial layer of connective tissue, and a layer of elastic tissue, the internal elastic membrane. The second coat, the *tunica media,* contains smooth muscle fibers and elastic and collagenous tissues in varying proportions. The outer coat, the *tunica adventitia,* essentially consists of fibroelastic tissue, the elastic component of which commonly concentrates next to the media as an external elastic layer or membrane. In large veins and certain muscular arteries, this coat also contains longitudinally running smooth muscle fibers. Small blood vessels, known as vasa vasorum, are found in the tunica adventitia.

Arterial Vessels. Arterial blood vessels are classified into three groups: (1) large arteries, containing a preponderance of elastic fibers; (2) small to medium-sized arteries, containing numerous muscular elements; and (3) arterioles, the smallest arterial vessels. Blood is ejected from the heart in a pulsatile fashion (i.e., during systole), and the large elastic arteries (the pulmonary arteries, the aorta, and its principal branches) expand to receive the output of the ventricles. The passive elastic recoil of these arteries during diastole smooths the flow of blood within them. The small and medium-sized (muscular) arteries, also termed *arteries of distribution,* regulate the flow of blood to the different organs and tissues of the body depending upon need. There is a gradual transition from elastic to muscular artery, and vessels possessing characteristics intermediate between the two types are seen. Arterioles, with a diameter of 100 μm or less, possess one to five layers of muscle cells within their tunica media. They have relatively thick walls and narrow lumina, and they control the distribution of blood to different capillary beds by vasodilation and vasoconstriction in localized regions. They are the prime controllers of systemic blood pressure, and most of the fall in blood pressure occurs within them, so that only a gentle stream passes into the delicate capillary beds.

Venous Vessels. Venous blood vessels also are classified into three groups: (1) venules, (2) small to medium-sized veins, and (3) large veins. Since blood in the veins is under a pressure much less than that in the arteries, they must accommodate a greater volume of blood. Hence, veins generally are larger in diameter than their corresponding arteries, and their walls are thinner, chiefly because of a reduction of muscular and elastic components. The transition from capillary or venous capillary to venule is a gradual one and involves the acquisition of connective tissue elements first and smooth muscle fibers later. Venules can be recognized as such when they are about 20 μm in diameter and possess an endothelial lining and an outer sheath of collagenous fibers. When the vessel attains a diameter of about 50 μm, elastic fibers appear in the tunica intima and smooth muscle fibers are present between the intima and the outer fibrous sheath. In venules of 200 μm or more, the circular muscle fibers form a continuous layer (media), one to three cells thick. Small and medium-sized veins show a distinct intima, media, and adventitia. The intima and media are thin, and the adventitia is well developed and forms the bulk of the wall. In large veins, the intima may contain some longitudinal smooth muscle and the media is poorly developed. Smooth muscle elements within it are reduced or absent. The adventitia is the thickest of the three coats and contains many longitudinal muscle fibers, separated by collagenous fibers. Many small and medium-sized veins, particularly those of the lower limb, possess *valves* that prevent retrograde blood flow. The valves are paired folds or pockets of the intima that project into the lumen with their free margins directed toward the heart. Both surfaces of the valve are covered with endothelium. In these veins, blood flow against gravity and toward the heart is aided by contraction of neighboring skeletal muscles and the system of valves. Blood travels along the larger veins of the trunk by a sucking effect generated during respiratory movements, and these vessels are devoid of valves.

The Heart. The heart, a highly specialized portion of the vascular system that propels blood through the blood vessels, has three layers—an inner endocardium, a middle myocardium, and an outer epicardium. These correspond roughly to the three tunics of larger blood vessels. The endocardium is continuous with the intima of blood vessels and is composed of an endothelial lining, a layer of relatively dense connective tissue, and an outer layer of loose connective tissue. The latter contains numerous blood vessels and nerves and branches of the conducting system of the heart. The myocardium is composed of cardiac muscle and its thickness varies in different parts of the heart, being thinnest in the atria and thickest in the left ventricle. The muscle is arranged in sheets that wind around the chambers in complex, spiraling courses and mostly attach to the central supporting structure of the heart, the cardiac skeleton. The external coat, the epicardium, is a serous membrane (the visceral pericardium). It is covered externally by a single layer of mesothelial cells, beneath which is a relatively thick layer of areolar or adipose tissue containing the coronary blood vessels and nerves. The atrioventricular valves of the heart and the semilunar valves of the aorta and pulmonary artery are reduplications of endocardium containing a core of dense connective tissue continuous with that of the cardiac skeleton. A system of specialized cardiac muscle fibers, the Purkinje fibers, coordinates the heart beat. Purkinje fibers generally have a larger diameter than ordinary cardiac muscle fibers and contain relatively more sarcoplasm. Myofibrils are reduced in number and usually are limited to the periphery of the fibers. An impulse begins at the sinoatrial node, which consists of a dense network of small Purkinje fibers that are in continuity with atrial cardiac muscle fibers. The impulse spreads via these muscle fibers to the atrioventricular node, a dense mass of Purkinje fibers located in the median wall of the right atrium. The node continues into a common stem, the atrioventricular bundle, which divides into two trunks that lie beneath the endocardium on either side of the interventricular septum. These trunks terminate in a system of Purkinje fibers that connects with ordinary cardiac muscle fibers of the ventricles.

LYMPH VASCULAR SYSTEM

The lymph vascular system commences as blindly ending capillaries which, like blood capillaries, are simple, endothelium-lined tubes, but which are some-what larger and not uniform in caliber. They lack a complete basal lamina and are surrounded by a thin layer of reticular and collagenous fibers. They form richly anastomosing plexuses that drain into larger lymphatic vessels. These vessels structurally resemble veins but their walls tend to be thinner than those of veins of equal caliber. The vessels contain numerous valves that are more closely spaced than those found in veins. Between valves, the vessels are swollen; thus they have a beaded appearance. The lymphatic vessels finally join to form the main lymphatic trunks—the thoracic and right lymphatic ducts—that empty into veins at the root of the neck. In structure, the main lymphatic trunks are much like a vein of equal size, except for a greater concentration of smooth muscle fibers within the media.

Figure 8–1. Fenestrated capillary: freeze-etch preparation.

A surface view of portions of two endothelial cells is shown. The interface between the two cells runs obliquely across the figure. In both cells, circular fenestrations, each closed by a diaphragm, are frequent. $\times$ 40,000.

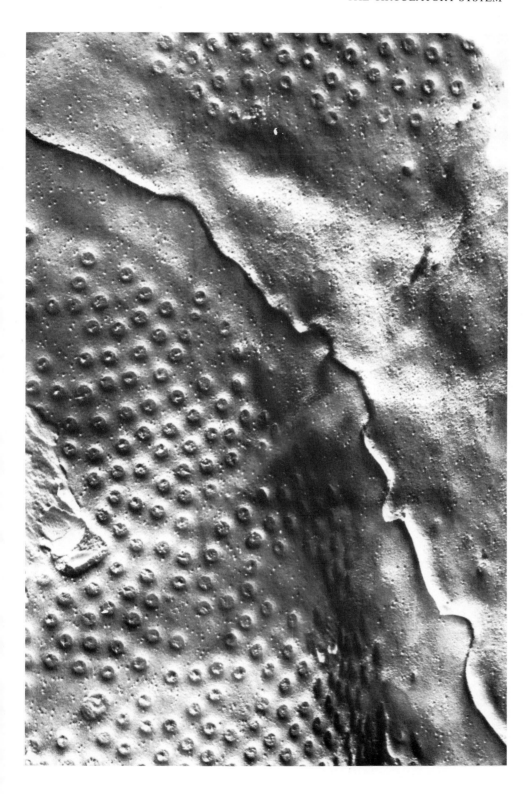

Figure 8–2. Conducting system of the heart.

Drawing of the heart, with the interior of the ventricles exposed, to show the main components of the conducting system. S.A.N. = sinoatrial node; A.V.N. = atrioventricular node; A.V.B. = atrioventricular bundle (of His); R. and L.B.B. = right and left branches of the bundle.

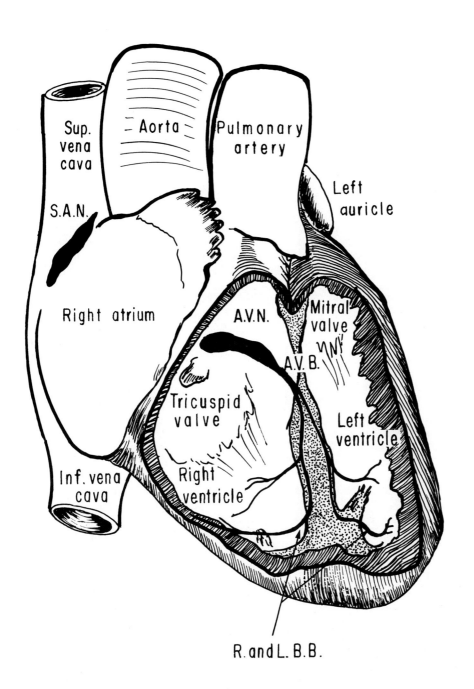

Sup.
vena
cava

Aorta

Pulmonary
artery

Left
auricle

S.A.N.

Right atrium

A.V.N.

Mitral
valve

A.V.B.

Tricuspid
valve

Left
ventricle

Inf. vena
cava

Right
ventricle

R. and L. B.B.

Figure 8–3. Endothelium. Spread preparation. Silver method. Medium power.

In this spread preparation of mesentery, a portion of a small vein is shown. The lining endothelial cells have been outlined with silver. Note that the cells are elongated in the long axis of the vessel and show simple intercellular boundaries.

Figure 8–4. Blood capillaries. Mallory-Azan. High power.

Two capillaries, sectioned longitudinally, are present in this section of a pulmonary lymph node. Nuclei of endothelial cells (arrows) lining the vessels are elongated and protrude into the lumen. The cytoplasm of these cells is attenuated and difficult to define. Each capillary is surrounded by a thin sheath of delicate reticular and collagenous fibers (blue). The surrounding tissue contains concentrations of lymphocytes, with densely staining spherical nuclei and no apparent cytoplasm.

Figure 8–5. Capillaries. Spread preparation. Nuclear fast red. Medium power.

In this spread preparation of mesentery, there is a network of small blood vessels that contain packed erythrocytes within their lumina. A small arteriole (A) branches into numerous capillaries (C). The walls of the blood vessels are not stained. The background connective tissue, which is adipose in character, is indistinct and contains a mast cell (arrow).

Figure 8–6. Capillaries. Plastic section. H and E. High power.

In this section of tendon, a portion of peritendineum appears between two fiber bundles. The peritendineum contains a capillary, sectioned both transversely (above) and longitudinally (below). Endothelial nuclei (arrows) project into the lumen, and the cytoplasm of these cells is attenuated. The capillary is embedded in delicate connective tissue (pink).

Figure 8–7. Aorta. Verhoeff's elastic stain. Low power.

In this elastic artery, sectioned transversely with the lumen to the left, the thin tunica intima cannot be defined at this magnification. The tunica media is thick and composed principally of concentrically arranged laminae of elastic tissue. The narrow spaces between the laminae contain some collagenous fibers and smooth muscle cells. The tunica adventitia (TA) is relatively thin and consists mainly of collagenous fibers. It merges into the surrounding adipose tissue (arrows).

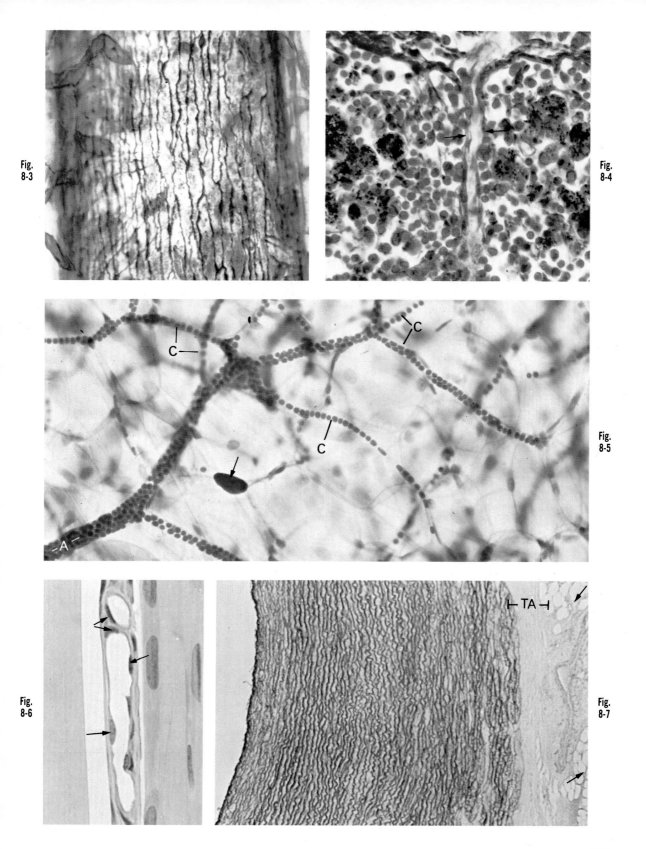

Fig. 8-3

Fig. 8-4

Fig. 8-5

Fig. 8-6

Fig. 8-7

Figure 8–8. Aorta. Plastic section. Methylene blue. Low power.

The concentrically arranged laminae of elastic tissue within the thick tunica media are unstained and appear wavy in this preparation. The stained material between the laminae contains fibroblasts, an amorphous ground substance, collagenous fibers, and scattered smooth muscle cells. The tunica adventitia (TA) contains numerous small blood vessels (vasa vasorum). The thin tunica intima in relation to the lumen (L) cannot be defined at this magnification.

Figure 8–9. Large muscular artery. Plastic section. Methylene blue. Medium power.

The tunica intima exhibits three definite layers. Beneath the endothelium, there is a prominent subendothelial layer (arrows) and a thick, wavy internal elastic lamina (unstained). In the underlying tunica media, numerous elastic fibers course between groups of smooth muscle cells.

Figure 8–10. Muscular artery. Mallory. Low power.

This artery is sectioned transversely and shows a lumen (L) full of erythrocytes. The endothelium cannot be discerned at this magnification. A thin subendothelial layer of delicate connective tissue (blue) lies internal to the prominent internal elastic membrane (red), which shows a wavy outline. The thick tunica media (light blue) is composed of numerous layers of circularly disposed smooth muscle cells, between which are a few elastic fibers (red). The tunica adventitia (dark blue) is almost as thick as the tunica media and is composed principally of collagenous fibers. It contains a small blood vessel (arrow), one of the vasa vasorum.

Figure 8–11. Muscular artery. Weigert's elastic stain. Low power.

This large muscular artery, sectioned transversely and with the lumen to the left, shows the internal elastic membrane (I) and elastic fibers within the tunica adventitia concentrated in relationship to the tunica media (TM) as the external elastic layer (E). Elastic fibers also are present in the tunica media, between the concentrically arranged smooth muscle cells.

Figure 8–12. Muscular artery. Gridley's reticulin. Medium power.

The thick tunica media is bounded internally by the internal elastic lamina (unstained) and externally by a concentration of reticular fibers (specifically stained) in the tunica adventitia. Smooth muscle cells within the tunica media are outlined by staining of the delicate reticular fibers that surround them.

Figure 8–13. Muscular artery. Plastic section. Toluidine blue, safranin. High power.

This small muscular artery is sectioned longitudinally. The tunica intima is composed principally of endothelium (E) and a distinct internal elastic membrane (red). Muscle cells, circularly arranged and here sectioned transversely, compose the tunica media. A nucleus is visible in most cells. A small portion of the external elastic layer of the tunica adventitia appears at lower right.

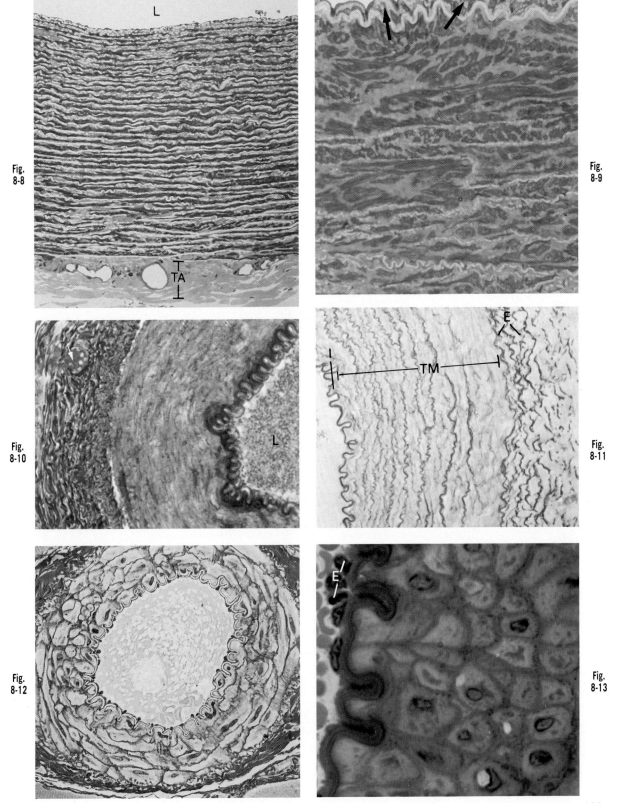

Fig. 8-8

Fig. 8-9

Fig. 8-10

Fig. 8-11

Fig. 8-12

Fig. 8-13

Figure 8–14. Muscular artery and medium-sized vein. Plastic section. Methylene blue, azure A. Low power.

Comparison of vein (*left*) and artery (*right*) within loose areolar connective tissue. The artery is identified by the overall thickness of its wall, the thick tunica media, and the prominent internal elastic lamina (unstained). Smooth muscle cells in the thin tunica media of the vein are separated by connective tissue, principally collagenous fibers.

Figure 8–15. Arteriole and venule. Plastic section. Methylene blue, azure A. High power.

The loose connective tissue between bundles of smooth muscle cells, sectioned transversely, contains a small arteriole (*left*) which shows a tunica intima, consisting of endothelium (arrows) and a narrow internal elastic lamina (unstained), and a tunica media composed of a single layer of smooth muscle cells. The tunica adventitia is narrow and ill-defined and blends with the surrounding connective tissue. The venule (*right*) has a wall that consists of endothelium (arrows) and a thin outer sheath (adventitia) of collagenous fibers that merge with those of the surrounding connective tissue. Also present are a lymph capillary (L), which appears as an irregular cleft within the connective tissue lined by endothelial cells, and an arterial capillary (arrowhead, *lower left*).

Figure 8–16. Arteriole. Plastic section. H and E. High power.

This arteriole, within the capsule of the suprarenal gland, is sectioned both transversely (*below*) and longitudinally (*above*). In the intermediate portion, the section passes through the wall and shows the circular arrangement of smooth muscle cells. Nuclei of endothelial cells (E) appear elongated, and the tunica media consists of a single layer of smooth muscle cells (M).

Figure 8–17. Neurovascular bundle. Plastic section. H and E. Medium power.

This section shows a venule (V), an arteriole (A), and a nerve fascicle (N) within dense, irregular connective tissue. The small venule possesses an endothelial lining and a delicate sheath of connective tissue (adventitia). The arteriole shows an endothelium, a distinct internal elastic membrane (red, arrows), and a thin tunica media. The nerve fascicle, surrounded by delicate connective tissue (perineurium), contains cross-sectioned nerve fibers. The nuclei are those of neurilemma (Schwann) cells.

Figure 8–18. Medium-sized vein. Weigert's elastic stain. Low power.

The concentration of elastic fibers as the internal elastic layer (I) marks the boundary between the narrow tunica intima and the tunica media (M). The latter is composed of small bundles of smooth muscle cells separated by delicate networks of elastic fibers. A portion of the adventitia (A), composed of thick collagenous fibers interspersed with delicate elastic fibers, lies to the right.

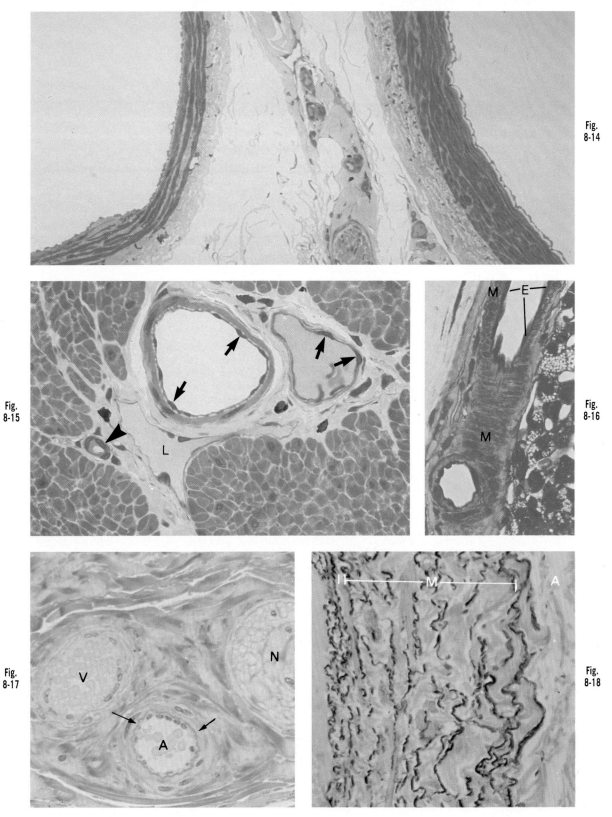

Fig.
8-14

Fig.
8-15

Fig.
8-16

Fig.
8-17

Fig.
8-18

Figure 8–19. Inferior vena cava. Plastic section. H and E. Low power.

In this large vein, the tunica media is thin and contains only a few smooth muscle cells, circularly arranged. The tunica adventitia is thick and contains numerous bundles of longitudinally arranged smooth muscle cells, here sectioned transversely, that are separated by collagenous fibers.

Figure 8–20. Inferior vena cava. Plastic section. Methylene blue, azure A. Medium power.

This is a section of the inferior vena cava immediately prior to its entry into the right atrium. The thin tunica media is composed principally of connective tissue elements, but it does contain a few smooth muscle cells that are circularly arranged. The thick tunica adventitia contains principally cardiac muscle.

Figure 8–21. Epicardium. Azan. Low power.

The epicardium is covered by a single layer of mesothelium (arrows). Beneath this, there is a thin layer of collagenous connective tissue (blue) and a wide subepicardial layer composed principally of adipose tissue. This layer, which attaches to the myocardium (M), contains a large tributary of the coronary sinus that shows a thick tunica intima (gray), no obvious tunica media, and a distinct tunica adventitia (blue).

Figure 8–22. Sinoatrial node. Phosphotungstic acid, hematoxylin. Low power.

The node, which lies within the subepicardial layer, consists of an irregular nework of small Purkinje fibers (purple) separated by bundles of collagenous fibers (red). At the lower border of the node, there is a large branch of the coronary artery. A small portion of the myocardium of the right atrium is present at the extreme right.

Figure 8–23. Atrioventricular bundle. Phosphotungstic acid, hematoxylin. Low power.

The bundle appears as an indefinite group of fibers extending from top left to bottom right. It is composed of small Purkinje fibers (purple) and of loose connective tissue that is continuous at the periphery of the bundle with the connective tissue of the cardiac skeleton. A small portion of the myocardium of the left ventricle is present at the upper right.

Figure 8–24. Purkinje fibers. Plastic section. Methylene blue, azure A. High power.

Purkinje fibers, sectioned transversely, are shown within the ventricular subendocardium. The fibers are large, with clear sarcoplasm centrally that contains an occasional nucleus and with peripheral concentrations of myofibrils. The Purkinje fibers may be identified readily from the ordinary cardiac musculature of the myocardium (above).

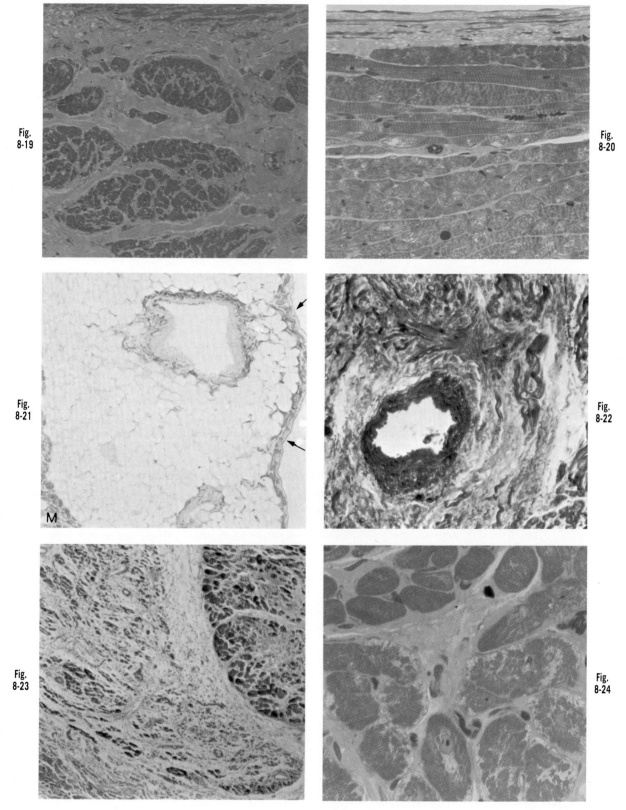

Fig.
8-19

Fig.
8-20

Fig.
8-21

M

Fig.
8-22

Fig.
8-23

Fig.
8-24

Figure 8–25. Purkinje fibers. H and E. Medium power.

A small bundle of Purkinje fibers, sectioned longitudinally, occupies the center of the field. The fibers are large and possess pale nuclei situated in a clear central mass of sarcoplasm. Myofibrils are relatively sparse and are limited to the periphery of the fibers. The features of the Purkinje fibers should be compared with those of ordinary cardiac muscle fibers of the myocardium (left). In the latter, the fibers are small and stain more densely, owing to the concentration of myofibrils within them. A small portion of the connective tissue of the endocardium lies to the right.

Figure 8–26. Thoracic duct. Plastic section. Methylene blue, azure A. Medium power.

The thin tunica intima of main lymphatic trunks consist of an endothelial lining, a delicate subendothelial layer, and a thin, inconstant elastic membrane; however, only the endothelial lining can be defined at this magnification. The tunica media contains smooth muscle cells, usually arranged concentrically. The tunica adventitia, which consists of coarse collagenous fibers, contains a few small blood vessels (vasa vasorum, arrows).

Figure 8–27. Lymph capillary. Plastic section. Methylene blue, azure A. High power.

A small lymph capillary within the myocardium of the heart is shown. It presents as an irregular cleft within the delicate connective tissue between cardiac muscle cells. It is lined by endothelial cells, the nuclei of which are apparent (arrows).

Figure 8–28. Lymphatic vessel. Plastic section. H and E. Medium power.

A lymphatic vessel, sectioned obliquely, lies within the connective tissue at the hilum of a lymph node. The section has passed through the roots of two valve leaflets. The wall of the vessel consists of endothelial cells, a few nuclei of which are apparent (arrows), and a thin outer sheath (adventitia) of collagenous fibers. Also present within the connective tissue are a venule (V) and an arteriole (A).

Figure 8–29. Lymphatic vessel: valve. Spread preparation. Nuclear fast red. Medium power.

A lymphatic vessel is shown within this spread preparation of connective tissue. Only nuclei, both within the vessel wall and within the surrounding connective tissue, are stained. A pair of valves within the lumen of the vessel is seen clearly, with the free ends of the valves directed centrally (to the right). The vessel expands in diameter beyond the attachment of the valves.

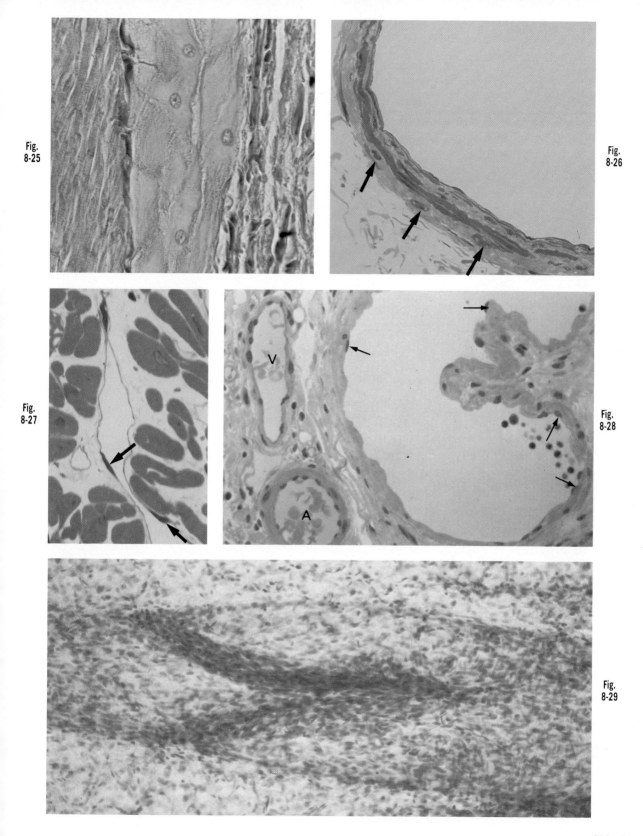

Fig.
8-25

Fig.
8-26

Fig.
8-27

Fig.
8-28

Fig.
8-29

129

CHAPTER
NINE

Lymphoid Organs

Several organs and structures within the body consist largely of *lymphoid (lymphatic)* tissue, which has two principal components:

1. *Reticular tissue* comprises a framework of reticular fibers and reticular cells. The reticular cells may be relatively undifferentiated (primitive reticular cells), or they may have acquired phagocytic properties to become fixed macrophages.

2. The *free cells*, which lie within the interstices of the reticular tissue, are of several types. Most common are the small lymphocytes. Medium-sized lymphocytes and large lymphocytes, which are actively dividing elements, are less abundant. Free macrophages, plasma cells, monocytes, and granulocytes are found within the meshes of the stroma.

In many regions the lymphoid tissue is not sharply delineated from the surrounding connective tissue and is termed *diffuse lymphoid tissue*. It occurs principally as an infiltration of the lamina propria of mucous membranes, particularly those of the digestive and respiratory systems. It is characterized by a loose organization of lymphocytes. This form of lymphoid tissue grades into a more dense form, termed *lymph nodules*, in which the component cells, principally lymphocytes, are concentrated into dense spherical masses. Each nodule may appear homogeneous or may exhibit a darker cortex and a lighter central area, the germinal center. Lymph nodules are not constant features, either in structure or in position. They appear, remain for a time, and then disappear. New nodules may arise in diffuse lymphoid tissue at any time, since they are an expression of the cytogenetic and defense functions of lymphoid tissue.

The development of lymphocytes and monocytes occurs within the lymphoid tissue and, to some degree, within myeloid tissue as well. The process of differentiation of these cells cannot be followed as readily as that of myeloid elements, however, since morphological evidence of differentiation is not marked. Both lymphocytes and monocytes retain the cytoplasmic basophilia and generally primitive nuclear shape of the stem cell. The latter cell, the *hemocytoblast* (or lymphoblast), divides actively to give rise to large and medium-sized lymphocytes which, in turn, multiply and differentiate into small lymphocytes. The development of small lymphocytes occurs principally in the lymph nodes and spleen, whereas monocytes develop mainly within the spleen and bone marrow, either directly from hemocytoblasts or via a lymphocyte stage.

Lymph nodules may occur as isolated nodules, such as the solitary nodules of the digestive tract, or they may be aggregated, forming the unencapsulated *Peyer's patches* of the intestine. Other nodules are components of specific lymphoid organs such as the lymph nodes, tonsils, and spleen, where they constitute the structural units. Lymph nodes are the only lymphoid organs that are interposed in the course of lymphatic vessels—thus, they possess both afferent and efferent lymphatic vessels. The tonsils, thymus, and spleen have efferent vessels, but they are not associated with afferent lymphatic vessels.

LYMPH NODES

Lymph nodes are covered by a definite capsule that is continuous with *septa* or *trabeculae*, in the substance of each organ. The capsule is pierced by numerous afferent lymphatic vessels and at the *hilum* by a few efferent lymphatic vessels.

The parenchyma of each node is specialized into two regions: an outer *cortex* containing lymph nodules, and an inner *medulla*, in which the lymphoid tissue is arranged chiefly in the form of irregular, anastomosing cords.

Internal to the major cortical zone, which contains nodules that are responsible for the production of specific humoral antibody, there is a zone composed principally of small lymphocytes, the *paracortex*. The latter is concerned with cell-mediated immune responses.

The lymph sinuses, through which lymph circulates, are subdivided into *subcapsular, cortical* (paratrabecular), and *medullary* groups. They are incompletely lined by reticular cells and by fixed macrophages whose cytoplasmic processes form a network supported by reticular fibers.

TONSILS

The *palatine, lingual,* and *pharyngeal* tonsils form a ring of lymphoid tissue around the pharynx. They show greater organization than aggregated nodules in that they are encapsulated and possess epithelial inpocketings and a coarse internal framework of collagenous and reticular fibers. The epithelium covering the tonsils is extensively infiltrated by lymphocytes. Plexuses of lymph capillaries occur around the lymphoid tissue and drain into efferent lymphatic vessels.

THE THYMUS GLAND

The thymus varies in size and attains its maximum development at about puberty, after which it involutes. It is bi-lobed, and each lobe contains thousands of *lobules*, each with *cortical* and *medullary* components. Extensions from the thin capsule delineate the lobules, which are not completely separate since the medulla constitutes a central core that sends prolongations into each lobule. The cortex lacks lymph nodules and consists of lymphocytes *(thymocytes)* that are densely packed, obscuring the sparse reticular framework. Lymphocytes are less numerous in the medulla, and consequently the epithelial reticular cells are prominent. The medulla also contains *thymic corpuscles* (of Hassall)—spherical or ovoid bodies composed of concentrically arranged epithelial cells.

There are no afferent lymphatic vessels and no lymph sinuses in the thymus. Efferent lymphatics run mainly in the interlobular connective tissue.

THE SPLEEN

The spleen, the largest lymphoid organ, is specialized for filtering blood. The capsule, covered by a serosa, consists of collagenous and elastic fibers and some smooth muscle. Thick trabeculae, which contain large branches of the splenic artery and vein, pass from the capsule into the interior of the organ. Between the trabeculae there is a network of reticular fibers that supports the *splenic parenchyma*. The latter is of two types:

1. *White pulp,* typical lymphoid tissue that surrounds and follows the arteries.
2. *Red pulp*, which often occurs in irregular masses, the *pulp cords*.

The distribution and organization of the white and red pulp depend upon the complex vascular arrangement. Splenic arteries branch within the trabeculae and leave them to enter the splenic parenchyma. As they do so, the tunica adventitia of the arteries becomes infiltrated with lymphocytes. At various points along the course of the vessels, the lymphatic sheath is increased in amount to form the *splenic* (or *malpighian*) *nodules*. The vessels, which are termed *central arteries* or *arterioles,* although they are eccentric with reference to the nodules, supply capillaries to the white pulp. After numerous divisions, the arterioles lose their investment of white pulp and enter the red pulp. Here each arteriole subdivides into several branches called *penicilli*. These small vessels show three distinct regions:

1. Pulp arterioles.
2. Sheathed arterioles.
3. Terminal capillaries

The termination of the capillaries is the subject of considerable controversy, and discussion of this can be found in textbooks of histology. The capillaries open either directly into venous sinuses or into the pulp reticulum, from which blood gradually filters back into the *venous sinuses*. The venous sinuses, which form a system of irregular, anastomosing tunnels through the red pulp, are lined by specialized reticular cells supported by reticular fibers. These sinuses eventually empty into pulp veins, lined by endothelium, that leave the pulp and unite to form larger veins that pass into the trabeculae as *trabecular* or *interlobular veins*. Like the thymus, the spleen has no afferent lymphatic vessels and no lymph sinuses.

Figure 9–1. Splenic lobule.

In this diagrammatic representation, the white pulp consists of nodules and aggregations of lymphocytes that surround and follow the arterial blood vessels. The red pulp is an open mesh with sinusoids.

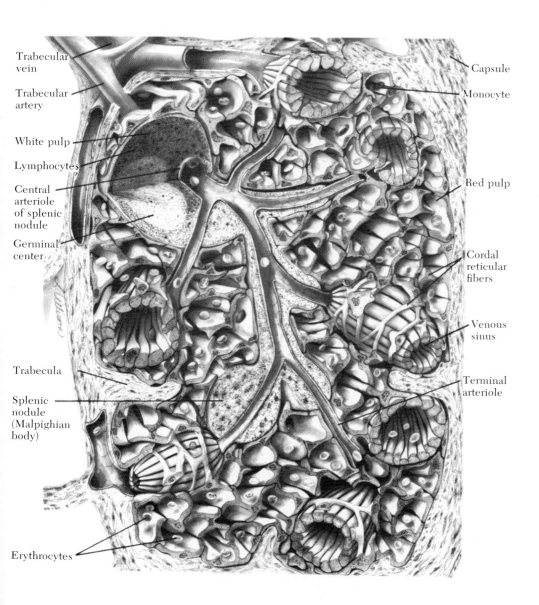

Trabecular vein

Trabecular artery

White pulp

Lymphocytes

Central arteriole of splenic nodule

Germinal center

Trabecula

Splenic nodule (Malpighian body)

Erythrocytes

Capsule

Monocyte

Red pulp

Cordal reticular fibers

Venous sinus

Terminal arteriole

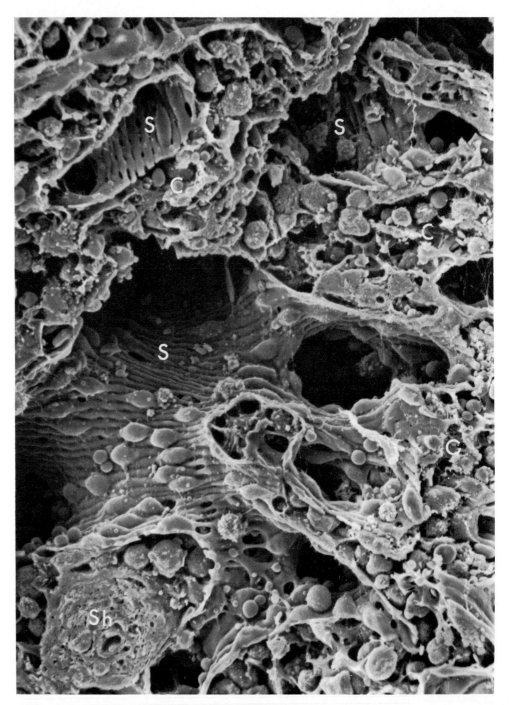

Figure 9–2. Scanning electron micrograph of the red pulp of the spleen.

The walls of the venous sinuses (S) are seen mainly in surface view. Also shown are splenic cords (C) and a sheathed arteriole (Sh). × 700. (Courtesy of Dr. T. Fujita.)

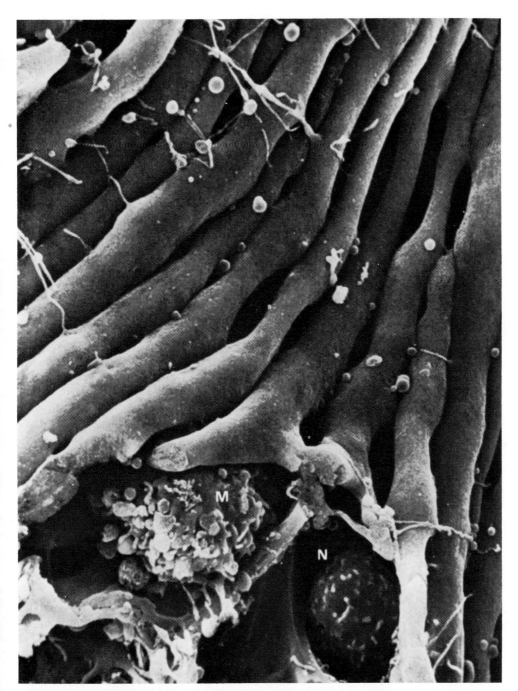

Figure 9–3. Scanning electron micrograph of a venous sinus.

The littoral (rod) cells show deficiencies between them. Also present are a macrophage (M) and a neutrophil leukocyte (N). × 3700. (Courtesy of Dr. T. Fujita.)

Figure 9–4. Ileum: Peyer's patch. H and E. Low power.

Peyer's patches are aggregations of lymph nodules within the antimesenteric wall of the ileum. Here, each nodule shows a pale germinal center and a darker periphery. Over the patch, villi (V) are present in reduced numbers and appear somewhat irregular in outline. the muscularis mucosae (arrows) is interrupted by the nodules, which extend into the submucosa (SM). The muscularis externa (M) limits the submucosa externally.

Figure 9–5. Lymph node. H and E. Low power.

The lymph node is surrounded by a definite capsule (arrows), composed principally of densely packed collagenous fibers. The parenchyma of the node is specialized into two regions, an outer cortex (C) and an inner medulla (M). The cortex consists of lymph nodules, most of which show pale germinal centers. The nodules are separated from the capsule by a narrow space, the subcapsular sinus, through which lymph circulates. The medulla appears pale, and the lymphoid tissue within it is arranged in dense, irregular anastomosing strands or medullary cords. The cords are surrounded by medullary lymph sinuses.

Figure 9–6. Lymph node. Azan. Medium power.

The capsule (blue) contains numerous blood vessels, and from its inner aspect small bundles of fibers extend as trabeculae into the interior of the node. The cortex (C) contains lymphocytes closely packed into nodules, some of which show pale germinal centers. The lymph spaces between the cortex and the capsule constitute the subcapsular sinus. The medulla (M) contains irregular lymph (medullary) cords that are surrounded by wide medullary lymph sinuses. A few blood vessels (red) are present in both cortex and medulla.

Figure 9–7. Lymph node: cortex. Reticular fibers. Bielschowsky's method. High power.

The capsule (top) contains collagenous fibers (yellow-brown) and scattered delicate reticular fibers (black). Small lymphocytes are present within the subcapsular sinus (S), which is bridged by a few reticular fibers. Below this, there is a portion of a cortical lymph nodule in which there is a delicate meshwork of reticular fibers between the massed lymphocytes. Concentrations of reticular fibers also are present around small blood vessels (V), sectioned obliquely.

Figure 9–8. Lymph node: cortical nodule. Plastic section. H and E. Oil immersion.

The germinal center (outlined) contains principally medium-sized lymphocytes. A few cells (arrows) show large nuclei with distinct nucleoli. These are large lymphocytes and lymphoblasts. Occasional plasma cells (P) also occur in this zone. Small lymphocytes, produced within the germinal center, are pushed to the periphery and constitute the cortex of the nodule (C).

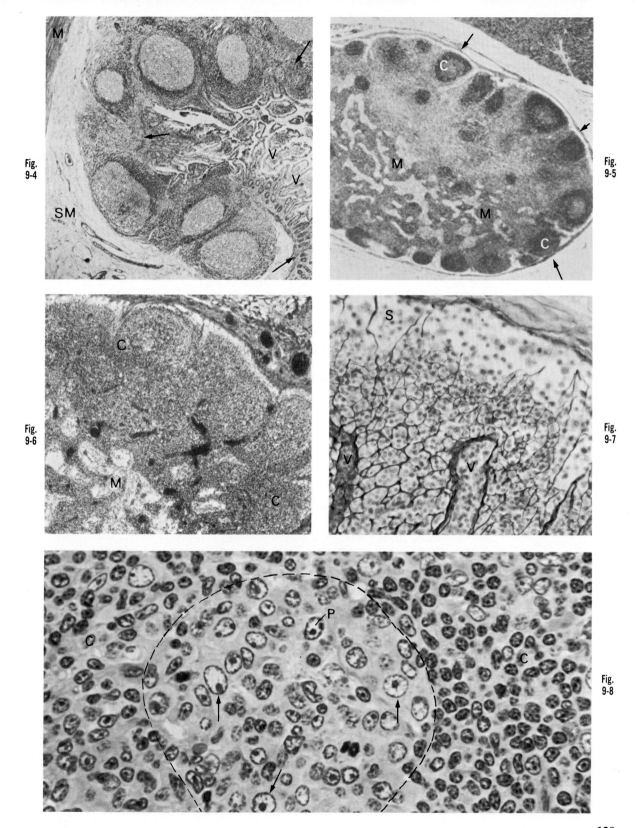

Fig.
9-4

Fig.
9-5

Fig.
9-6

Fig.
9-7

Fig.
9-8

139

Figure 9–9. Bronchial lymph node: carbon particles. Plastic section. H and E. High power.

A portion of the capsule is present at the top. Immediately beneath it is the subcapsular sinus, lined by endothelium (arrow) and containing a few cells, principally small lymphocytes. Below this, there is a portion of the cortex of a lymph nodule. The collections of black material are carbon particles that have been taken up by the actively phagocytic cells associated with the reticulum. The carbon particles were inhaled and passed via the pulmonary lymphatic vessels to the node.

Figure 9–10. Lymph node: medulla. H and E. Medium power.

Portions of several medullary cords occupy the lower half of the field. They appear densely stained owing to the concentrations of lymphocytes within them. A small arteriole (A) shows elongated nuclei of the endothelium lining the narrow lumen and nuclei of smooth muscle cells circularly arranged. The vessel lies within connective tissue of a trabecula. Medullary sinuses (S) occupy the interval between the medullary cords and the trabecula. They are incompletely lined by fixed macrophages and reticular cells and contain numerous free cells, principally small lymphocytes.

Figure 9–11. Lymph node: medulla. Azan. High power.

The dark, irregular masses of small lymphocytes shown here are medullary cords. In addition to lymphocytes, the cords contain a few collagenous fibers (blue) and small blood vessels (red). The wide, irregular spaces are medullary lymph sinuses (S), which contain a few small lymphocytes. The sinuses are lined by reticular cells and fixed macrophages, which are irregular in shape and have long cytoplasmic extensions that appear to join with those of neighboring cells. The supporting reticular network has not been stained specifically.

Figure 9–12. Lymph node: medulla. Plastic section. H and E. High power.

Portions of two medullary cords (M), composed mainly of small lymphocytes, are shown. Between them, there is a medullary sinus (S) containing numerous small lymphocytes. A small blood vessel (V) is associated with one medullary cord.

Figure 9–13. Palatine tonsil. Masson. Low power.

Palatine tonsils are masses of lymphoid tissue within the mucosa and are covered by nonkeratinizing stratified squamous epithelium. Here, the surface epithelium (E) invaginates into the underlying lymphoid tissue to form an irregular crypt (C). Lymphoid tissue surrounds the crypt as a diffuse mass in which are embedded lymph nodules, some with germinal centers. Connective tissue septa (arrows) surround the lymphoid tissue associated with the crypt.

Figure 9–14. Palatine tonsil. H and E. Medium power.

The tonsillar tissue consists of a diffuse mass of lymphoid tissue that contains circumscribed lymph nodules with large germinal centers. At the top, the tissue is covered by stratified squamous epithelium.

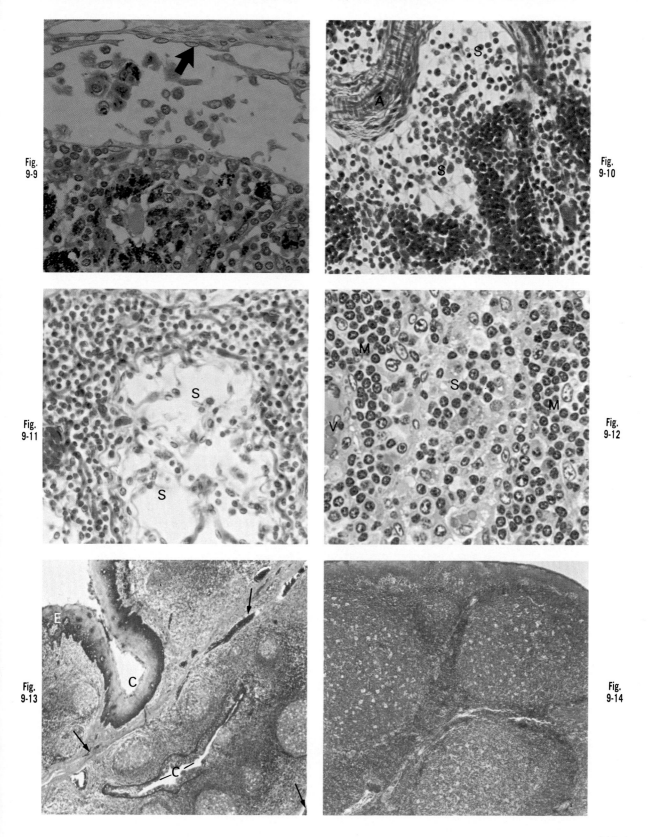

Figure 9–15. Pharyngeal tonsil. H and E. High power.

The pharyngeal tonsil is an accumulation of lymphoid tissue within the posterior wall of the nasopharynx. The epithelium over the free surface generally is pseudostratified with cilia and goblet cells, but in the adult there often are extensive islands of stratified squamous epithelium, as shown here. The boundary between the epithelium and the underlying lymphoid tissue is indistinct because of the extensive invasion of epithelium by lymphocytes.

Figure 9–16. Thymus. Plastic section. H and E. Low power.

A portion of one lobule from the thymus of a child is shown. It is surrounded by a delicate capsule composed of collagenous fibers. Lymphocytes (thymocytes) are densely packed within the cortex (C) and are less numerous in the medulla (M). The pale-staining bodies within the medulla are thymic corpuscles (T).

Figure 9–17. Thymus. Azan. High power.

The cortex, which occupies the left half of the field, contains densely packed lymphocytes within a meshwork of delicate connective tissue (pale blue). In the medulla (right half of field), lymphocytes are less densely packed and a thymic corpuscle of Hassall (T) is present. A portion of a trabecula (arrow) also is shown.

Figure 9–18. Thymus: Hassall's corpuscle. H and E. High power.

A large Hassall's corpuscle, within the medulla, occupies the center of the field. It shows a dense, hyalinized core surrounded by concentrically arranged, flattened epithelial cells.

Figure 9–19. Thymus: medulla. Plastic section. H and E. High power.

Scattered between the small lymphocytes are epithelial reticular cells (arrows) that possess pale, vesicular nuclei. Also present is a small thymic corpuscle (T) with a hyalinized core surrounded by flattened epithelial cells.

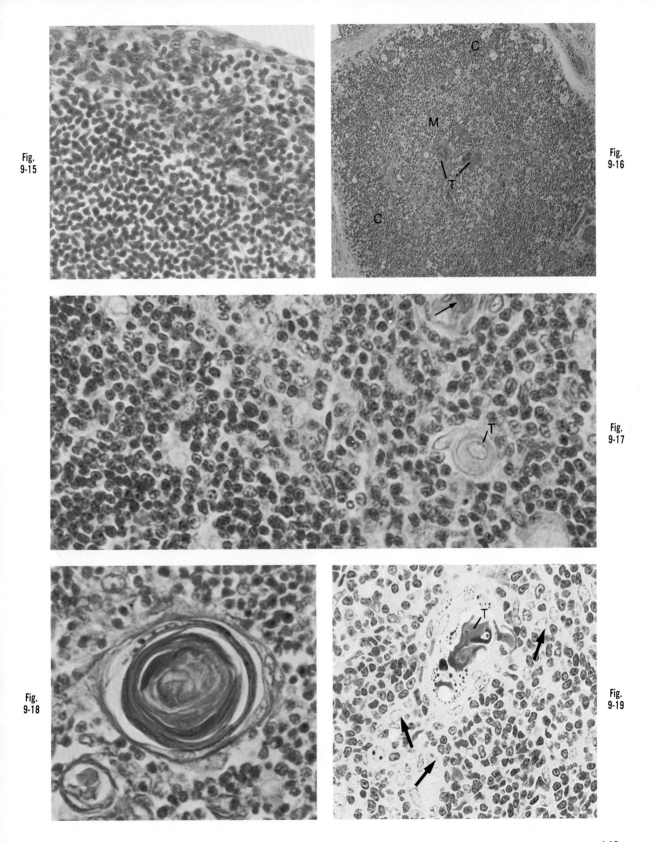

Fig.
9-15

Fig.
9-16

Fig.
9-17

Fig.
9-18

Fig.
9-19

143

Figure 9–20. Spleen. H and E. Low power.

The capsule (above) is thick and from it a trabecula (T) runs into the interior of the organ. Red pulp forms the bulk of the parenchyma and within it are accumulations of lymphoid tissue, the white pulp, forming splenic nodules or malpighian bodies (W), many with germinal centers.

Figure 9–21. Spleen. Azan. Low power.

The capsule, covered by a layer of mesothelial cells (not visible), and a trabecula (T) passing into the interior consist principally of collagenous fibers (blue). The majority of the parenchyma is red pulp, consisting of cellular cords and numerous venous sinuses. Two splenic nodules (W) of white pulp are dense accumulations of lymphocytes, each associated with a small artery (blue).

Figure 9–22. Spleen. Plastic section. H and E. Medium power.

A central arteriole (A) is surrounded by densely packed lymphocytes that constitute a splenic nodule. The arteriole is somewhat eccentric in position with regard to the nodule. Above the nodule, there is a trabecula (T) associated with a small vein. The right half of the field is occupied by red pulp, consisting of loose lymphatic tissue in the form of irregular, anastomosing cords (C) separated by venous sinuses (V). Nuclei of the specialized reticular cells that line the sinuses project into the lumina.

Figure 9–23. Spleen: trabecular vein. Plastic section. H and E. High power.

A pulp vein (lower left) passes into a trabecula to join a trabecular (or interlobular) vein. Note the numerous smooth muscle fibers (M), here sectioned transversely, within the trabecula.

Figure 9–24. Spleen: reticular fibers. Bielschowsky's method. High power.

In this section of red pulp, reticular fibers have been stained specifically (black), outlining clearly the venous sinuses within the parenchyma. The walls of the sinuses are supported by reticular fibers that are circularly arranged: thus, in sections that pass obliquely through the sinus walls, the reticular fibers appear as short dark profiles. Nuclei of reticular cells lining the sinuses are interposed between the fibers and the lumen. The remainder of the red pulp between the sinuses is composed of irregular cords of lymphatic tissue. A trabecula (T) contains delicate reticular fibers and collagenous fibers (brown).

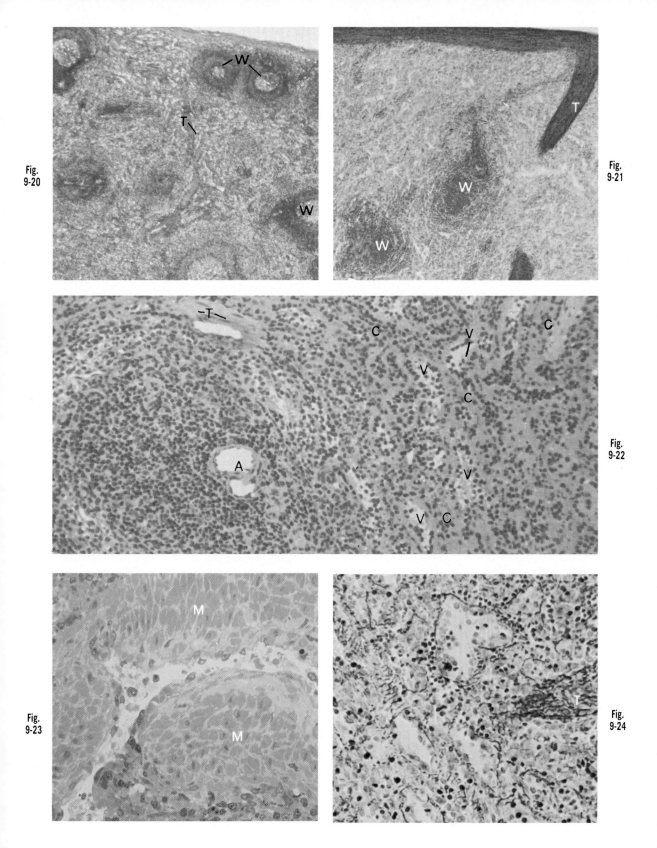

Fig. 9-20

Fig. 9-21

Fig. 9-22

Fig. 9-23

Fig. 9-24

The Skin and Its Appendages (The Integument)

The integument comprises the skin that covers the surface of the body and specialized derivatives of it. These include nails, hairs, and several kinds of glands.

THE SKIN

The skin is composed of two layers: (1) the *epidermis*, a specialized epithelium derived from ectoderm, and (2) the *dermis*, a vascular connective tissue derived from mesoderm. These two layers are firmly adherent to each other and form a membrane that varies in thickness from about 0.5 to 4 mm. The *hypodermis*, the superficial fascia of gross anatomy, lies beneath the dermis. It is a layer of loose connective tissue, either areolar or adipose in character, and it permits considerable mobility of the skin over most regions of the body. The free surface of the skin exhibits numerous *ridges* that correspond to similar patterns on the surface of the dermis. Thus, in sections, the boundary between epidermis and dermis usually appears uneven. Skin commonly is classified as thick or thin, terms that refer not to thickness of the skin as a whole, but only to the epidermis.

Epidermis

The epidermis, a *keratinizing* stratified squamous epithelium, varies in thickness in different regions, but generally it is about 0.1 mm thick. In the skin of the palms and soles, however, it may be 0.7 to 1.5 mm in thickness. It is composed of four distinct cell types:

1. Keratinocytes.
2. Melanocytes.
3. Langerhans cells.
4. Merkel cells.

Keratinocytes. The bulk of the epidermis, of ectodermal origin, undergoes a process of keratinization, resulting in the formation of the dead superficial layers of the skin.

Melanocytes. The second component, comprising the melanocytes, which produce melanin, does not undergo keratinization.

The superficial keratinized cells are continuously lost from the surface and must be replaced by cells that arise as a result of mitotic activity of cells of the basal layers of the epidermis. In the palm and sole, the epidermis ("thick" skin) may be divided into five distinct layers:

1. The *stratum germinativum* is a single layer of columnar or cuboidal cells, each with short cytoplasmic processes on its basal surface. The processes fit into pockets of the basal lamina and appear to anchor the epithelium to the underlying dermis. Mitotic figures occur frequently in this layer.

2. The *stratum spinosum* is several cells thick and is composed of irregular polyhedral keratinocytes. The surface of the cells (prickle cells) is covered with short cytoplasmic spines, or projections, that meet with similar projections of adjacent cells to form "intercellular bridges." The strata germinativum and spinosum commonly are grouped together as the *malpighian layer*. It is this layer that is responsible for proliferation and for initiation of the keratinization process.

3. The *stratum granulosum* consists of three to five layers of flattened cells that contain basophilic granules of *keratohyalin*. At this level death of epidermal cells commences.

4. The *stratum lucidum* consists of a tightly packed layer of cells without nuclei and is strongly acidophil.

5. The outermost layer, the *stratum corneum*, is composed of clear, dead, scale-like cells without nuclei. The cytoplasm is replaced with keratin. The surface cells of this layer are desquamated constantly. Over most of the body, the epidermis ("thin" skin) is much thinner and simpler; all layers of the epidermis are reduced, and the stratum lucidum is usually absent.

The color of the skin is dependent upon three factors:

1. The presence of carotene, which is yellow in color.

2. Blood showing through from the underlying vascular dermis.

3. The accumulation of melanin pigment, brown in color. Melanin is present mainly in the stratum germinativum and in the deeper layers of the stratum spinosum. It is produced by *melanocytes*, which are scattered within the basal layer of the epidermis and which send numerous cytoplasmic processes between the cells of the stratum spinosum. The melanin they produce is liberated and distributed to the keratocytes. Melanocytes cannot be identified in normal preparations, but they can be made visible with a special reagent, "dopa," which they oxidize; the reaction causes them to turn black.

Langerhans Cells. These constitute the third cellular population within the epidermis. These star-shaped cells, with numerous dendritic processes, are found mainly within the stratum spinosum. Although they appear as "clear" cells on light microscopy, they can be sharply delineated after impregnation with gold chloride. They are thought to be of immunological importance.

Merkel Cells. The fourth cellular population within the epidermis is composed of Merkel cells, which commonly are found in or near the stratum germinativum. They possess irregularly shaped nuclei, and their cytoplasm is less dense than that of adjacent keratinocytes. They occur frequently in association with intraepithelial nerve endings and possibly play a role in cutaneous sensation.

Dermis

The dermis is a layer of connective tissue containing vascular and nervous elements, and the glands and hairs of the skin lie embedded within its structure. It can be subdivided into two layers:

1. The *papillary layer* includes the papillae and ridges that protrude into the epidermis. Some papillae contain special nerve terminations (nervous papillae); others possess loops of capillary blood vessels (vascular papillae).

2. The *reticular layer* is composed of coarse, dense, interlacing collagenous fibers, in which are intermingled a few reticular fibers and numerous elastic fibers.

APPENDAGES

Nails

Nails are horny plates that form a protective covering on the dorsal surface of the terminal phalanges of the digits. Each nail lies upon a *nail bed* and is contained within a U-shaped *nail groove*, which itself is bordered by a fold of skin, the *nail wall*. The nail bed consists of the deeper layers of the epidermis and the underlying dermis, which is grooved longitudinally. The nail plate is formed by intimately fused epidermal scales, and the body of the plate is translucent, transmitting the pink color of blood vessels in the underlying dermis of the nail bed. The root of the nail plate, which is more opaque, becomes continuous with the body over a crescentic margin, the *lunule*. Cells from the horny layer of the nail wall extend over the proximal surface of the nail plate as the *eponychium*, or cuticle, and are thickened below the free margin of the nail to form the *hyponychium*.

Hair

Hairs are elastic keratinized threads that develop from the epidermis. They are present over the entire skin except for the palms, soles, and region of the anal and urogenital apertures. Each hair has a free *shaft* and a *root* enclosed within a tubular *hair follicle* that consists of epidermal and dermal portions. The epidermal portion is divided into inner and outer epidermal root sheaths. At the lower end, the follicle expands into a *hair bulb* that is indented at the basal end by a connective tissue *papilla*. Associated with the hair follicle are one or more sebaceous glands and a bundle of smooth muscle, the *arrector pili*. These structures constitute the *pilosebaceous unit*.

Glands of the Skin

Sebaceous Glands. With few exceptions, the sebaceous glands are connected with hair follicles. They lie within the dermis and are alveolar (or saccular) in form. The secretion (sebum) is composed of degenerated cells desquamated from the lining of the alveolus. Thus, the secretion is *holocrine* and is passed along a short wide duct into the neck of a hair follicle. The duct is lined by a stratified squamous epithelium continuous with that of the hair follicle below and the epidermis above.

Sweat Glands. The ordinary sweat glands *(eccrine)* are unbranched, coiled tubular glands distributed throughout the skin except for the nail bed, margins of the lips, glans penis, and eardrum. The secretory portion is situated deeply, either in the dermis or hypodermis, and is coiled into a discrete mass. It is lined by a simple columnar or cuboidal epithelium that contains two distinct cell types: (1) principal (clear) cells and (2) mucigenous (dark) cells. Spindle-shaped myoepithelial cells wind in longitudinal spirals around the tubule, and are interposed between the bases of the secretory cells and the bounding basal lamina. The excretory portion, or duct, rises to the epidermis and opens on the surface by a minute pit, the *sweat pore*. It is lined by a double layer of darkly staining cuboidal cells. Certain large sweat glands in the axilla, areola of the nipple, labia majora, and circumanal region produce a thicker secretion than the ordinary sweat glands and are said to be *apocrine* in type.

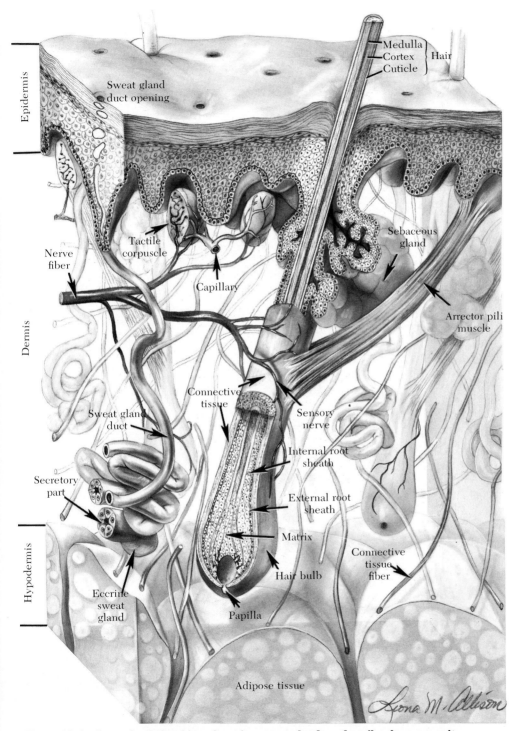

Figure 10–1. General relationships of eccrine sweat glands and a pilosebaceous unit.

In this diagram, the pilosebaceous unit consists of a hair follicle and its associated sebaceous glands and arrector pili muscle.

Figure 10–2. Scanning electron micrograph of a hair from monkey scalp.

Note the way in which cells of the cuticle overlap; the irregular skin surface results from desquamating cells of the stratum corneum. × 1200. (Courtesy of Dr. P. M. Andrews.)

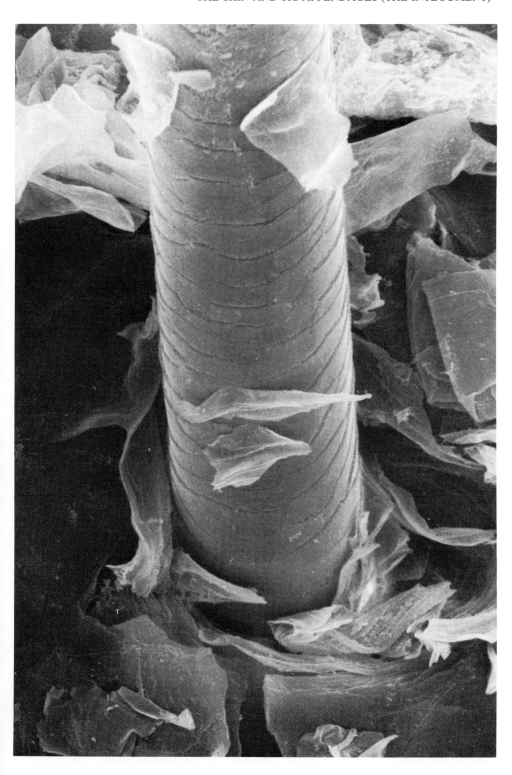

Figure 10–3. Thick skin of the sole of the foot. H and E. Low power.

The skin is composed of the epidermis (A) and of the dermis (B), with an uneven boundary between the two. Note that the epidermis consists chiefly of keratin (stratum corneum). Beneath the dermis is the hypodermis, here adipose in character and containing sweat glands (arrows) and a Vater-Pacini corpuscle (P).

Figure 10–4. Thick skin of sole of foot. H and E. Medium power.

The epidermis shows the malpighian layer (strata germinativum and spinosum), the stratum granulosum (arrows), and the stratum corneum, traversed by the duct of a sweat gland. The stratum lucidum is not apparent on this section. A small portion of the papillary layer of the dermis is present at lower left.

Figure 10–5. Thick skin. Plastic section. H and E. High power.

The stratum germinativum is a single row of columnar cells, each cell of which has short cytoplasmic processes on its basal surface (arrows). The stratum spinosum, several layers thick, is composed of irregular, polyhedral cells, slightly separated from each other. The surface of the cells is covered with short cytoplasmic spines that meet with similar projections of adjacent cells to form intercellular bridges. The stratum granulosum consists of four to five layers of flattened cells that contain basophil keratohyalin granules. Small portions of the stratum lucidum (L) and the stratum corneum (C) are present at upper right.

Figure 10–6. Epidermis: stratum spinosum. Masson. Oil immersion.

The prickle cells have large nuclei with distinct nucleoli and show intercellular cytoplasmic bridges. In two regions (arrows), the cytoplasmic processes are shown in cross section.

Figure 10–7. Thin skin of a black person. H and E. Medium power.

Note the scattered cells representative of the stratum granulosum (arrows) and the thinness of the stratum corneum. There is marked deposition of pigment (melanin) in the malpighian layer, particularly in the stratum germinativum.

Figure 10–8. Thin skin. Plastic section. H and E. High power.

Keratohyalin granules (arrows) are seen clearly in cells of the stratum granulosum.

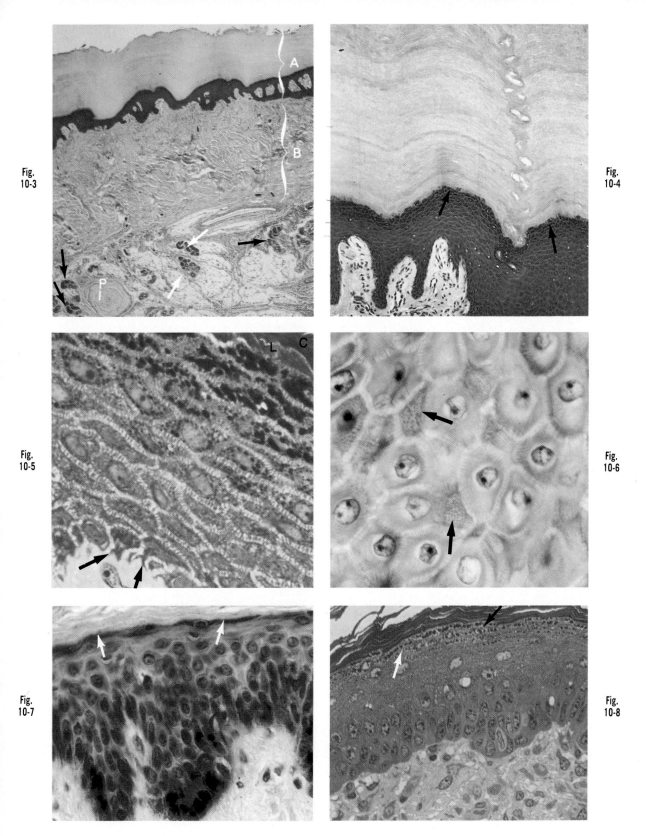

Fig. 10-3

Fig. 10-4

Fig. 10-5

Fig. 10-6

Fig. 10-7

Fig. 10-8

155

Figure 10–9. Nail: transverse section. H and E. High power.

The nail plate (NP) appears homogeneous, since it consists of intimately fused horny scales. The nail bed, which underlies the nail plate, consists of the deeper layers of the epidermis (dark red) and the dermis (D), which lacks sweat glands and hair follicles. The dermis is grooved longitudinally, and thus in transverse sections the junction between dermis and epidermis appears markedly irregular.

Figure 10–10. Fingertip: nail. Longitudinal section. H and E. Low power.

Shown in this section is the distal phalanx of a finger (P) and the nail bed (NB), with the nail plate (NP) above. A portion of the proximal nail wall extends onto the free surface of the nail plate as the eponychium (E), and a portion of distal nail wall is thickened below the free margin of the nail to form the hyponychium (H).

Figure 10–11. Skin of the scalp. Masson. Low power.

Numerous hair follicles (arrows), sectioned transversely, lie within the dermis and hypodermis. One follicle near the surface of the dermis is associated with alveoli of sebaceous glands (S).

Figure 10–12. Hair follicle: longitudinal section. H and E. High power.

This section shows portions of the hair root (right half of field) and the hair follicle. The hair exhibits the medulla (M), the cortex (C), and the cuticle (HC), a single row of cornified cells with their free edges directed upward. The inner component of the epidermal root sheath consists of: the cuticle of the root sheath (RC), similar in structure to the hair cuticle but with the free edges projecting downward; Huxley's layer (Hu), the cells of which contain trichohyalin granules (deep red); and Henle's layer (He), a single row of clear cells (pale pink). The outer component of the epidermal root sheath contains several rows of polyhedral cells internally (P) and a single row of tall cells externally (T). The dermal root sheath shows an inner glassy membrane (G), and two strata of connective tissue (1 and 2) that correspond to the papillary and reticular layers of the dermis.

Figure 10–13. Hair follicle: longitudinal section. Iron hematoxylin, aniline blue. Medium power.

The hair follicle is expanded into a hair bulb, where the root of the hair (HR) and its sheath blend into a mass of primitive cells, the matrix (M). The base of the bulb is indented by a connective tissue papilla (P). The hair root is surrounded by the hair follicle, composed of the inner (I) and outer (O) epidermal root sheaths and the dermal root sheath (D).

Figure 10–14. Developing hair follicles: transverse section. H and E. Medium power.

Numerous hair follicles, sectioned transversely or obliquely, lie within the dermis. The hair root exhibits only cortex (C) and cuticle (arrows). The inner epidermal root sheath, here sectioned on a deep level, consists of the cuticle of the root sheath (arrowheads), Huxley's layer (Hu), and Henle's layer (He). The outer epidermal root sheath (O) at this level is poorly developed and is composed of a single row of cells. No dermal root sheath is apparent.

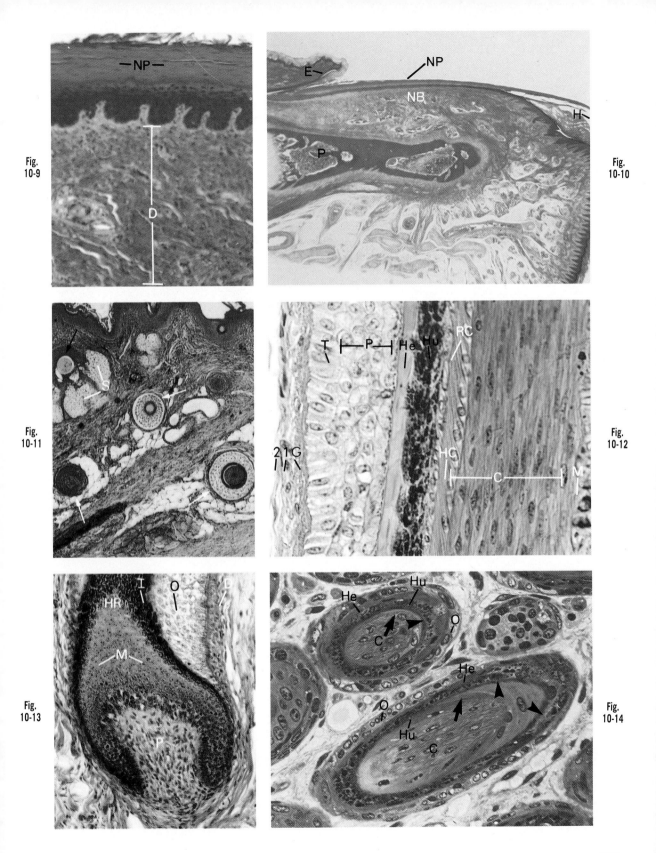

Fig.
10-9

Fig.
10-10

Fig.
10-11

Fig.
10-12

Fig.
10-13

Fig.
10-14

Figure 10–15. Sebaceous gland. Iron hematoxylin, aniline blue. Low power.

A hair follicle (above) is associated with two sebaceous gland alveoli, embedded within dense connective tissue of the dermis (blue). A single row of low cuboidal cells (arrows), continuous with the basal cells of the epidermis at the neck of the hair follicle, surrounds the central alveolus. The alveolus is filled with a stratified epithelium and, toward the center, cells become progressively larger and the cytoplasm appears vacuolated (owing to the loss of fat droplets during preparation).

Figure 10–16. Sebaceous gland. Plastic section. H and E. Medium power.

A single row of low cuboidal cells (arrows), surrounding the alveolus, is separated from the embedding dermal connective tissue by a wide, eosinophil basal lamina. Toward the center of the alveolus, cells become progressively larger and the cytoplasm is distended with fat droplets. Nuclei appear shrunken and pyknotic.

Figure 10–17. Sweat gland. Iron hematoxylin, aniline blue. Medium power.

Sweat glands, since they are coiled tubular glands, will be cut in numerous planes in sections. Here, the secretory portion is seen below and the excretory portion above. The former is lined by a simple epithelium; the clear and dark cells are not differentiated by this stain. The excretory portion is lined by two layers of darkly staining cuboidal cells. The gland is surrounded by collagenous connective tissue of the hypodermis (blue) and by fat cells.

Figure 10–18. Sweat gland. Plastic section. H and E. High power.

Below are profiles of the secretory portion of this eccrine gland. The lining cells are pyramidal or columnar and possess a pale cytoplasm. Between the bases of the cells and the bounding basal lamina, cytoplasmic processes of myoepithelial cells, deeply acidophil, are visible (arrows). The excretory duct (above), represented by four profiles, is lined by a double layer of darkly staining cuboidal cells.

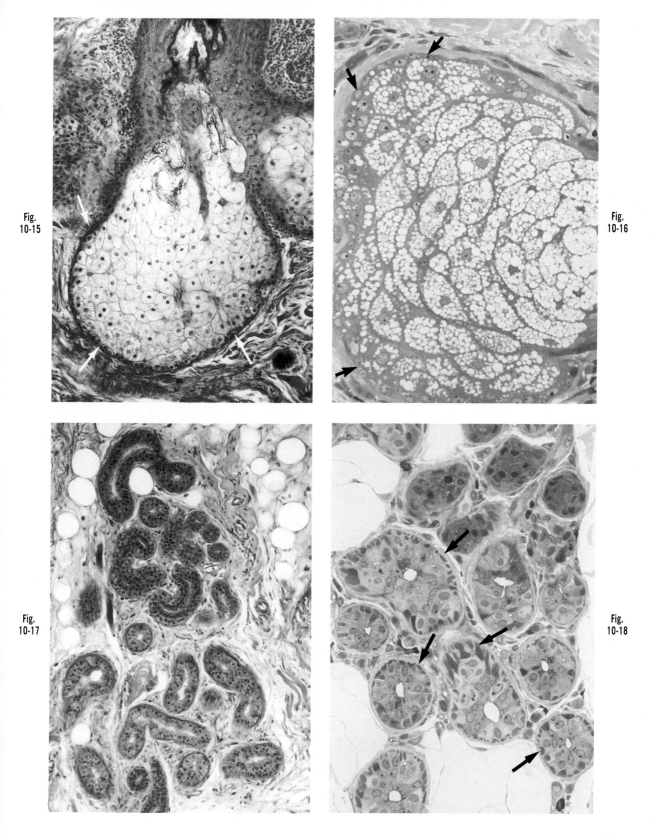

Fig.
10-15

Fig.
10-16

Fig.
10-17

Fig.
10-18

CHAPTER
ELEVEN

The Digestive System

The digestive system consists of a long tube, the alimentary canal, extending from mouth to anus, and the major glands—salivary glands, pancreas and liver—that, although situated outside the digestive tract, pass their secretions into it by duct systems. Digestion is the process whereby food material is converted into substances that can be absorbed into the circulation. Useless and toxic materials are eliminated by fecal excretion.

LAYERS OF THE DIGESTIVE TRACT

From esophagus to anus, the wall of the canal is composed of four layers or tunics:

1. The innermost layer is the *tunica mucosa*, a wet epithelial membrane lying on a basal lamina, supported by a cellular connective tissue, the lamina propria, and in most regions with a thin layer of smooth muscle, the muscularis mucosae.

2. The *tunica submucosa* lies external to the mucosa and is a coarse areolar connective tissue containing plexuses of larger blood vessels and nerves and ganglion cells (submucosal plexus of Meissner). In some regions, there are submucosal glands. The submucosa permits distention of the lumen.

3. The third layer, the *muscularis externa (tunica muscularis),* is composed of an inner layer of circular (tight spiral) and an outer layer of longitudinal (open spiral) smooth muscle, although in the esophagus there is striated, but involuntary, muscle. Between the layers are a vascular plexus and a nerve plexus with small ganglion cells (myenteric plexus of Auerbach). This layer propels food onward through the digestive tract by peristalsis, and churns and mixes food material in the lumen.

4. The outermost layer is the *tunica serosa*, a relatively dense areolar connective tissue that is covered by peritoneum (simple squamous epithelium or mesothelium). In the esophagus and some "bare" areas of the tube, there is no peritoneal covering and the connective tissue blends with surrounding tissue as an adventitia.

ORAL CAVITY

In the oral cavity and pharynx, which serve additional functions to digestion, there are special features. The lining epithelium is mainly stratified squamous in type, a "wear and tear" epithelium that resists abrasion by relatively coarse food material. This type of epithelium also lines the esophagus. It lies on a basal lamina. The submucosa generally is poorly delineated and blends deeply with striated muscle in the lips, cheeks, and pharynx. Mucous, serous, and mixed glands are common in this region and lie in the submucosa. The oral cavity also includes the teeth and tongue, structures involved in mastication, and sense organs for taste ("taste buds"). The tongue, a complex fleshy organ of muscle, glands, and lymphatic tissue, is covered by epithelium that is modified to form papillae of three types. Papillae are small surface protrusions that account for the "roughness" of the surface. Associated with some of the papillae are taste buds. Teeth too are complex, and this chapter includes micrographs to illustrate not only their structure but also their development.

THE STOMACH

At the *esophagogastric junction,* the lining epithelium changes abruptly to a simple columnar type. In the *stomach*, the epithelium is invaginated as masses of simple tubular, or branched tubular, glands in which several different cell types are present in addition to the surface epithelial cells. These include chief (enzyme-secreting) cells, parietal (acid-secreting) cells, enteroendocrine (hormone-secreting) cells, and mucous neck cells.

THE SMALL INTESTINE

The small intestine generally shows several modifications to increase surface area. Individual cells show a *microvillus,* or *brush border*. There are finger-like processes, or *villi*, formed by epithelium with a core of lamina propria, and epithelium is invaginated into the lamina propria as tubular *glands* or *crypts*. Additionally, in the upper part of the *small intestine*, there are transverse folds of the entire thickness of the mucosa with a core of submucosa, the *plicae circulares (valves of Kerckring)*. In addition to simple columnar (lining) epithelial cells, there are goblet cells, enteroendocrine cells, and Paneth cells that secrete enzymes. Additional cell types have been described, but are not recognized by light microscopy. In the small intestine, the lamina propria shows lymphoid tendencies. Lymphatic capillaries lie in the cores of villi within the lamina propria; in this location they are called lacteals because they contain absorbed fat. The upper part of the small intestine, the *duodenum*, is characterized by the presence of submucosal glands (of Brunner).

THE LARGE INTESTINE

In the large intestine, there are no villi but intestinal glands are packed tightly and goblet cells are numerous. Most of the large intestine has an incomplete layer of longitudinal muscle in the muscularis in that it is present as three bands, or *taenia*. In the appendix, there usually are massive accumulations of lymphoid tissue. At the distal end of the tract, i.e., at the rectoanal junction, the epithelium abruptly changes first to stratified squamous and then to keratinized (epidermis).

MAJOR DIGESTIVE GLANDS

Salivary Glands. The associated glands include the major salivary glands (paired), all opening via ducts to the oral cavity. All are compound tubuloalveolar: the parotid is serous; the submandibular gland is mixed, with serous, mucous, and mixed acini; and the sublingual gland is mucous, although a few serous acini may be present.

The Pancreas. The pancreas is a mixed gland in the sense that it is both exocrine and endocrine. The exocrine portion is compound, tubuloalveolar, and serous. Scattered among the acini are the endocrine islets of Langerhans with several cell types, including the insulin-secreting beta cells.

The Liver. The liver is the largest gland in the body, subserving many functions. Basically, it is divided into lobules but with very little connective tissue. The parenchymal cells are arranged in anastomosing cords and plates radiating outward from venous channels (central veins) and with sinusoidal blood spaces between the plates. At the periphery of the lobules are "portal canals," regions where branches of the hepatic artery, the portal vein, bile duct tributaries, and lymphatic vessels lie close together.

Figure 11–1. Gastrointestinal tract.

This diagram illustrates the general plan of the gastrointestinal tract.

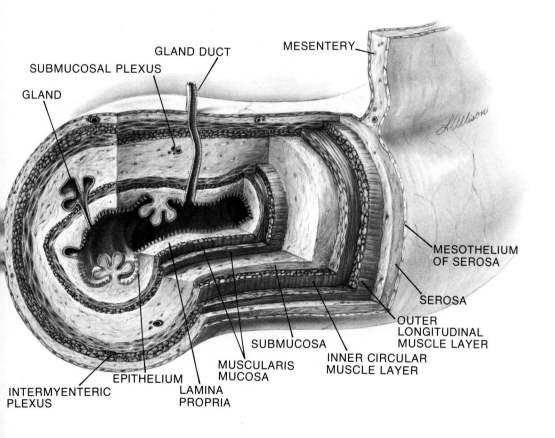

GLAND DUCT

MESENTERY

SUBMUCOSAL PLEXUS

GLAND

MESOTHELIUM
OF SEROSA

SEROSA

OUTER
LONGITUDINAL
MUSCLE LAYER

INNER CIRCULAR
MUSCLE LAYER

SUBMUCOSA

MUSCULARIS
MUCOSA

EPITHELIUM

LAMINA
PROPRIA

INTERMYENTERIC
PLEXUS

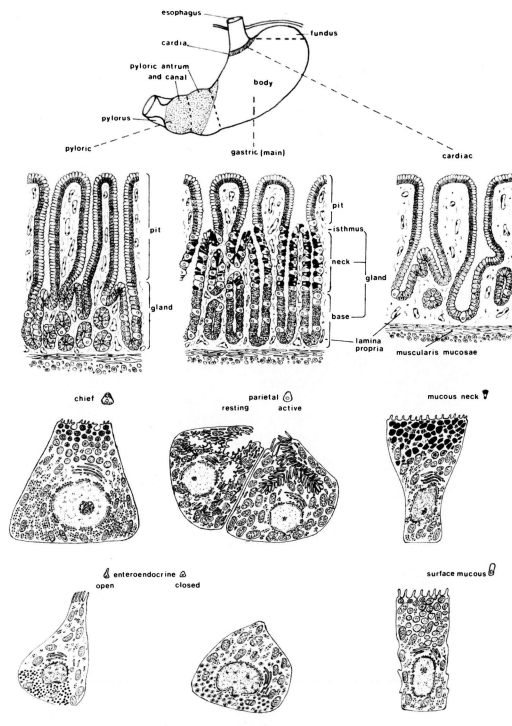

Figure 11–2. *See legend on opposite page.*

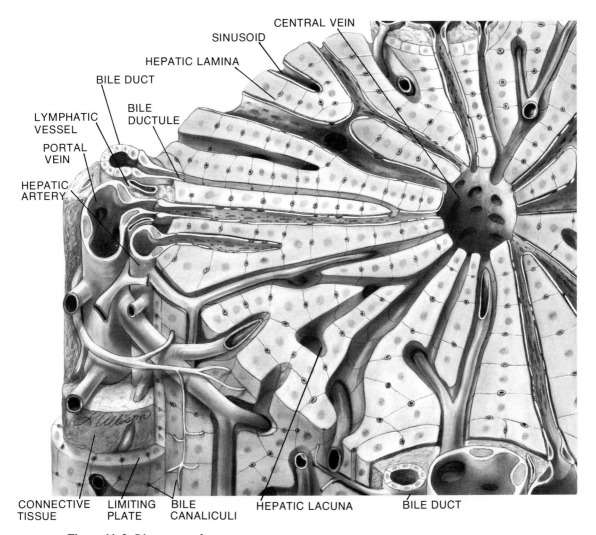

CENTRAL VEIN

SINUSOID

HEPATIC LAMINA

BILE DUCT

BILE
DUCTULE

LYMPHATIC
VESSEL

PORTAL
VEIN

HEPATIC
ARTERY

CONNECTIVE   LIMITING   BILE   HEPATIC LACUNA   BILE DUCT
TISSUE   PLATE   CANALICULI

Figure 11–3. Liver parenchyma.

The diagram shows part of one lobule and the blood supply.

Figure 11–2. Summary of the main features of the gastric mucosa.

At the top of the diagram, the three main histological regions (types of gastric glands) are shown in relation to the gross anatomy of the stomach. At center, the light microscopic appearance of the three regions is shown. Note in all the relation between depth of pit and gland, the relative tortuosity of the glands (more in the pyloric region), and the cell composition. At bottom, the appearance of most of the cell types as seen by electron microscopy is illustrated. The main mucous cell of the pyloric region is similar to the mucous neck cell. The main cell of the cardiac region also is mucus-secreting, but differs from the other cell types. (These two cells are not illustrated.)

Figure 11–4. Lip. Iron hematoxylin, aniline blue. Low power.

This vertical section shows the external skin surface (S), the internal mucosal surface (M), and the free margin (right). The external surface is covered by thin skin with obvious hair follicles, sebaceous glands, and sweat glands; the epithelium is stratified, squamous, and keratinizing in type. As the free margin is approached, hairs and glands disappear and dermal papillae become tall. At the free margin, there are no glands and the surface is kept moist by licking. The epithelium of the mucous membrane on the internal surface is nonkeratinizing and is supported by a lamina propria (blue) with high papillae. Within the connective tissue here are several small mucous (labial) glands (G, pink). In the core of the lip are masses of striated muscle arranged in bundles (arrows) and here cut transversely. This is muscle of the orbicularis oris. (See also Figure 2–1.)

Figure 11–5. Tongue. H and E. Low power.

This is a section through the tip of the tongue with upper (U) and lower (L) surfaces covered by stratified squamous epithelium with very irregular connective tissue papillae. This irregularity is greater on the upper surface owing to the presence of fungiform papillae. Papillae are small protuberances responsible for the "furred" or roughened appearance of the tongue. Fungiform papillae are shaped like a mushroom (fungus) with a short stalk and a broader cap (arrow). The connective tissue core usually shows secondary papillae over which the epithelium is quite thin. A rich vascular plexus in the core imparts a reddish tinge to the structure. Within the tongue are striated muscle fibers, running vertically, transversely, and longitudinally, and some mixed salivary glands (G).

Figure 11–6. Tongue, rabbit. Plastic section. Methylene blue. Low power.

This is a section of the upper surface and shows filiform (F) and foliate (O) papillae. The filiform papillae have conical, pointed cores of connective tissue with a covering epithelium which, while not fully keratinized, is hard. (In some animals it is keratinized.) Foliate papillae, similar to circumvallate papillae of the human, are large, with a core of connective tissue and a surrounding depression or trench. Taste buds are located in the sides of the papillae, that is, in the walls of the trench, and appear as pale-staining, barrel-shaped structures. Serous glands (S) lie in the connective tissue with their ducts (D) opening into the floors of the trenches (arrow).

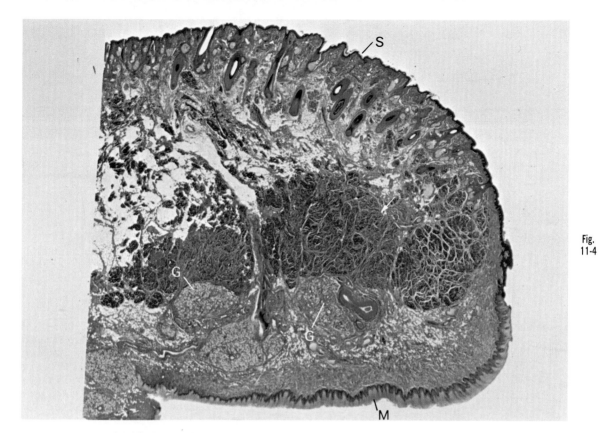

Fig. 11-4

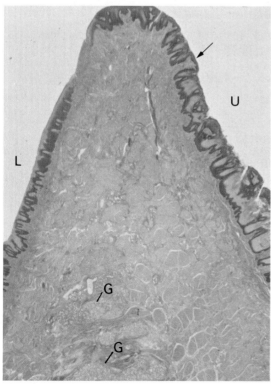

Fig. 11-5

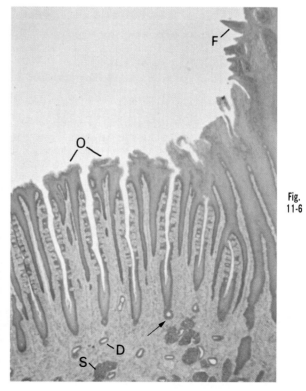

Fig. 11-6

Figure 11–7. Filiform papilla. H and E. Medium power.

The conical form of the connective tissue core (C) of the filiform papilla with covering epithelium is seen. Note that papillae protrude for 2 to 3 mm from the surface.

Figure 11–8. Circumvallate papilla. H and E. Medium power.

These number only 10 to 14 in man and are located along the V-shaped sulcus between the anterior and posterior parts of the tongue on its upper surface. Each protrudes slightly from the surface and is surrounded by a moat-like, circular furrow (arrows; a vallum is a wall). Secondary papillae are seen with taste buds on the lateral wall (arrowheads).

Figure 11–9. Taste bud. Plastic section. H and E. Oil immersion.

This is the lining epithelium from the side of a circumvallate papilla and is clearly stratified squamous in type. Located in the epithelium is a taste bud. This is barrel-shaped and composed of cells that are curved, fusiform, and arranged like the staves of a barrel. Apically, a taste pore is present (arrow), filled with hair-like processes, the taste hairs. Within the taste bud are sustentacular or supporting cells and neuroepithelial taste cells. The former are pale-staining, with ovoid, pale-staining nuclei (S). The latter are more slender and darker-staining, and they have darker, ovoid nuclei (N). A third cell type, the basal cell (B), is present and may be a stem cell for the other two types.

Figure 11–10. Tongue, glands. Plastic section. H and E. High power.

The bulk of the tongue is composed of striated muscle fibers (F), serous glands (S), and mucous glands (M). (See also Figures 1–29 and 2–14.)

Figure 11–11. Tooth, ground section. Medium power.

This is the neck region, i.e., the junction of the crown and root, and shows dentin (D) covered by enamel (E) over the crown and acellular cementum (C) over the root. A regular, radial striation in the dentin is due to the presence of fine dentinal tubules. The striation in the enamel represents enamel prisms—each unit of hexagonal outline extending through the entire thickness of enamel and formed by a single ameloblast. Between prisms is interprismatic, calcified matrix. Both prisms and interprismatic substance are composed of apatite crystals with a little organic matrix. Cementum is similar to bone and is noncellular near the neck of the tooth.

Figure 11–12. Tooth, dentinoenamel junction. High power.

This also is a ground section. Within the enamel (E) are curved, slightly sinuous enamel prisms. Only peripheral dentin (D) is seen. The thin dark lines within it are dentinal tubules, in life occupied by dentinal fibers or processes of odontoblasts. Between the tubules is a meshwork of collagenous fibers (not seen here) embedded in a calcified matrix. Note that some dentinal tubules branch (arrows) at their extremities.

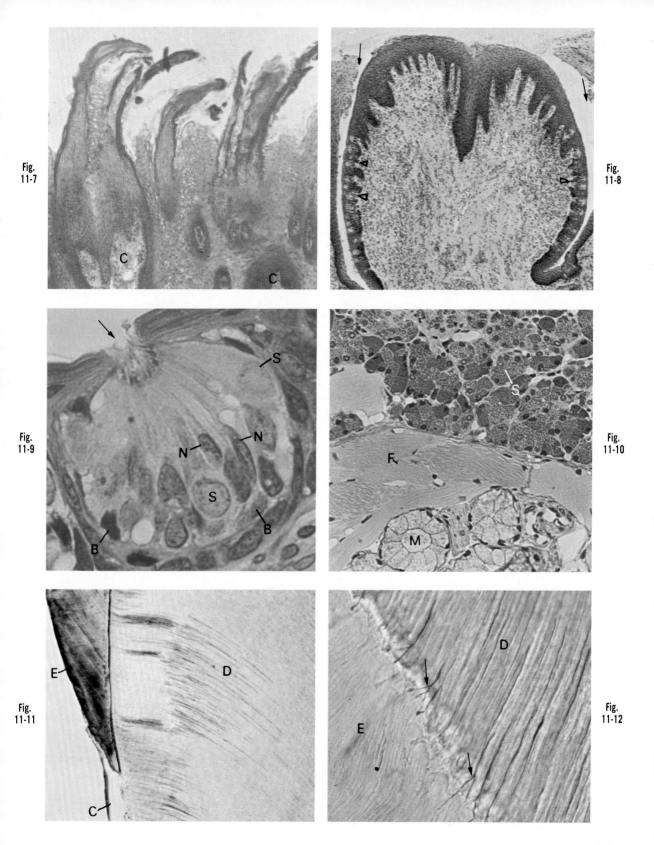

Fig. 11-7

Fig. 11-8

Fig. 11-9

Fig. 11-10

Fig. 11-11

Fig. 11-12

Figure 11–13. Tooth, pulp. Romanes' stain. Medium power.

In this section of decalcified tooth, dentin lies to the left, pulp to the right. The pulp is composed of connective tissue with small, stellate cells, a few fine collagen fibrils, and relatively large amounts of mucoid intercellular substance. It resembles embryonic mesenchyme, but lacks the potentiality of mesenchyme. It also contains blood vessels and nerves, which enter and leave the tooth through the apical canal. The periphery of the pulp shows a single row of tall columnar epithelium-like cells. These are odontoblasts, which have slender apical processes (Tomes' dentinal fibers) entering dentinal tubules (arrows). The paler (pink)-staining of dentin adjacent to odontoblasts represents predentin.

Figure 11–14. Dentinal fibers. Mallory. High power.

Dentin stains dark blue with paler-staining dentinal tubules passing through it. Odontoblasts (O) are partially destroyed, but show apical, pink, slender dentinal fibers or processes extending into dentinal tubules (arrows).

Figure 11–15. Dentin, ground transverse section. High power.

The small, dark spherical dots are dentinal tubules, in life occupied by dentinal fibers. Immediately surrounding them is a lightly stained area called the sheath of Neumann (peritubular sheath). This area of the matrix contains less collagen and is more highly calcified than the remainder of the dentin matrix. The visible striation in the matrix indicates bundles of collagenous fibers, oriented in the long axis of the tooth at right angles to the dentinal tubules.

Figure 11–16. Cementum, ground section. High power.

Cementum of the root is thicker toward the apex, and cellular. The cells or cementocytes (arrows) occupy lacunae within the matrix, with delicate processes extending from them and lying in slender canaliculi in the matrix. This arrangement is similar to that of bone, and Haversian canals with blood vessels may occasionally be found in regions or conditions where cementum is very thick. Dentin (D) with dentinal tubules also is seen.

Figure 11–17. Periodontal membrane. Plastic section. H and E. High power.

To the left is a small part of dentin (D, pink) covered by acellular cementum (C), here quite thin. To the right is alveolar bone (B), with osteocytes in lacunae. Between cementum and bone is the periodontal membrane, consisting of collagen fibers and fibroblasts and with numerous small blood capillaries. Note that bundles of collagen fibers run obliquely between bone and cementum, thus "slinging" the tooth in its socket, and that these fibers extend into matrix of both bone (arrows) and cementum (arrowheads) as Sharpey's fibers.

Figure 11–18. Embryo, dental laminae. H and E. Low power.

This coronal section through the head of an embryo shows nasal cavities (N), oral cavity (O), tongue (T), and developing mandible (M) with Meckel's (first arch) cartilage (C). In each half jaw, at the angles of the mouth, an early enamel organ and dental lamina are seen (arrows). The dental lamina appears as a thickening of the oral ectoderm with a bud-like enamel organ, embedded in condensing mesenchyme (connective tissue) termed the dental sac. (Please see Figure 11–19.)

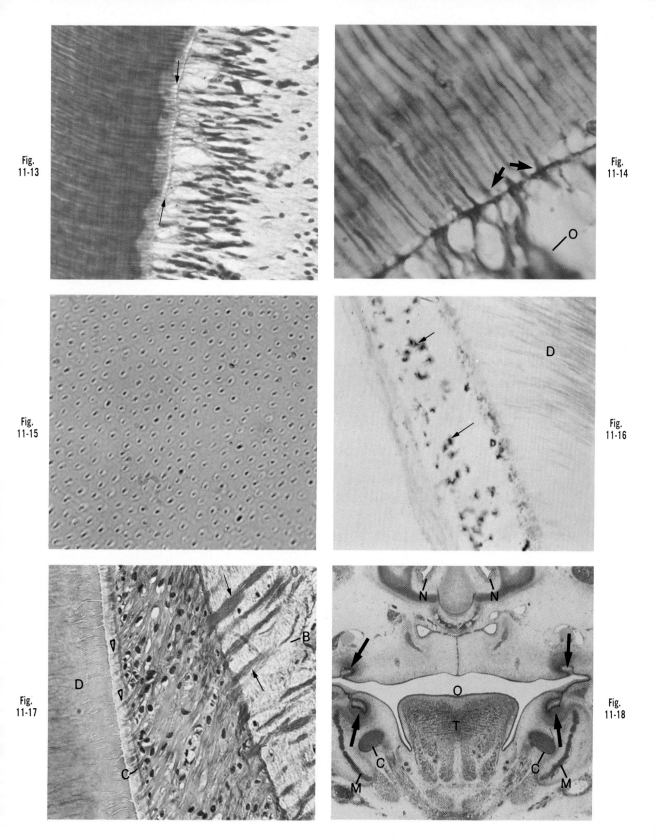

Fig.
11-13

Fig.
11-14

Fig.
11-15

Fig.
11-16

Fig.
11-17

Fig.
11-18

173

Figure 11–19. Dental lamina. H and E. Medium power.

To the left is stratified epithelium (ectoderm) lining the oral cavity, thickened to form the dental lamina (arrow). This extends deeply (to the right) into mesenchyme to form a bell- or cap-like expansion, the tooth germ. The central, pale area of the germ will become the stellate reticulum; the deepest cells (right) are the inner enamel epithelium. Cells here differentiate into ameloblasts (A) and later will form enamel. Note too the "condensation" of mesenchyme around the tooth germ. Those mesenchymal cells in relation to ameloblasts will differentiate into odontoblasts and later form dentin.

Figure 11–20. Developing tooth. H and E. Low power.

This section shows part of an erupted tooth of the "milk," or deciduous dentition (T), and, enclosed in alveolar bone, a developing tooth in the late "bell" stage. Identifiable are outer enamel epithelium (E), stellate reticulum (S), inner enamel epithelium (I), or ameloblasts, odontoblasts (O), and mesenchyme of the developing pulp (P). Predentin is seen as a thin, pink-staining layer (arrow) between odontoblasts and ameloblasts.

Figure 11–21. Developing tooth. H and E. High power.

Ameloblasts (A) are seen as a row of tall columnar cells with basal nuclei and extensive, granular apical cytoplasm, lying on a (pink) basal lamina that separates them from a layer of small cuboidal cells (the stratum intermedium) and the stellate reticulum (S). A thin layer of dark, purple-stained enamel (E) lies adjacent to pink-staining dentin (D) in which dentinal tubules are seen. Predentin (P) stains pale and is opposed to a row of odontoblasts (O).

Figure 11–22. Parotid gland. Plastic section. H and E. Medium power.

The parotid, one of the major salivary glands, is a compound, tubuloalveolar serous gland. Most of the field is occupied by serous acini, the cytoplasm of the cells filled with pink secretory droplets or granules. Also present are small intralobular ducts (D) lined by simple high cuboidal epithelium.

Figure 11–23. Submandibular gland. Plastic section. Azan trichrome. Medium power.

This major salivary gland is compound, mixed, acinar in type with serous (s), mucous (m), and mixed (x) acini, the last showing a serous crescent or demilune (arrows). Also seen are an intralobular duct (d) and blood vessels containing erythrocytes (arrowheads) in the interacinar connective tissue. (See also Figures 2–15 and 2–18.)

Figure 11–24. Sublingual gland. Mallory. Low power.

The sublingual salivary gland is really a collection of several small glands, each with a separate duct opening into the floor of the oral cavity. It is a compound, acinar, mucous gland, although a few mixed acini and, rarely, a few serous acini may be present. This section shows portions of several lobules separated by interlobular connective tissue (blue). Secretory units are mucous, with an interlobular duct (D) lying in relatively dense connective tissue and accompanied by small blood vessels. Fat cells (F) also are present.

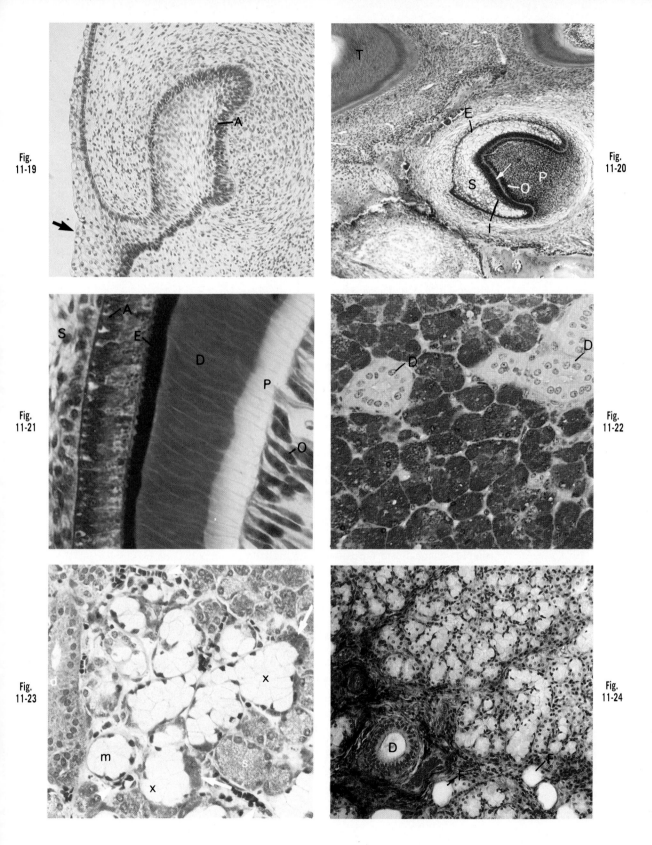

Fig.
11-19

Fig.
11-20

Fig.
11-21

Fig.
11-22

Fig.
11-23

Fig.
11-24

175

Figure 11–25. Esophagus. H and E. Low power.

This is a vertical section and shows the four tunics, or coats, found throughout the gastrointestinal tract. The mucosa (M) is formed by a stratified squamous epithelium and its lamina propria with a thin muscularis mucosae. Note the irregular but deep papillae of the lamina propria. The submucosa (S) is formed by quite dense areolar connective tissue and does contain glands, not seen here. The muscularis (F) shows a thick inner circular layer and outer longitudinal layer of muscle. Here the muscle is smooth, but striated muscle forms the muscularis in the upper esophagus. Externally there is an adventitia (A) of loose connective tissue.

Figure 11–26. Esophagus. H and E. Medium power.

Similar to Figure 11–25, this transverse section shows mucous glands (G) in the submucosa and nerve fibers of the myenteric (Auerbach's) plexus, between the layers of muscle in the muscularis (arrow).

Figure 11–27. Esophagogastric junction. H and E. Low power.

This longitudinal section passes through esophagus (E), cardiac orifice of the stomach, and the cardiac portion of the stomach (S). Only the mucosa and submucosa are seen. The esophageal epithelium is stratified squamous, and this changes abruptly (stars) at the esophagogastric junction to a simple, columnar, mucus-secreting cell type with simple tubular or branched tubular glands (arrows). In the submucosa of both terminal esophagus and upper cardia are collections of mucus-secreting glands (G). These are called cardiac glands of the esophagus because they resemble the cardiac glands of the stomach. (Please see Figures 11–28 and 11–29.) Similar glands are found in the lamina propria of the upper esophagus and in the submucosa of the esophagus throughout its length.

Figure 11–28. Stomach, cardia. Plastic section. H and E. Low power.

The mucosa (M), submucosa (S), and muscularis (F) are seen. The lining epithelium is simple columnar and mucus-secreting, and shows invaginations or pits (arrows). Simple tubular and branched tubular glands open into the pits and extend the full depth of the mucosa, i.e., deeply to the muscularis mucosae (arrowhead). The lamina propria is a cellular, loose (areolar) connective tissue. In the submucosa are some blood vessels. The muscularis is thick and in basically three layers—outer longitudinal, middle circular, and inner oblique. The cardiac glands are mucus-secreting, but a few parietal (acid-secreting) cells are present, interspersed among the mucus-secreting columnar cells.

Figure 11–29. Stomach, cardiac glands. Plastic section. Methylene blue, azure A, basic fuchsin. High power.

The bases of cardiac glands are coiled and thus cut in oblique-transverse section, rather than through their lengths. The major cell type is mucus-secreting, with apical secretory, mucin granules (arrowheads). A few parietal cells (arrows) also are seen. The lamina propria contains numerous capillary blood vessels (c).

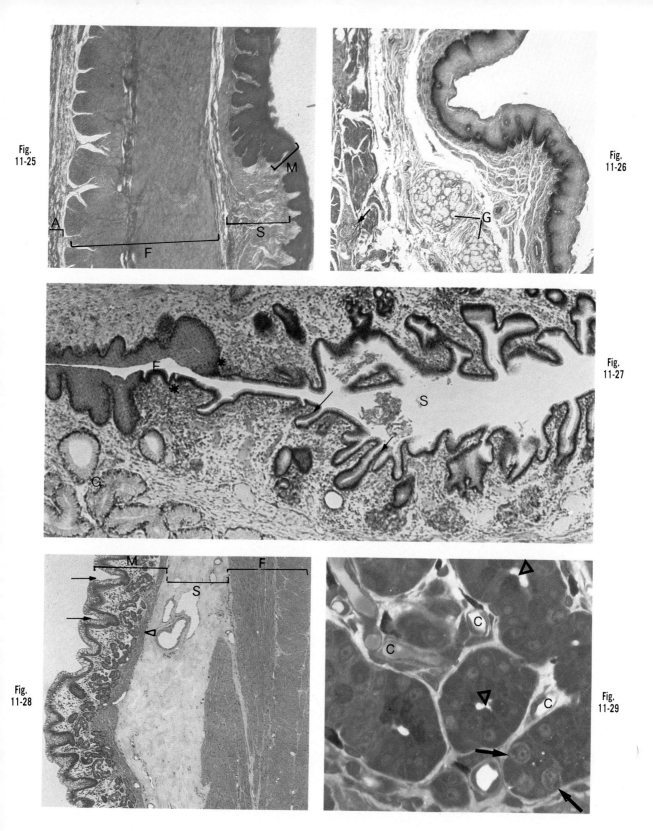

Fig.
11-25

Fig.
11-26

Fig.
11-27

Fig.
11-28

Fig.
11-29

Figure 11–30. Stomach, main glands. Plastic section. H and E. Low power.

The full thickness of the stomach is seen with muscularis (M) covered by serosa (right), submucosa (S), and mucosa (left). In the mucosa, note the thick muscularis mucosae (m) at its base, the remainder occupied by glands between which are slips of lamina propria. The surface epithelium is simple columnar and shows shallow pits (P). (Compare with Figure 11–35.) Opening into the pits are long, simple tubular glands divided into base (B), neck (N), and isthmus (I). Dark-staining chief or zymogenic cells are confined to the bases of glands, and scattered among them are pink-staining parietal cells. Other cell types are not clearly identifiable at this magnification.

Figure 11–31. Stomach, base of main (fundic) glands. Plastic section. Alcian blue, nuclear red. High power.

The bases of the main gastric glands show chief (zymogenic) cells (C) with basophil cytoplasm, apical (unstained) secretory droplets, and prominent nucleoli—features of protein (enzyme)-secreting cells. Interspersed among them are pale-staining parietal cells (P), some showing clear, intracellular canaliculi (arrowheads). Enteroendocrine cells also are present (arrows) and, in the neck region of the glands (above), mucous neck cells (N). Between glands are slips of lamina propria (L) with the muscularis mucosae (M) below. (See also Figure 11–2.)

Figure 11–32. Stomach, necks of main glands. Plastic section. Alcian blue, nuclear red. High power.

The glands are cut longitudinally (indicating that they are straight and not coiled) and show parietal cells (P), some showing clear intracellular canaliculi (arrowheads), and mucous neck cells (N)—cells of irregular outline, "squashed" between the adjacent cells, and with clear, unstained, apical secretory droplets.

Figure 11–33. Stomach, pits and apex of main glands. Plastic section. Toluidine blue and safranin. High power.

This shows mucus as dark purple secretory droplets present in surface epithelial cells (arrows) at the surface and in pits, and in mucous neck cells (arrowhead) in the necks of gastric glands. Parietal cells (P) are seen in both isthmus (I) and neck (N). The meshwork of clear, intracellular canaliculi within the cytoplasm of parietal cells is seen clearly.

Figure 11–34. Stomach, pits and apex of main glands.

This is a higher magnification of Figure 11–30. The simple, tall columnar surface epithelium is mucus-secreting and extends to line pits (arrows). Opening into the bases of the pits are gastric glands at the isthmus (I), where parietal cells (P) are interspersed with surface epithelial cells. Slips of connective tissue of the lamina propria (L) are seen.

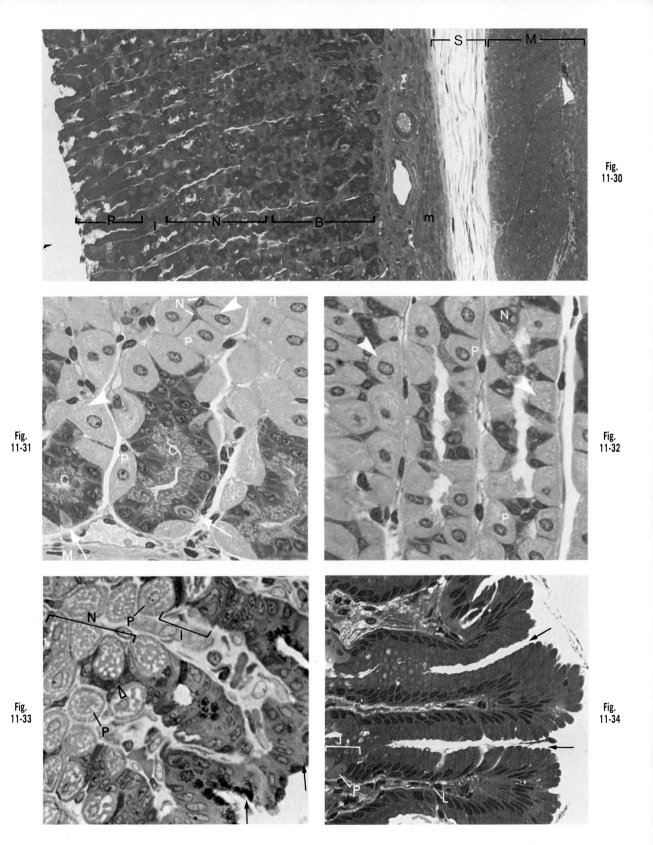

Fig. 11-30

Fig. 11-31

Fig. 11-32

Fig. 11-33

Fig. 11-34

Figure 11–35. Stomach, pyloric glands. Plastic section. Methylene blue, azure A, basic fuchsin. Low power.

The mucosa only is seen. In comparison with main gastric glands (see Fig. 11–30), the pits (P) are deep and the glands (G) are short and coiled. The main cell type in the glands is mucus-secreting, similar to the mucous neck cell. Between glands and pits is the lamina propria (L) with a thick muscularis mucosae (M) at right. (See also Figure 11–36.)

Figure 11–36. Stomach, pyloric glands. Plastic section. Methylene blue, azure A, basic fuchsin. High power.

A higher magnification of Figure 11–35, this shows the surface epithelial cells (S) with clear, apical secretory material. This cell extends to line the gastric pits (P). The pyloric glands are formed by mucus-secreting cells with apical mucin droplets, but a few parietal cells (arrows) and enteroendocrine cells (not seen here) also are present.

Figure 11–37. Gastroduodenal junction. H and E. Low power.

To the right is the terminal part of the stomach (pyloric canal) with the duodenum on the left. At the pyloric antrum, the middle (circular) layer of smooth muscle of the muscularis is thickened to form the pyloric sphincter (star). The submucosa of the stomach (S) is thin, and the mucosa shows complex folds or rugae, one of which is sectioned in such a manner that it appears to protrude through the pyloric orifice (arrow). The duodenal mucosa is thick and shows numerous villi (V), finger-like processes with a core of lamina propria, and intestinal glands (G), or crypts of Lieberkühn. The submucosa of the duodenum is thick and contains pale-staining glands (of Brunner, B). Two small lymphoid follicles (L) are seen.

Figure 11–38. Duodenum. H and E. Low power.

This transverse section also shows part of the pancreas (G) and the common bile duct (D). In the duodenum, the serosa (P), muscularis (F), submucosa (S), and mucosa (M) are seen. In the submucosa are glands of Brunner (B), and the mucosa shows villi protruding from the suface and intestinal glands (darkly staining).

Figure 11–39. Jejunum. H and E. Low power.

Cut in transverse section. This shows all layers. Villi (V) are long, and glands stain dark in the mucosa. A plica circularis (arrow), bifid at its apex, is seen and has a core of submucosa (S). The muscularis (F) is quite thin.

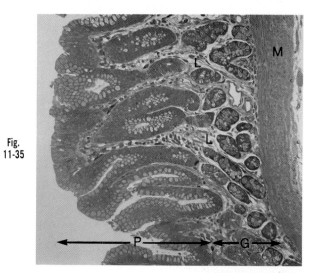

Fig.
11-35

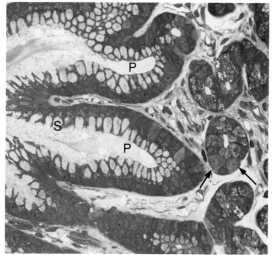

Fig.
11-36

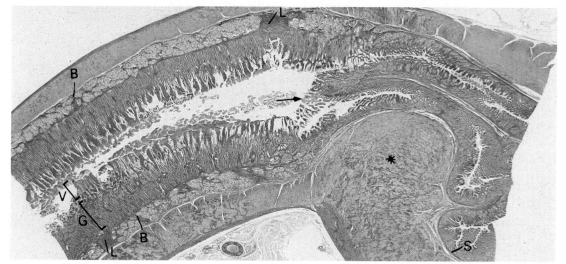

Fig.
11-37

Fig.
11-38

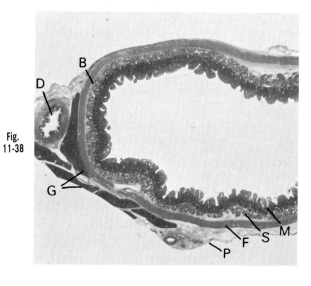

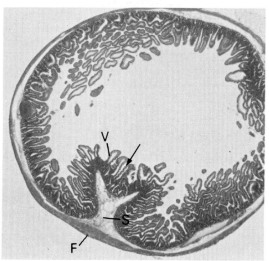

Fig.
11-39

Figure 11–40. Duodenum, Brunner's glands. Plastic section. Methylene blue, azure A, basic fuchsin. Medium power.

Above are the bases of intestinal glands or crypts (G), below are the submucosal glands of Brunner (B). This gland secretes a neutral or alkaline mucus with a high bicarbonate content. The ducts of the gland pass through the muscularis mucosae (M) to drain into the bases of the crypts, as seen at arrow. (See also Figure 11–72.)

Figure 11–41. Duodenum, Brunner's glands. Plastic section. Methylene blue, azure A, basic fuchsin. Oil immersion.

A higher magnification of Figure 11–40, this section shows smooth muscle (M) of the muscularis mucosae in transverse section with parts of two secretory acini of Brunner's glands. The cells are tall columnar in type, nuclei are basally located, and the extensive apical cytoplasm is pale-staining and filled with mucous droplets.

Figure 11–42. Jejunum. Mallory. Low power.

This is a longitudinal section of the upper jejunum. The submucosa is quite thick and extends into the cores of two plicae circulares (arrows). In the mucosa, villi (V) and glands (G) are seen clearly. It is obvious that the surface of the gut lining is increased greatly by plicae, villi, and glands.

Figure 11–43. Jejunum. Plastic section. H and E. Low power.

All four layers are seen—the serosa at arrow, outer (O) and inner (I) layers of the muscularis, the submucosa (S), and, as parts of the mucosa, the muscularis mucosae (m) and lamina propria (L) lying between intestinal glands (G) and in the cores of villi (V). In the epithelium of glands and villi, clear-staining goblet cells are present (arrowheads).

Figure 11–44. Ileum, villus. Plastic section. Methylene blue, azure A, basic fuchsin. Medium power.

The connective tissue core of lamina propria (L) contains blood capillaries (c) and a variety of connective tissue cells. Also present is a small bundle of smooth muscle (m). On the surface, the simple columnar (absorptive) cells show a brush border (arrowheads). Scattered among them are goblet or mucous (g) cells of characteristic shape, filled with secretory droplets. Enteroendocrine cells also are present in this epithelium. Arrows indicate cells that may be of this type.

Figure 11–45. Intestinal epithelium. Plastic section. H and E. Oil immersion.

The simple columnar (absorptive) epithelium here is seen covering villi of the duodenum. Note that no goblet cells are visible (although they are present); this indicates that the section was from the duodenum. Goblet cells increase in number from duodenum to terminal ileum. The columnar cells or enterocytes show elongated nuclei, the cytoplasm is basophilic, and in a supranuclear position the Golgi apparatus is seen as a negative image (arrowheads). Apically, there is a brush border (b) and on some lateral cell interfaces near the lumen, a dense pink dot indicates a junctional complex or terminal bar (arrows). The basally located cell with dark irregular nucleus at bottom may be an enteroendocrine cell.

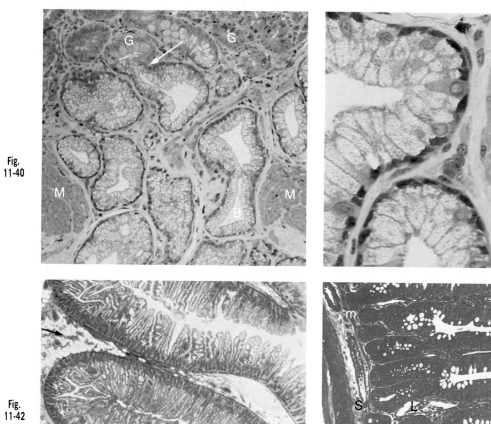

Fig.
11-40

Fig.
11-41

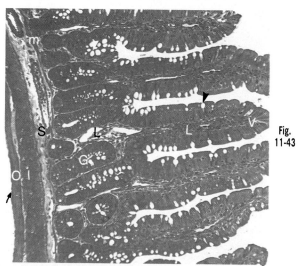

Fig.
11-42

Fig.
11-43

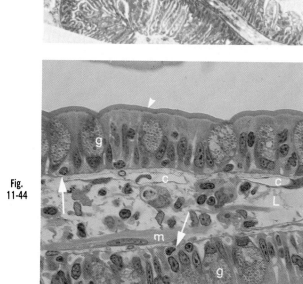

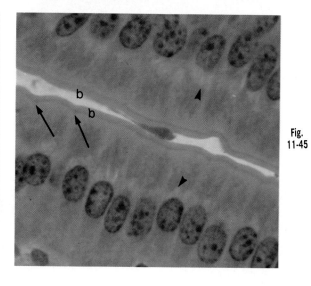

Fig.
11-44

Fig.
11-45

Figure 11–46. Jejunum, glands. Plastic section. H and E. High power.

Outer (O) and inner (I) layers of the muscularis are covered by a thin serosa (s), with submucosa (S) internally. In the bases of intestinal glands or crypts there are immature columnar (stem) cells (c) that show negative Golgi apparatuses in a supranuclear position, some in mitosis (a telophase is indicated by arrow); immature goblet (oligomucous) cells (o); and Paneth cells (p), clearly distinguished by apical, eosinophilic, secretory droplets. (See also Figure 11–47.) Note the plasma cell (arrowhead) in the lamina propria.

Figure 11–47. Paneth cells. Plastic section. H and E. Oil immersion.

The base of one jejunal gland or crypt contains Paneth cells, serozymogenic in type and with spherical, apical, secretory droplets, varying in size. These cells produce lysozyme. The cell indicated by the arrow, lying higher in the crypt with a few, small secretory droplets, probably is an immature Paneth cell formed in the "stem cell zone." Columnar epithelial cells, where cut obliquely through their apices, show prominent terminal bars (arrowheads).

Figure 11–48. Intestinal nerve plexuses. Plastic section. Toluidine blue, aldehyde fuchsin. Medium power.

This is a section through the outer portion of the ileum to show the myenteric (Auerbach's) and submucosal (Meissner's) plexuses. At top left is serosa (P) covering the outer longitudinal (L) and inner circular (C) layers of smooth muscle of the muscularis. To the right is submucosa (S) extending up to the muscularis mucosae (M). Between the two layers of the muscularis is a collection of ganglion cells and nerve fibers of Auerbach's plexus (arrow), with a similar collection of Meissner's plexus (arrowhead) in the submucosa.

Figure 11–49. Goblet cells. Plastic section. PAS. Oil immersion.

The epithelium of an ileal villus shows goblet cells, with the "stem" containing the nucleus (n) and the apex expanded to the goblet shape with mucous secretory granules. The mucus is an acidic glycoprotein. Also staining positively (magenta) with the periodic acid–Schiff (PAS) technique is the brush border of the columnar cells (arrow) as a result of the glycocalyx and, faintly, the basal lamina (arrowhead).

Figure 11–50. Ileum. H and E. Low power.

All layers are seen with the mesentery (arrow). Compare with Figures 11–38 and 11–39. Villi here are short and closely packed, and the lumen is smaller than that of the duodenum or jejunum.

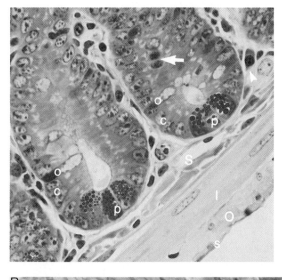

Fig.
11-46

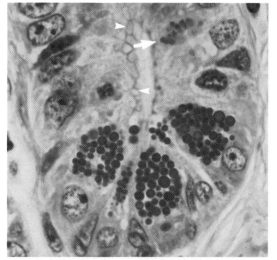

Fig.
11-47

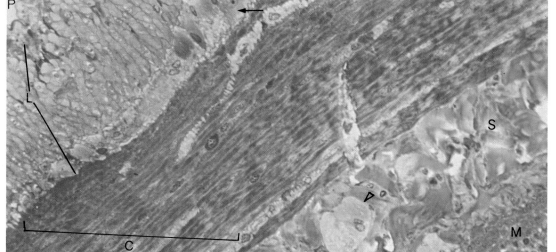

Fig.
11-48

Fig.
11-49

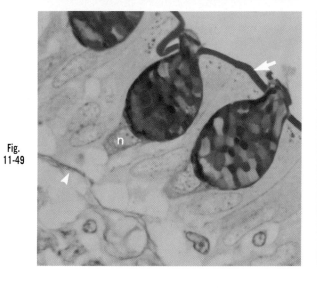

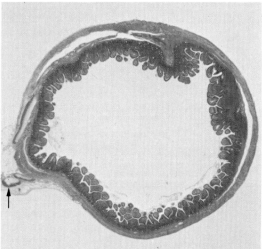

Fig.
11-50

Figure 11–51. Ileum, Peyer's patches. H and E. Medium power.

Here, masses of lymphoid tissue occupy the lamina propria and infiltrate the submucosa (arrowhead). Such masses may be visible to the naked eye. They are located on the antimesenteric border. Where follicles are large, there are no villi and there may be no glands, the follicles being separated from the lumen only by a simple columnar epithelium (arrow).

Figure 11–52. Peyer's patch, ileum. Plastic section. Methylene blue, azure A, basic fuchsin. High power.

Lymphatic tissue in the Peyer's patch infiltrates the lamina propria (L) and muscularis mucosae (M) and forms follicles (F) in the submucosa. Above, the bases of intestinal glands (g) are visible, but villi and glands may not be present over a Peyer's patch. (See Figure 11–51.)

Figure 11–53. Appendix. Plastic section. Methylene blue, azure A, basic fuchsin. Low power.

Shown here are lumen (L), mucosa (M), submucosa (S), and part of the muscularis (F). In the mucosa, there are no villi and the glands (arrows) are few and lined by a simple columnar epithelium in which goblet cells (clear-staining) are numerous. The lamina propria is very cellular because of lymphoid infiltration with lymph nodules (arrowheads) extending into the submucosa through an incomplete muscularis mucosae. Note fat cells (a) in the submucosa.

Figure 11–54. Colon. Plastic section. PAS. High power.

The simple tubular glands of the mucosa contain numerous goblet cells. The secretory mucin granules are stained magenta. (See also Figure 11–49.) The mucus is discharged to lie in the lumen near the surface (arrow). The surface epithelium is simple columnar with interspersed (and dying) goblet cells. There are no villi in the large intestine.

Figure 11–55. Rectoanal junction. H and E. Low power.

In the terminal rectum, there are a few simple tubular glands (G) with a simple columnar epithelial lining. The columnar epithelium then changes abruptly (arrow), in this longitudinal section, to a stratified squamous epithelium lining the anal canal. This is short, and at the anal orifice the epithelium changes again to epidermis. At the anus, the epithelium is keratinized, and deep to it are the branched, tubular, circumanal glands (darkly staining).

Figure 11–56. Small intestine, blood vessels injected. Low power.

This is a transverse section of the jejunum. The arterial system was injected with red gelatin to demonstrate the blood supply. Terminal branches (vasa recta) of arterial arcades from the superior mesenteric artery lie in the connective tissue of the serosa (P). They give a few branches to serosa and muscularis and then pass through the muscularis (F) to form an extensive submucosal plexus (S). In the muscularis, blood vessels run parallel to muscle fibers; i.e., they are circular in the inner layer (arrow). From the submucous plexus, vessels run radially and extend into villi (V) to form extensive capillary networks. Indeed, capillary plexuses here are so extensive as to clearly outline villi. Venous return, not demonstrated here, starts in mucosal plexuses and then passes to an extensive submucosal plexus. Large veins drain this plexus and pass through muscularis and serosa to run with arteries and join the portal vein to pass to the liver.

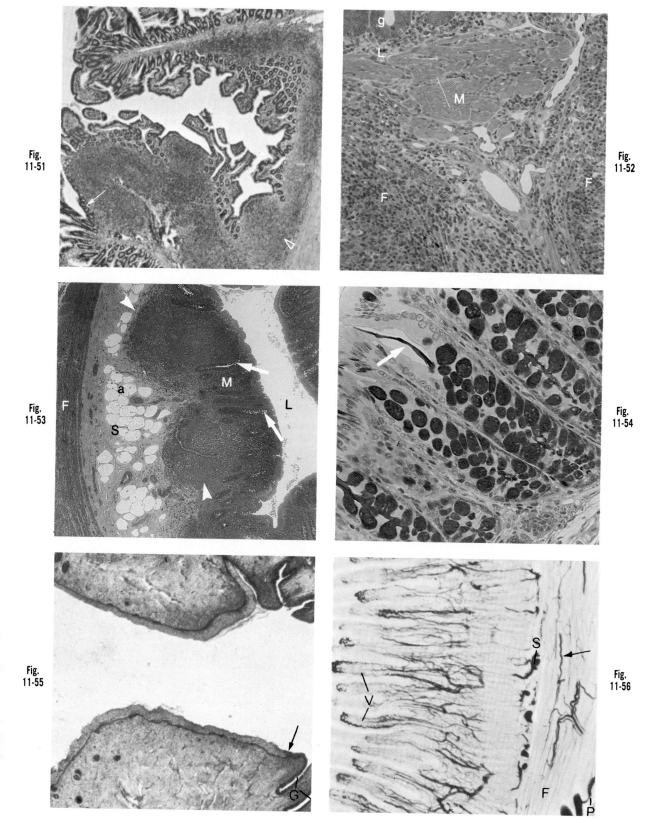

Fig.
11-51

Fig.
11-52

Fig.
11-53

Fig.
11-54

Fig.
11-55

Fig.
11-56

Figure 11–57. Pancreas. Plastic section. H and E. Low power.

The pancreas is both exocrine and endocrine. Parts of several lobules are seen, with fine connective tissue between lobules. The secretory units or acini are not clearly distinguished at this magnification, but are formed by cells with basophil cytoplasm and pink-staining secretory droplets. In the more extensive connective tissue are some large blood vessels (V). Located in lobules among the acini are two pale-staining, spheroidal clumps of cells (L). These are the endocrine islets of Langerhans. The exocrine pancreas is classified as a compound acinar serous gland, secreting digestive enzymes. The islets secrete insulin, the antidiabetic hormone, and glucagon, which increases the level of blood sugar. (See also Figures 1–8 and 1–13.)

Figure 11–58. Pancreas, exocrine. Plastic section. Methylene blue, basic fuchsin. Oil immersion.

Several acini are seen with sparse connective tissue between them in which there is a blood capillary (c). Acinar cells show the features of protein (enzyme) secretion with vesicular nuclei with prominent and often multiple nucleoli, intense cytoplasmic basophilia, and discrete, apical secretory droplets (pink). A centroacinar cell (arrowhead) is seen in one acinus, and beneath it is an intercalated duct lined by simple, low cuboidal epithelium, the cells with pale-staining nuclei (n), and the lumen containing pink-staining secretory material (arrow).

Figure 11–59. Pancreas, exocrine. Plastic section. Methylene blue, basic fuchsin. Oil immersion.

The exocrine cells show features similar to those in Figure 11–58; note, however, that the lumina of two acini show continuity with intercalated ducts at the arrows, the ducts lined by squamous–low cuboidal epithelium. A capillary (c) also is seen.

Figure 11–60. Endocrine pancreas. Plastic section. H and E. High power.

The field mainly is occupied by an islet of Langerhans, surrounded by exocrine acini. (See Figures 11–58 and 11–59.) In the islet, the endocrine cells are large, polygonal, pale-staining with centrally located nuclei and are arranged in cords and clumps between blood capillaries (c) containing erythrocytes (red). Most of the cells are insulin-secreting B cells. Cells with pinker cytoplasm at the periphery of the islet are glucagon-secreting A cells (arrows).

Figure 11–61. Endocrine pancreas. Plastic section. Methylene blue, basic fuchsin. Oil immersion.

A portion of an islet of Langerhans shows large polygonal cells with fine secretory granules, much smaller than the pink-staining granules in the adjacent exocrine cells (above). Most of the islet cells stain purple and are insulin-secreting B cells (B), but a few at the periphery show more red-colored granules and are glucagon-secreting A cells (A) and perhaps D (somatostatin-secreting) cells. All endocrine cells contact a capillary blood vessel, of which two are seen in the area. (The nuclei of lining endothelial cells are arrowed.)

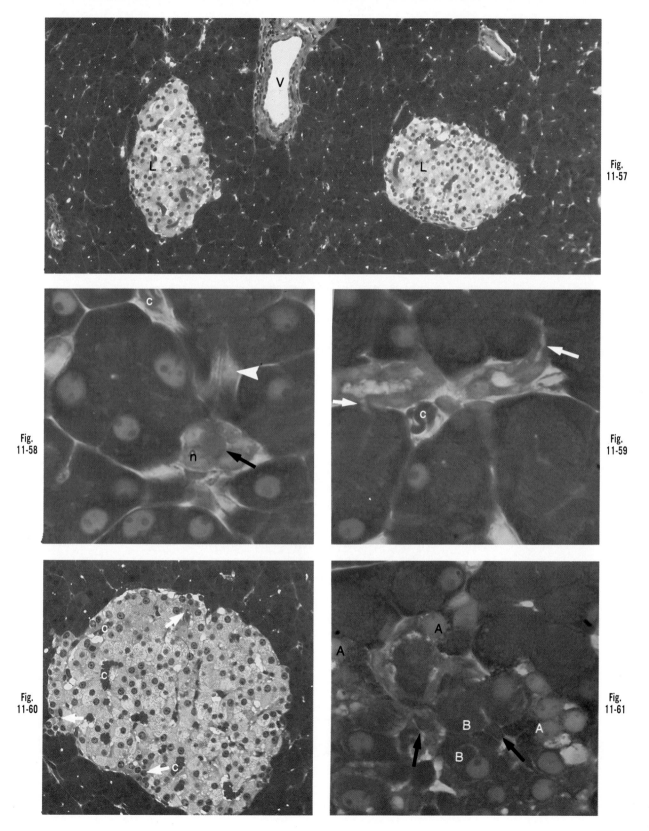

Figure 11–62. Liver. H and E. Low power.

Liver parenchymal cells are arranged as cords of cells with vascular sinusoidal spaces between the cords. The cords radiate from central veins (C)—tributaries of the hepatic veins—and these are the centers of classical hepatic lobules. Lobules are polygonal prisms, and at their peripheries are portal canals (P), these composed of branches of the portal vein, hepatic artery, bile duct, and lymphatics. Lobules are not delineated by connective tissue. In a lobule, blood enters the periphery from portal vein and hepatic artery radicles and passes radially in the sinusoidal channels between cords of parenchymal cells to the central vein, and then to hepatic veins and the inferior vena cava. (See also Figures 1–3 and 1–15.)

Figure 11–63. Liver. Kull method. Low power.

This technique demonstrates blood vessels and sinusoidal spaces (black). Most of the field is occupied by part of one lobule. At its center is a central vein (C) with portal canals (P) at its periphery. Note the radial arrangement of the sinusoidal spaces (arrows) draining to the central vein. Parenchymal cells are arranged as cords or plates between the sinusoidal spaces.

Figure 11–64. Liver. Plastic section. Methylene blue, azure A, basic fuchsin. High power.

Liver parenchymal cells are arranged in anastomosing plates and cords. Their nuclei are vesicular, often with prominent nucleoli, and polyploidal or binucleate cells (arrowhead) are common. The cytoplasm is basophil and here shows several small, clear, spherical spaces that represent lipid as a cytoplasmic inclusion. Between the plates of parenchymal cells are blood sinusoids containing red and white blood corpuscles lined by cells of the endothelial (e) or phagocytic (Kupffer) types. The latter cannot be recognized with certainty in this preparation, but probable phagocytic cells are arrowed. (See Figure 11–68.) Between each arrowed cell and the adjacent parenchymal cell is a slender space, the perisinusoidal space of Disse (also visible in other areas).

Figure 11–65. Liver, central vein. Silver stain. High power.

This stain demonstrates reticular fibers (black). Parenchymal cells stain brown with black nuclei and are arranged in cords radiating from a central vein (C). Note that reticular fibers are found in the wall of the central vein and in the walls of liver sinusoids (arrows), the sinusoids draining into the central vein (arrowheads).

Figure 11–66. Liver, portal area. H and E. High power.

Portal areas or canals are surrounded by small amounts of connective tissue and contain the "portal triad" of hepatic artery (A), portal vein (V), and bile duct (D), usually with a lymphatic vessel (L). The bile duct is lined by simple cuboidal epithelium; the branch of the hepatic artery is an arteriole lined by endothelium and with a single layer of smooth muscle in its wall; and the branch of the portal vein is a large venule. Parenchymal cells lie as a plate around the portal area, this being called the limiting plate (arrows), and as radiating cords in adjacent liver lobules.

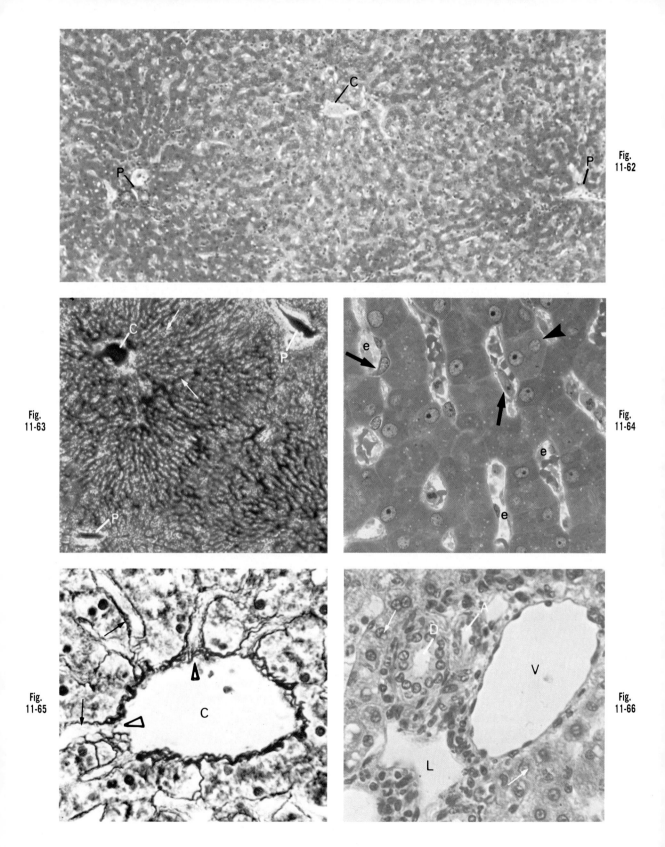

Figure 11–67. Liver, bile canaliculi. Injected specimen.

The liver parenchymal cells stain green and are arranged in cords with clear spaces of sinusoidal channels between. Bile canaliculi are seen as fine tubular channels arranged in a three-dimensional network, between the parenchymal cells. Their walls are formed by adjacent parenchymal cells, that is, they are simply spaces between cells and have no intrinsic cellular lining of their own. Drainage of bile in a classical lobule is from the center to the periphery.

Figure 11–68. Liver phagocytosis. Lithium carmine, toluidine blue. High power.

Before death, an animal was injected with lithium carmine, a particulate, red dye. Here, part of a central vein (C) is seen with radiating cords of liver cells and sinusoidal spaces between them. Associated with liver sinusoids are endothelial-type cells and phagocytic (stellate) cells of Kupffer (K). The latter have picked up the dye material. Clearly, they are stellate in shape, with thin cytoplasmic arms, and lie in relation to sinusoidal spaces.

Figure 11–69. Fetal liver. Plastic section. Toluidine blue. High power.

In the fetus, the liver is a hemopoietic organ. Here, the normal architecture of the liver is obscured by masses of cells of the erythrocyte and myeloid series. Parenchymal cells can be distinguished between the arrows. (See also Figure 5–11.)

Figure 11–70. Gallbladder. Plastic section. Methylene blue, basic fuchsin. Medium power.

The lining mucosa of the gallbladder usually shows folds or rugae, as seen here, and is formed by a simple columnar epithelium with supporting lamina propria. In the lamina, small mucous glands (g) may be present, particularly at the neck region. There is no true submucosa. External to the lamina is the muscularis (M), composed of slips of smooth muscle with an external adventitia (A).

Figure 11–71. Gallbladder. Plastic section. Methylene blue, azure A, basic fuchsin. High power.

This is a higher magnification of Figure 11–70. Note the simple, tall columnar epithelium. In these cells, a "negative" Golgi apparatus is seen clearly in a supranuclear position (arrowhead). The lamina propria is loose (areolar) connective tissue, containing an arteriole (a), a venule (v), and capillaries (c), with mucous glands. The smooth muscle slips of the muscularis are cut longitudinally (right).

Figure 11–72. Ampulla of Vater. Masson. Low power.

This section is through the combined opening of the common bile duct and main pancreatic duct as it passes through the wall of the duodenum. The mucosa, with a simple columnar epithelium, is thrown into valve-like folds (arrowheads). Also seen are glands of Brunner (B) in the submucosa of the duodenum. Fluid flows in the combined duct in the direction of the arrow.

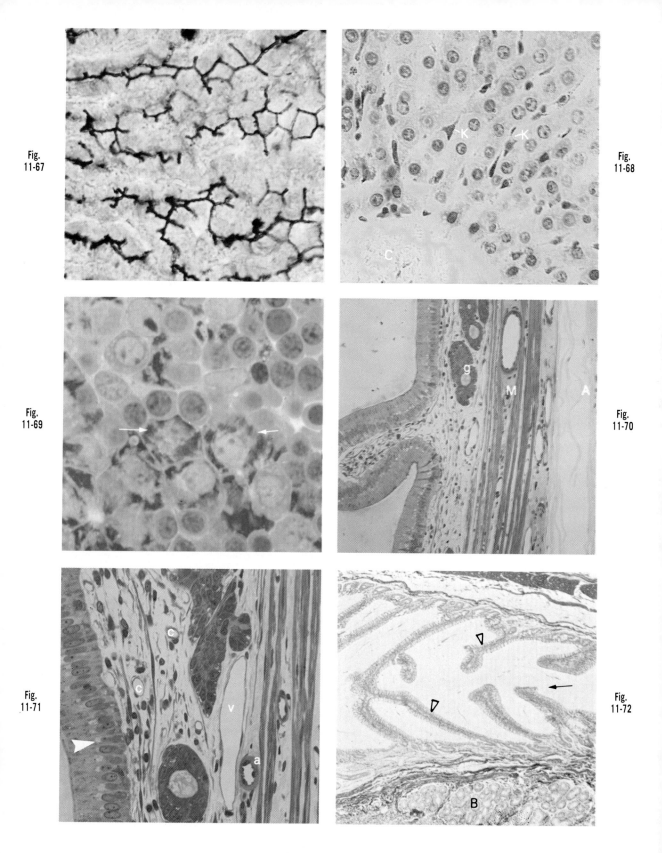

Fig.
11-67

Fig.
11-68

Fig.
11-69

Fig.
11-70

Fig.
11-71

Fig.
11-72

CHAPTER
TWELVE

The Respiratory System

ORIGIN AND FUNCTION

The respiratory system consists of the lungs and the respiratory passages that connect the lungs to the exterior. Usually, it is divided into a *conducting part* composed of nose, nasopharynx, larynx, trachea, bronchi, and bronchioles, and a *respiratory part* that includes the alveoli of the lung and the respiratory bronchioles. The main function of the system is to provide for gaseous exchange, that is, the transfer of oxygen to the blood and the elimination of carbon dioxide. To perform this function, the blood-air "barrier" is extremely thin in respiratory tissue in the lungs. This barrier, formed by structures interposed between air in alveoli and blood in pulmonary capillaries, consists of the very thin, attenuated, squamous epithelial lining of air spaces (pulmonary surface epithelium), its supporting basal lamina, and the basal lamina and attenuated endothelium of pulmonary capillaries. A narrow connective tissue space, the zona diffusa, lies between the two basal laminae and contains a few reticular and elastic fibers. The pulmonary surface epithelium is "wet," being covered by a thin fluid film containing a lipoprotein surface-active agent ("surfactant") that functions to prevent collapse of the small air spaces.

The respiratory system from nasal cavities to alveoli is a closed system open to the exterior only at the nasal orifices. The lungs lie within the pleural cavities, and, as the thorax expands on *inspiration,* a negative pressure is created within the respiratory system and air enters the lungs. In *expiration,* the rich elastic network found within the lungs, which was stretched on inspiration, undergoes elastic recoil as the thorax decreases in size. In the sense that water is lost in expired air, the lungs also are excretory organs.

The lungs have a double blood supply. Oxygenated blood for metabolism of lung tissue itself is carried in bronchial arteries—branches of the aorta—and deoxygenated blood passes to the lungs from the right side of the heart in pulmonary arteries. After circulation through the lungs, this blood is fully oxygenated and returns in pulmonary veins to the heart for circulation in the systemic system.

CONDUCTION

The Nose and Nasopharynx

The conducting part of the respiratory system is lined by respiratory epithelium of the pseudostratified ciliated columnar type with goblet cells. In addition to conveying air to respiratory tissue, this part has other functions. It strains out particulate matter in the inspired air (hairs in the nostrils, mucus, and ciliated cells), washes or humidifies inspired air (serous secretions) and warms or cools it, depending upon the ambient temperature (vascular plexuses in the walls). It is important that patency of the airway be maintained, i.e., that the respiratory passages do not collapse, and this rigidity is accomplished by the presence of cartilage in its walls. A variation in diameter of the passages is achieved by contraction of smooth muscle, also present in its walls.

The nasal apertures are lined by epidermis with coarse hairs and sebaceous glands. Then there is a narrow transitional zone lined by stratified squamous epithelium. The nasal cavities are lined by respiratory epithelium in which the cilia beat posteriorly to the nasopharynx. Externally, the cavities are supported by bone and cartilage from which three conchae or turbinate bones protrude into the cavities. In the roof of the cavities is located the olfactory mucosa, the receptor for smell. Connected to the nasal cavities are the paranasal air sinuses. These are bony cavities in the maxilla, frontal, ethmoid and sphenoid bones, and they too are lined by respiratory epithelium and contain air. Although their function is obscure, they do modify the tone of the voice.

The Larynx

At the opening of the larynx lies the epiglottis. This has a core of elastic cartilage covered by a mucous membrane with stratified squamous epithelium on its superior aspect and respiratory epithelium inferiorly. It also contains mixed mucous and serous glands. The larynx itself is lined by respiratory epithelium, except over the vocal cords where the epithelium is stratified squamous in type. Several hyaline cartilages support the wall, and the larynx functions principally in phonation.

The Trachea

The trachea is supported by about 20 horseshoe-shaped cartilages lying one above the other, connected by connective tissue, and with the deficiencies posteriorly. Here, there are slips of smooth muscle (the musculus trachealis), oriented mainly transversely, which on contraction diminishes the diameter of the trachea. In the submucosa of the trachea are small mixed glands, lying mainly posteriorly and between the cartilage rings. The mucosa is lined by respiratory epithelium and here the cilia beat upward to the nasopharynx. In the connective tissue of the trachea, as elsewhere in the respiratory tract, elastic fibers are prominent.

The Lung

Bronchi. Extrapulmonary bronchi closely resemble the trachea in structure, but bronchi within the lung differ from those outside it in several basic features. Within the lung, the cartilage in the wall is in the form of complete rings, although the rings are of irregular outline. At the junction of mucosa and submucosa, where in the trachea and extrapulmonary bronchi there is a condensation of elastic fibers, in intrapulmonary bronchi this elastic tissue is reinforced by smooth muscle fibers that spiral around the bronchus. These fibers vary lumen diameter.

Bronchioles. Bronchi in the lung branch to form *bronchioles*. Although there is no abrupt transition between small bronchi and bronchioles, a bronchiole is a conducting tube of 1 mm diameter or less, supported by very little connective tissue and surrounded by respiratory tissue. Cartilage, glands, and lymphatic tissue are not present; however, the lamina propria contains prominent bundles of smooth muscle and elastic fibers. In large bronchioles, the lining epithelium is ciliated columnar with some goblet cells. In smaller bronchioles (about 0.3 mm), the lining ciliated epithelium is low columnar or cuboidal in type. Goblet cells disappear at this level. (Cilia extend further down the bronchial tree than do goblet cells or glands.) Scattered in the bronchiolar epithelium are nonciliated, columnar cells, the apices of which protrude into the lumen. These are secretory *(Clara)* cells that add to bronchiolar secretion and may secrete some surfactant. In the smallest or terminal bronchioles, the epithelium shows only patches of ciliated cells among nonciliated cuboidal cells.

RESPIRATION

Respiratory Bronchioles

Arising from terminal bronchioles are *respiratory bronchioles,* so called because their walls are interrupted by saccular outpocketings, or *alveoli,* where gaseous exchange occurs. The lining epithelium of the larger respiratory bronchiole is ciliated cuboidal in type, becoming simple cuboidal in the smaller ones, and is continuous with the simple squamous alveolar lining at the openings of the alveoli. External to the epithelium the wall is formed by interlacing bundles of smooth muscle and elastic fibroconnective tissue. Respiratory bronchioles terminate by branching into two or more alveolar ducts.

Alveolar Ducts

Alveolar ducts are cone-shaped, thin-walled tubes with a squamous epithelial lining, and with many alveoli and alveolar sacs (clusters of alveoli) opening around their circumferences. Smooth muscle fibers with elastic and some collagen fibers support this epithelium and interweave between and around the openings of alveoli along the wall of an alveolar duct. Alveolar ducts terminate by opening into *atria,* which simply are vestibules or irregular chambers from which *alveolar sacs* and alveoli diverge. Usually, two or more alveolar sacs open from each atrium.

Alveolar Sacs, Alveoli, and the Interalveolar Septum

Alveolar sacs are multilocular, being a cluster of alveoli opening into a central, slightly larger chamber. Around the openings of atria, alveolar sacs, and alveoli is a supporting network of fine elastic and reticular fibers. *Alveoli* are polyhedral or hexagonal, packed tightly, and separated by *interalveolar septa* in which pulmonary capillaries are located. The septa contain reticular and elastic fibers and a few cells within the connective tissue space that is limited by the basal laminae surrounding the blood capillaries (lined by endothelium) and underlying the alveolar lining epithelium. The alveolar epithelium is formed mainly by squamous (alveolar or type I) surface epithelial cells, so thin (only 0.2 μm) that they are invisible by light microscopy.

Scattered singly or in small groups of two or three in this epithelium are the great alveolar (type II or septal) cells. They are cuboidal and may bulge into alveolar spaces, but usually they are situated in corners or angles of alveolar walls. The cytoplasm often appears vacuolated because of the presence of lipid-containing bodies (cytosomes), and this cell secretes surfactant, a detergent material (mainly dipalmitoyl lecithin) that diminishes the surface tension of alveolar fluid. In turn, this decreases the force necessary to inflate alveoli and facilitates breathing. Alveolar macrophages or phagocytes are found in the interstitium of interalveolar septa, free in alveolar spaces, and in the process of passing through the alveolar wall into the alveolar space. As already indicated, gaseous exchange occurs in alveoli.

Figure 12–1. The lung.

Top left: This photomicrograph shows the terminal bronchiole (Tb), which leads to respiratory bronchiole (Rb); this divides into two alveolar ducts (Ad). Also seen are alveolar sacs (S), alveoli (A), and branches of the pulmonary artery (e). The features of these structures are illustrated in the diagrams in both longitudinal and transverse sections. The main diagram *(top right)* shows a lung acinus (i.e., the parts supplied by a terminal bronchiole) and is an interpretation of the section with the left alveolar duct shown dividing further into two smaller ducts (asterisks) of which one terminates in an atrium (At) from which alveolar sacs and alveoli open. b = Type II cell; c = blood capillary; d = cell within an interalveolar septum; m = muscle; p = free alveolar phagocyte. Arrows indicate alveolar pores; numbers indicate section levels.

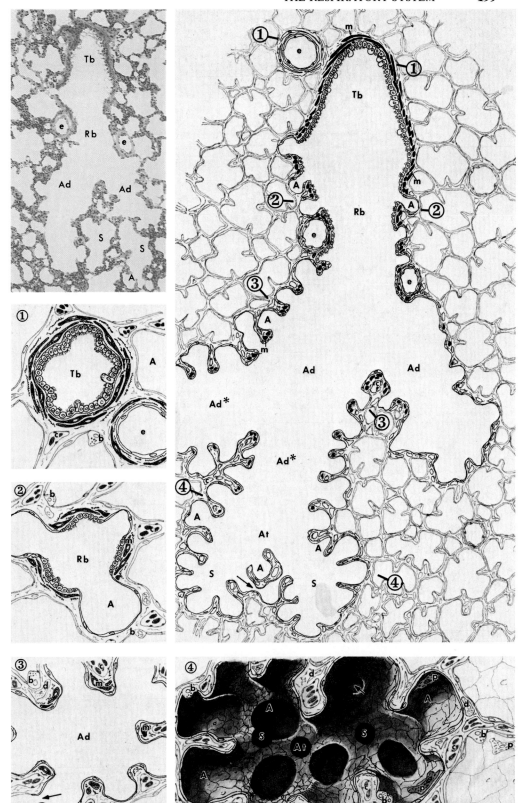

Figure 12–1. *See legend on opposite page.*

Figure 12–2. Rat lung.

This scanning electron micrograph shows a terminal bronchiole (T), respiratory bronchioles (R) with alveoli opening from their walls (arrows), alveolar sacs (S), and alveoli. Also present is a small blood vessel (V). × 100. (Courtesy of Dr. Peter Andrews.)

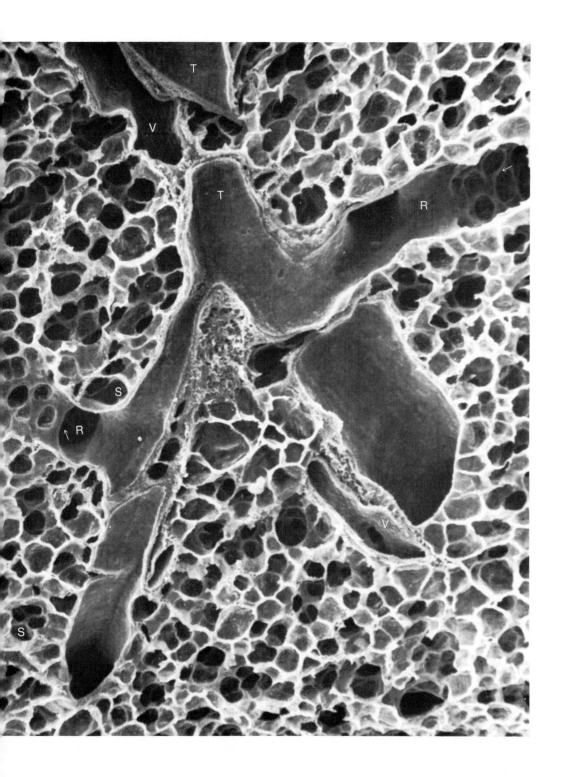

Figure 12–3. Nasal concha. H and E. Medium power.

This is a section through a nasal concha or turbinate bone and shows the respiratory mucosa (R), with its lamina propria blending with periosteum of the bone (B), and the olfactory epithelium (O). The latter is pseudostratified columnar in type, with nuclei in several rows. In the connective tissue underlying the olfactory epithelium are dilated venous channels (V) that constitute the so-called cavernous or erectile tissue, ducts (D), and small acini (A) of serous glands (of Bowman), and numerous small peripheral nerves (N).

Figure 12–4. Nasal cavity, respiratory mucosa. Methylene blue, azure A, basic fuchsin.
                Plastic section. High power.

The epithelium (above) is pseudostratified ciliated columnar in type with ciliated, goblet, and basal cells. In the supporting lamina propria are seromucous glands (g) (here two ducts open to the surface, arrows) and numerous venous channels (v). The lamina propria blends with periosteum of bone (arrowhead) to form a mucoperiosteum (or mucoperichondrium if nasal cartilage underlies it).

Figure 12–5. Olfactory mucosa. Methylene blue, azure A, basic fuchsin. Plastic section.
                High power.

The epithelium lacks a distinct basal lamina and is of the pseudostratified tall columnar type without goblet cells. Nuclei occur in several rows and are of three cell types: basal (b), probably the undifferentiated stem cell; sustentacular or supporting cells, their nuclei lying as a more superficial row (e); and olfactory or sensory cells, darker-staining cells with their nuclei (s), in several rows basal to those of sustentacular cells. These are spindle-shaped, bipolar nerve cells, apically with a small olfactory vesicle and six to eight olfactory hairs or modified cilia, and basally with a slender axon. The axons collect into small bundles, the fila olfactoria (f), lying in the lamina propria, which also contains serous glands of Bowman (g), their ducts (arrowheads) passing through the epithelium to the surface. Venous sinuses (v) also lie in the lamina propria.

Figure 12–6. Larynx, sagittal section. H and E. Low power.

Above (posteriorly) is the esophagus (E), and below (anteriorly) is the trachea (T). Note that the stratified squamous epithelium lining the esophagus is much thicker than the respiratory mucosa of the trachea. Also seen is the epiglottis (G) with a core of elastic cartilage, some mucous glands inferiorly (right) and covered above (left) by stratified squamous epithelium and below (right) by respiratory epithelium. Anteriorly (below) is a row of oval profiles of hyaline cartilage of tracheal rings and some of the laryngeal cartilages such as the cricoid (C) and arytenoid (A). Striated muscle of the larynx and esophagus also is present. The position of the vocal cord is indicated by the dotted line.

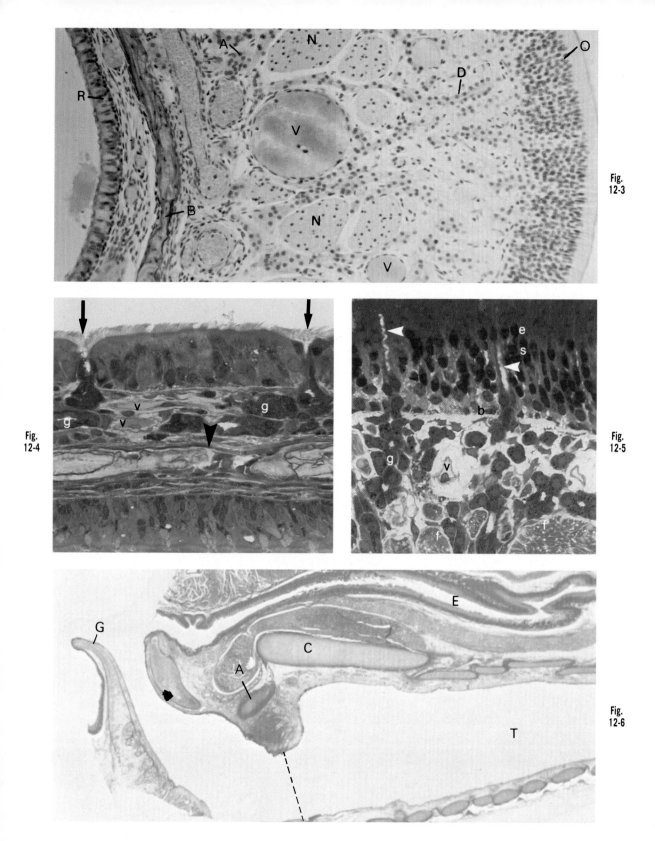

Fig. 12-3

Fig. 12-4

Fig. 12-5

Fig. 12-6

Figure 12–7. Trachea, transverse section. Mallory. Low power.

Part of one tracheal hyaline cartilage ring (C) is seen, with perichondrium and other collagenous material stained dark blue. The trachea is lined by pseudostratified ciliated columnar epithelium supported by a thin lamina propria, which blends with the submucosa. Posteriorly, tracheal rings are incomplete and here are slips of smooth muscle of the trachealis muscle (T) and some glands (G).

Figure 12–8. Trachea, longitudinal section. Van Gieson, orcein. Low power.

Portions of two tracheal rings (C) are seen and externally is relatively dense connective tissue containing a bundle of nerve fibers (F). In the lamina propria of the respiratory epithelium is a concentration of elastic fibers (arrow, brown), also present in the connective tissue around and between the cartilaginous "rings." Pseudostratified ciliated columnar epithelium with goblet cells (arrowhead) lines the trachea.

Figure 12–9. Trachea, transverse section. Mallory. Medium power.

The lining epithelium is pseudostratified ciliated columnar in type, with goblet cells (arrow). Note the relatively compact areolar connective tissue of the submucosa and the mucous glands (M) in the submucosa. Below is perichondrium and cartilage.

Figure 12–10. Trachea, epithelium. Plastic section. H and E. Oil immersion.

In this pseudostratified, ciliated, columnar epithelium, nuclei lie at various levels and show a variation in appearance, indicative of different cell types. Four cell types are recognizable by light microscopy: ciliated, goblet, columnar, and basal—all seen here. Most are ciliated with obvious apical cilia (arrow), with two goblet cells (g) containing apical secretory droplets (dark pink), basal cells (b), and a columnar cell (c).

Figure 12–11. Tracheal bifurcation. H and E. Low power.

In longitudinal section, the trachea (T) here is seen to branch into right and left main bronchi (RB and LB), with the carina (F) at the bifurcation. Profiles of cartilage rings (C) are present, both in the trachea and the bronchi. Externally are several large blood vessels, including the aorta (A), and some lymph nodes (L), the largest in the bifurcation (right).

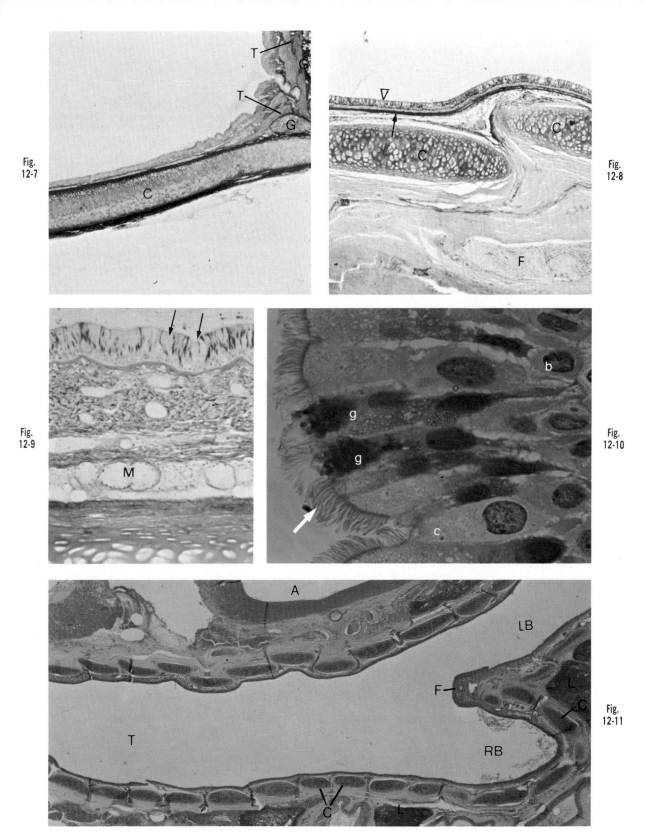

Fig. 12-7

Fig. 12-8

Fig. 12-9

Fig. 12-10

Fig. 12-11

Figure 12–12. Extrapulmonary bronchus. Van Gieson, orcein. Medium power.

This is similar in structure to the trachea (see Fig. 12–8) and shows the lining respiratory epithelium, a concentration of elastic fibers (brown) in the lamina propria beneath the epithelium, some venous channels (V), a small nerve (N) within the submucosa, and part of a cartilage ring and its perichondrium (C). (See also Figure 12–11.)

Figure 12–13. Lung, bronchus. H and E. Low power.

The major feature is a large intrapulmonary bronchus (B) with cartilage (c) and glands (g) in its wall, accompanied by a branch of the pulmonary artery (P), the two lying in connective tissue. Note that the lumen of the bronchus is regular and not collapsed. Also present is a terminal bronchiole (t) leading to a respiratory bronchiole (arrowhead indicates opening of an alveolus from the latter), alveolar ducts (d), alveolar sacs (s), and alveoli.

Figure 12–14. Intrapulmonary bronchus. Plastic section. Methylene blue, azure A, basic fuchsin. Medium power.

In this medium bronchus cartilage (c) is seen at right with the duct of a small gland (d) in the submucosa. At the junction of submucosa and mucosa, there is prominent smooth muscle (m) arranged in spiralling, interlacing bundles, most fibers here cut obliquely. The lamina propria of delicate connective tissue contains numerous small blood vessels (v), and the lining epithelium is pseudostratified, ciliated columnar in type (not as tall as that of the trachea) with goblet cells containing purple-stained secretory droplets. Note also the mast cells in the connective tissue (arrowheads).

Figure 12–15. Small bronchus. Plastic section. Methylene blue, basic fuchsin. Oil immersion.

The lining epithelium of this small bronchus is ciliated columnar in type with some nonciliated cells (arrowheads) and very few goblet cells at this level. None are present here. A small piece of cartilage appears at lower right.The attenuated slips of cytoplasm (arrow) are of smooth muscle cells, while the purple-stained material (e) just beneath the epithelium is elastic fibers.

Figure 12–16. Large bronchiole. Plastic section. Methylene blue, basic fuchsin, Weigert. Medium power.

The luminal outline characteristically is irregular in this transverse section with the mucosa thrown into longitudinal folds as a result of agonal contraction of smooth muscle in the lamina propria. The lining epithelium is ciliated (arrows), low columnar, and no goblet cells are present. Scattered among the ciliated cells are bronchiolar (Clara) cells, non-ciliated and with domed apices protruding into the lumen (arrowheads). Beneath the epithelium, elastic fibers (stained black) are prominent, as are bundles of smooth muscle (m). The bronchiole is supported by only a small amount of connective tissue and lies in respiratory tissue with alveoli (A, left) and interalveolar septa. (See also Figure 12–18.)

Figure 12–17. Bronchiole. Plastic section. Methylene blue, basic fuchsin. Medium power.

In this longitudinal section of a bronchiole slightly smaller than that seen in Figure 12–16, the lining epithelium is ciliated cuboidal in type with Clara cells (c). These Clara, or bronchiolar, cells are secretory cells, contributing to bronchiolar fluid and perhaps secreting some surfactant. The lamina propria contains bundles of smooth muscle cells (m), here cut mainly transversely, indicating that they run in a spiral around the bronchiole. Externally is a small amount of connective tissue. The bronchiole lies in respiratory tissue (alveoli, A) and adjacent to it is a branch of the pulmonary artery (P).

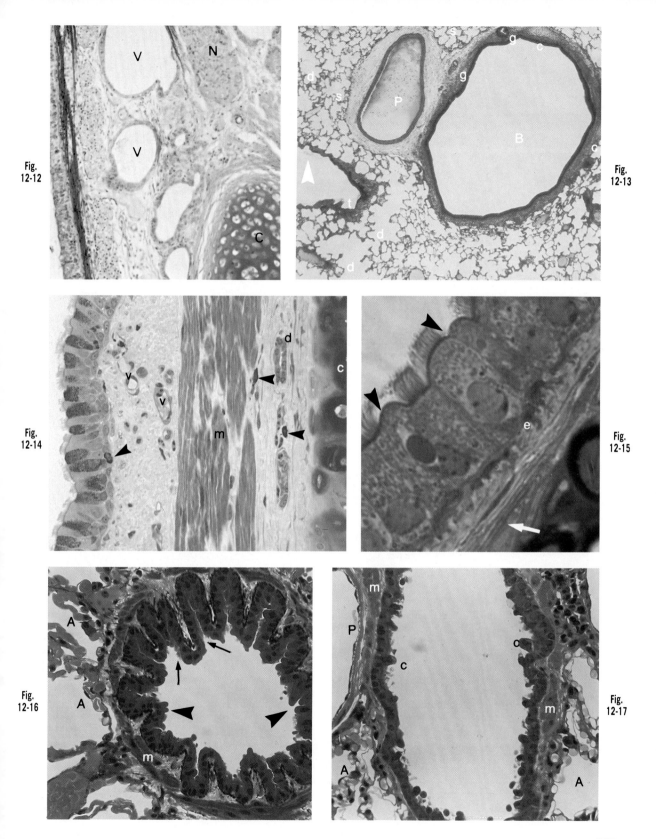

Fig. 12-12

Fig. 12-13

Fig. 12-14

Fig. 12-15

Fig. 12-16

Fig. 12-17

Figure 12–18. Lung, terminal bronchiole. Plastic section. Methylene blue, basic fuchsin, Weigert. Low power.

The portion of a bronchiole in transverse section (B, right) is the same as that in Figure 12–16. A terminal bronchiole (Tb), a branch of this bronchiole, is seen in longitudinal section at left, lying in respiratory tissue. Its lining epithelium is simple cuboidal with a few ciliated cells proximally (to the right) and with numerous Clara cells protruding into the lumen. Externally are slips of muscle and elastic fibers. This terminal bronchiole passes into a respiratory bronchiole at the marked lines (Rb, left), with outpocketing alveoli (arrowheads). Also seen are alveolar sacs (S) and alveoli (A), and below is a branch of the pulmonary artery (P).

Figure 12–19. Terminal-respiratory bronchiole. Plastic section. Toluidine blue. High power.

This figure shows the transition between the simple cuboidal epithelium (right) of a terminal bronchiole (arrows indicate Clara cells) and the squamous epithelium of a respiratory bronchiole. The change is abrupt here, and there are numerous capillary blood vessels in the wall of the respiratory bronchiole (arrowheads), with an indication of alveoli (A) opening from the wall of the respiratory bronchiole.

Figure 12–20. Lung; bronchioles, alveolar ducts, alveoli. H and E. Low power.

In the center of the field, a terminal bronchiole (Tb) passes to a respiratory bronchiole (Rb) (at the marked lines), with alveoli outpocketing from the latter (arrowheads). At the double asterisk, this respiratory bronchiole branches further into smaller respiratory bronchioles (rb), one of which terminates at the asterisk, passing to an alveolar duct (Ad). In turn, this duct terminates at an atrium (AT). Alveolar sacs, alveoli, and branches of the pulmonary artery (P,p), are seen. Note that in passing from terminal bronchiole to alveolar duct, not only does the epithelium change from (ciliated) cuboidal to squamous, but the amount of supporting tissue (smooth muscle and elastic fibroconnective tissue) decreases.

Figure 12–21. Respiratory bronchiole, transverse section. Plastic section. H and E. High power.

In transverse section, the "deficiencies" in the wall of a respiratory bronchiole that open into alveoli (A) are more apparent. Here, the lining of the respiratory bronchiole is low cuboidal with slips of smooth muscle (M) in the wall, but this epithelium changes abruptly to the squamous epithelium lining alveoli which occur as outpocketings of its wall.

Figure 12–22. Respiratory bronchiole. Plastic section. Methylene blue, azure A, basic fuchsin. High power.

Above is the lumen of a respiratory bronchiole, its lining simple cuboidal epithelium (C) interrupted by openings (arrows) to two alveoli (A). Supporting this epithelium are strands of smooth muscle (m). The cuboidal epithelium at arrowheads is continuous with squamous epithelium lining alveoli. Note numerous capillaries (c) in the interalveolar septum and nuclei of the following cell types: s = squamous (surface) epithelium (type I); e = endothelium; g = alveolar type II cell; w = white blood cell in capillary; o = unidentified cell in the septum.

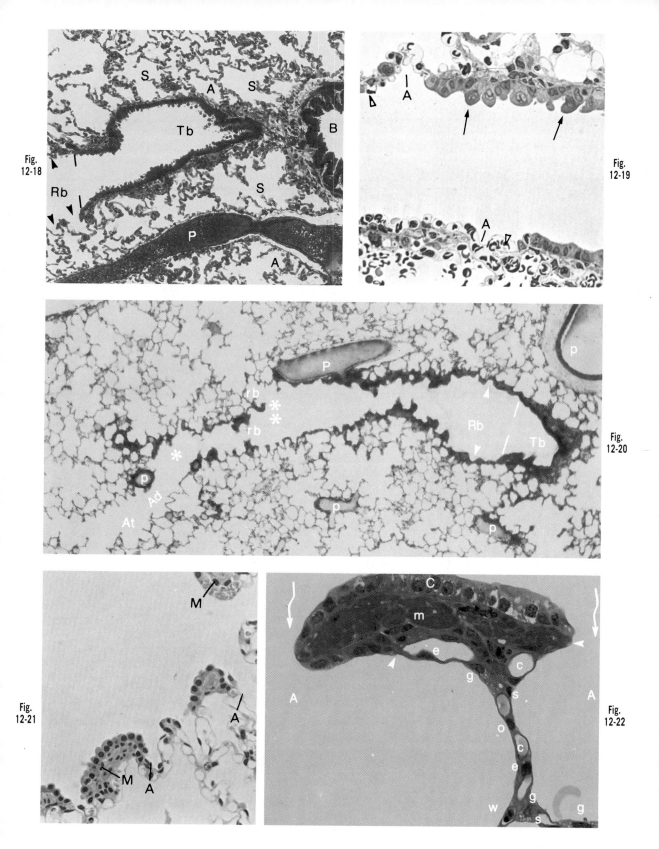

Figure 12–23. Interalveolar septa. Plastic section. Methylene blue, basic fuchsin, Weigert. Oil immersion.

Several alveoli (A) are seen with interalveolar septa between them. Prominent in the septa are numerous blood capillaries (c) containing erythrocytes (pink). Cell types identifiable are (nuclei labeled): endothelial cell (e) lining a capillary; type I squamous alveolar cells (s) lining alveoli; type II alveolar cell (g), with vacuolated cytoplasm; and a cell within the interstitium of a septum (o) that may be a plasma cell. Also seen is a free alveolar phagocyte (p). Note too the small strands of elastin (arrowheads, stained black) and the thickness of the blood-air barrier (between arrows). (See also Figures 12–24 and 12–25.)

Figure 12–24. Interalveolar septa. Plastic section. Methylene blue, basic fuchsin, Weigert. Oil immersion.

Labeling is the same as that in Figure 12–23. Note again the extreme vascularity of interalveolar septa and the thinness of the blood-air barrier. This figure and Figure 12–23 give an indication of the large surface area available for gaseous exchange.

Figure 12–25. Interalveolar septa. Plastic section. Methylene blue, basic fuchsin, Weigert. Oil immersion.

In this figure, a pulmonary venule (V) is seen at the top, lying in a septum that is supported by more prominent elastic tissue (large arrowheads) than seen in Figures 12–23 and 12–24. While there are small elastic fibers in the wall of the venule (small arrowheads), obviously the blood-air barrier still is thin.

Figure 12–26. Lung, injected. Low power.

The blood capillaries of the lung were injected with colored (red) gelatin via the pulmonary artery, and a thick section was prepared. It demonstrates the rich vascularity in interalveolar septa (I) and the extent of the capillary "net," seen particularly well where two alveoli have been sectioned tangentially (arrows).

Figure 12–27. Pleura, interalveolar septa. Plastic section. Methylene blue, azure A, basic fuchsin. High power.

Flattened, dark-staining nuclei (arrowheads) of the squamous pleural epithelium (mesothelium, visceral pleura) are seen at right. This is supported by elastic fibroconnective tissue in which a mast cell (m) is seen. Two interalveolar septa show capillaries (c) containing erythrocytes, type II alveolar cells (g) with vacuolated cytoplasm, a type I squamous alveolar cell (s), and an endothelial nucleus (e) of a cell lining a capillary.

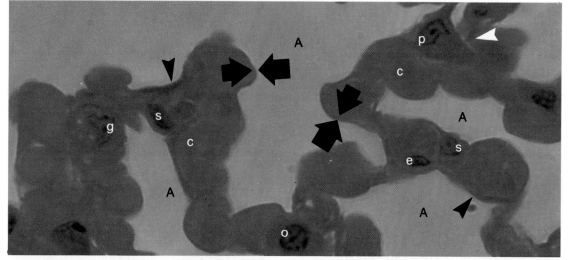

Fig. 12-23

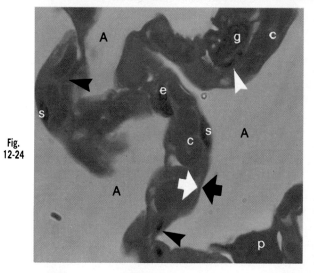

Fig. 12-24

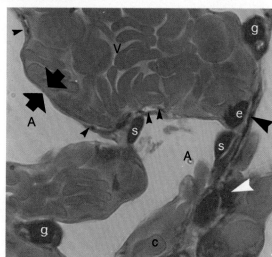

Fig. 12-25

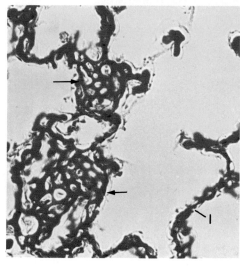

Fig. 12-26

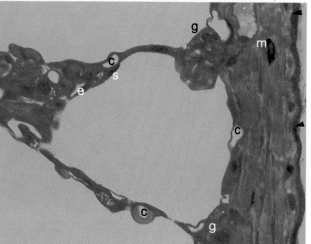

Fig. 12-27

Figure 12–28. Fetal lung. Hematoxylin, phloxin, saffranin. Low power.

The lung develops basically from two components—an endodermal diverticulum from the pharynx, which forms the lining epithelium of the respiratory "tree," and mesoderm which forms all other components. At first, the lung is "gland-like," as seen here, with a developing bronchus (B), an artery (A) (these two located in connective tissue), and branches of the original endodermal diverticulum having the appearance of a compound gland. Between the endodermal branches is mesenchyme. Lumina of terminal branches form alveoli, the mesoderm between them becoming compressed and forming interalveolar septa.

Figure 12–29. Lung at birth, unexpanded. H and E. Low power.

The lung remains gland-like and unexpanded until birth. In this secton of lung at birth, there are two large bronchioles (B) lined by cuboidal epithelium; the remainder of the field is occupied by respiratory tissue that is unexpanded. Also seen is the lobular nature of the lung at this stage, with connective tissue "septa" containing tributaries of the pulmonary vein (V).

Figure 12–30. Lung at birth, expanded. H and E. Low power.

With birth of the baby, inspiration occurs and this causes dilatation of respiratory passages. Compared with Figure 12–29, this section shows expansion of alveoli, alveolar ducts, and bronchioles, although dilatation is not complete. Seen here are a large bronchiole (B), a terminal bronchiole (T), respiratory bronchiole (R), alveolar ducts (D), and alveoli (A).

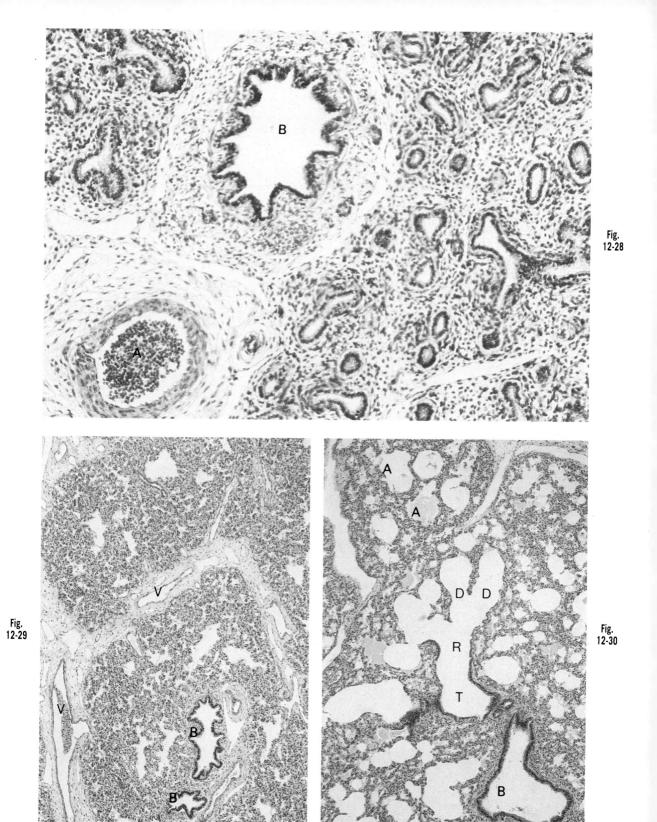

Fig.
12-28

Fig.
12-29

Fig.
12-30

213

CHAPTER
THIRTEEN

The Urinary System

THE KIDNEYS

The urinary system consists of the paired *kidneys* and their *ureters*, the *bladder*, and the *urethra*. The kidneys produce urine that passes via the ureters to the bladder for temporary storage and, eventually, periodic evacuation to the exterior via the urethra.

The kidneys function in the elimination of waste materials, particularly nitrogenous compounds such as creatinine and urea, resulting from metabolism of food by the body, and also foreign substances and their breakdown products. They also regulate water and electrolyte balance. Additionally, they secrete *renin*, involved in regulating blood pressure and sodium ion concentration, and *erythropoietin* (hemopoietin), concerned in the production of erythrocytes. The kidneys are essential to life.

The kidneys are bean-shaped organs located in the lumbar region. Basically, they are compound tubular glands concerned with filtering waste material from the body. Each kidney has a thin fibrous capsule, attached only weakly to the underlying parenchyma, and shows a medial concavity, or *hilum,* through which blood vessels enter and leave and which also contains the expanded upper extremity of the ureter, called the *pelvis.* Within the hilum, the pelvis usually divides into two major *calyces,* each of these subdividing to form a total of 8 to 12 cup-shaped minor calyces. Each minor calyx fits like a cap over a conical protuberance, or *papilla,* of renal substance. Within the kidney, there is a division into a darker, granular *cortex* and a paler-staining *medulla* that shows a distinct radial striation. Each papilla is the tip of a pyramidal area of the medulla (a *medullary pyramid)* extending from the hilum toward the capsule. The junction between cortex and medulla is not clear-cut because medullary substance extends into the cortex as thin, radially orientated rays (the *medullary rays)* and cortical substance extends centrally between adjacent medullary pyramids as renal columns (of Bertin). Each medullary pyramid plus its associated cortical tissue constitutes a lobe. Hence, the kidney is multipyramidal or multilobar.

The renal artery enters the kidney at the hilum, divides into several large branches, and these then pass in *renal columns* between pyramids and arch over the bases of pyramids between cortex and medulla. From these arcuate arteries, small vessels (interlobular arteries) enter the cortex radially, at the peripheries of *lobules,* and give rise to numerous arteriolar branches. These arterioles (afferent arterioles) form glomeruli (capillary tufts) which drain to efferent arterioles. Efferent arterioles from glomeruli of the outer cortex then form capillary plexuses to supply other cortical structures, while those of glomeruli near the medulla (the *juxtamedullary glomeruli*) pass into the medulla as straight, radial vessels (the vasa recta). Here, they form capillary networks to supply medullary tissue. Venous radicals from both cortex and medulla drain to the corticomedullary region to form *arcuate veins,* which in turn drain through renal columns to form the renal vein in the hilum.

Each lobe of the kidney is subdivided into lobules. Each lobule comprises a medullary (cortical) ray, the *kidney units*, or *nephrons*, that drain into it, and the continuation of the ray in a medullary pyramid. Thus, in the cortex, a lobule has a medullary ray at its center and its outer limits are indicated by interlobular arteries.

The individual unit of the kidney is the *uriniferous tubule,* composed of two continuous parts. These are the nephron and the *collecting tubule,* the former being responsible for urine secretion, the latter being the excretory duct carrying urine to the renal pelvis. In each kidney there are a million or more nephrons, each a long, epithelium-lined tube that starts blindly and terminates by joining a collecting duct.

THE NEPHRON

The first part of the nephron lies in the cortex; it is blind, dilated, and lined by very thin epithelium *(Bowman's capsule)*. This expansion is invaginated into the form of a cup by a tuft of capillaries called a *glomerulus*, the entire structure (Bowman's capsule and the glomerulus) being called a *renal corpuscle*. In the renal corpuscle, an ultrafiltrate of plasma is formed and passes down the renal tubule where it is altered by resorption and secretion to form urine. In order, the nephron then is formed by convoluted and straight portions of the proximal tubule, a thin segment, and straight and convoluted portions of the *distal tubule.* The distal tubule is continuous with a collecting tubule or duct. The *proximal convoluted tubule* (convoluted part of the proximal tubule) and the *distal convoluted tubule* (convoluted part of the distal tubule) lie adjacent to the renal corpuscle in the cortex (Fig. 13–1). Between these tubules, the remaining parts form the *loop of Henle,* which lies in a medullary ray and passes for a varying distance from the cortex into the medulla.

Nephrons are classified by the location of their renal corpuscles in the cortex, e.g., as *subcapsular* (superficial), *midcortical,* or *juxtamedullary*. Two types of nephrons are recognized based on the length of the loop of Henle:

1. Short (cortical) nephrons extend only into the outer zone of the medulla with a short thin segment in the descending limb.

2. Long (juxtamedullary) nephrons pass deeply into the inner zone of the

medulla with a thin limb that lies in both descending and ascending limbs and forms the loop.

Midcortical nephrons show features common to the long and short types. This variation in nephrons accounts for the zonation in the medulla. In the medulla, collecting tubules join to form large collecting ducts that pass radially in medullary pyramids to open at the apices of renal papillae and thus drain to the calyces.

As the distal tubule (ascending limb of the loop of Henle) passes back into the cortex, it travels to its renal corpuscle of origin and becomes specialized as the *macula densa* before continuing as the distal convoluted tubule. The macula densa is related intimately at the vascular pole of the corpuscle to afferent and efferent arterioles of the glomerulus and to a group of cells termed the *extraglomerular mesangium (Lacis cells)*. This association of arterioles, the macula, and the Lacis cells is termed the *juxtaglomerular apparatus* or complex. Here, smooth muscle cells in the media of the afferent arteriole become "epithelioid" in character—the juxtaglomerular (JG) cells—and contain granules. The macula densa, where nuclei lie close together (hence the term "dense-spot"), appears to act as a sensor of osmolarity of the fluid in the distal tubule and perhaps transmits this information to the JG cells. The JG cells produce and release the enzyme renin which, in the blood, acts on angiotensinogen to produce angiotensin I. This is inactive, but is converted to angiotensin II, a potent vasoconstrictor that also acts on the adrenal cortex to cause the release of aldosterone. Aldosterone acts on renal tubules (mainly the distal tubule) to increase the reabsorption of sodium, with a consequent increase in plasma volume and extracellular fluid. The role of the extraglomerular mesangium is uncertain, although it has been suggested that these cells may secrete erythropoietin.

In the proximal convoluted tubule, glucose, amino acids, and some sodium, chloride, and bicarbonate ions are resorbed from the glomerular filtrate together with water and passed to peritubular capillaries. Fluid leaving the proximal tubule is isotonic with respect to blood plasma, but in the descending limb of the loop of Henle it becomes increasingly hypertonic owing to loss of water and an addition of sodium ions. In the ascending limb of the loop of Henle, sodium actively is pumped from the tubule to the interstitium so that the fluid becomes first isotonic and then hypotonic. In the distal convoluted tubule, more sodium is actively resorbed and water is passively resorbed. Together with the collecting duct, the distal tubule is concerned in the regulation of blood pH and potassium balance. In collecting ducts, as they pass through the medulla, more water is resorbed.

EXCRETORY PASSAGES

Except for the terminal urethra, the remainder of the urinary tract from renal pelvis down to urethra is lined by transitional epithelium. This type of stratified epithelium is resistant to pH variation and permits distention. It is supported by connective tissue and smooth muscle. Urine released from the kidneys passes rapidly down the ureters to the bladder, where it is stored before voiding at intervals through the urethra. The urethra differs in male and female; in the male it is much longer, traversing the penis as the final duct for both urine and seminal fluid.

Figure 13–1. The human kidney.

Top: Diagrams of the human kidney, sectioned vertically, with a single nephron *(right)* to illustrate its component parts and blood supply. *Bottom*: Diagram showing zones of the kidney in relation to segments of outer cortical (A) and juxtamedullary (B) nephrons. *Note*: The outer cortical nephron has a loop of Henle barely penetrating the inner stripe of the medulla with a short, thin segment (black) in the descending limb; in contrast, the juxtamedullary nephron penetrates deeply into the inner zone and has an extensive thin segment in both descending and ascending arms of the loop. PCT = Proximal convoluted tubule; DCT = distal convoluted tubule; CD = collecting duct.

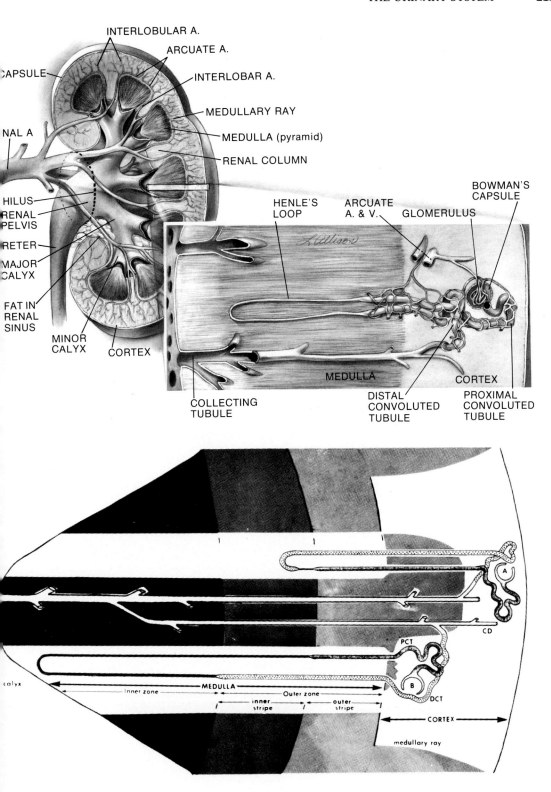

INTERLOBULAR A.

ARCUATE A.

INTERLOBAR A.

CAPSULE

MEDULLARY RAY

MEDULLA (pyramid)

NAL A

RENAL COLUMN

HENLE'S LOOP

ARCUATE A. & V.

GLOMERULUS

BOWMAN'S CAPSULE

HILUS

RENAL PELVIS

RETER

MAJOR CALYX

FAT IN RENAL SINUS

MINOR CALYX

CORTEX

MEDULLA

CORTEX

COLLECTING TUBULE

DISTAL CONVOLUTED TUBULE

PROXIMAL CONVOLUTED TUBULE

calyx

Inner zone

MEDULLA

Outer zone

inner stripe

outer stripe

PCT

CD

DCT

A

B

CORTEX

medullary ray

Figure 13–2. Renal corpuscle.

This scanning electron micrograph shows the nucleated cell bodies (N) of several podocytes, or visceral epithelial cells of Bowman's capsule. These cells show major processes (M) with side branches from which extend the foot processes, or pedicels (P). Pedicels of adjacent processes interlock and between them are narrow spaces, the filtration slits (arrows). The podocytes cover glomerular capillaries. Note also a cilium (C) and some microvillous processes (B). × 4850. (Courtesy of Dr. P. M. Andrews.)

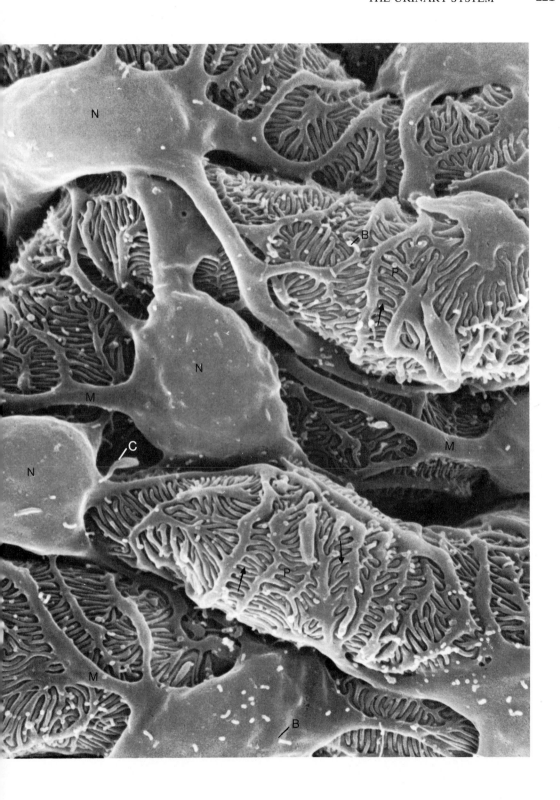

Figure 13–3. Kidney, rabbit. H and E. Low power.

The rabbit kidney differs from that of man in that it is a unilobar or unipyramidal kidney. Below is the hilum (H) with the lining of the pelvis (V). Protruding into the pelvis is the renal papilla of the single medullary pyramid (P). The medulla is pale-staining and is divided into outer (O) and inner (I) zones and appears to be radially striated. Large (red) blood vessels lie at the corticomedullary junction. The cortex (C) is granular and stains darker than the medulla. The thin renal capsule is not apparent.

Figure 13–4. Kidney, lobules. Mallory. Low power.

This section shows the deeper part of the cortex adjacent to the medulla, i.e., the juxtamedullary cortex, with the medulla lying to the left but out of the picture. Passing into the cortex from the medulla are three medullary rays (R) formed by radially orientated collecting tubules or ducts, here cut nearly longitudinally. Lobules are demarcated by interlobular arteries (A); the arteries are also cut mainly longitudinally (top and bottom). The cortex in each lobule is composed of many nephrons, with their renal corpuscles (C) appearing as large spherical profiles and their coiled tubules cut in all planes of section, mainly transverse and oblique. Thus, each lobule is bounded by interlobular arteries, has a medullary ray formed by collecting tubules at its center, and is composed of the nephrons (renal corpuscles and tubules) that drain into those collecting tubules.

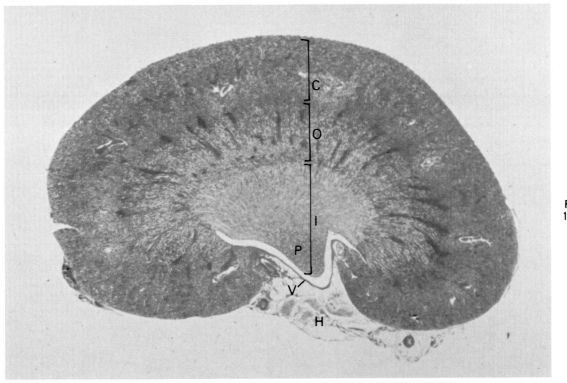

Fig.
13-3

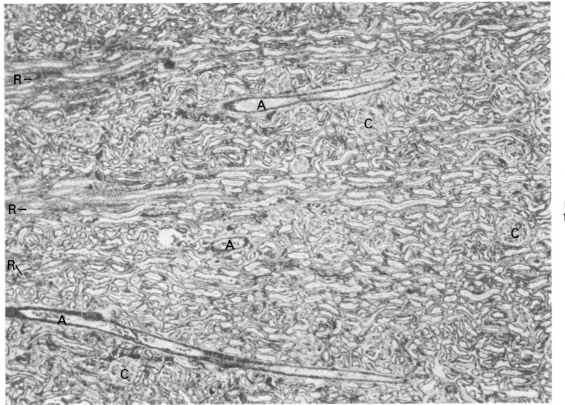

Fig.
13-4

Figure 13–5. Kidney, cortex. Masson. Medium power.

Cut longitudinally is part of an interlobular artery (L), and branching from it on each side is an afferent arteriole (A). Each afferent arteriole passes to the vascular pole (V) of a renal corpuscle to form a renal glomerulus. Each corpuscle also shows a urinary pole (U) where the thin squamous parietal epithelium of Bowman's capsule changes abruptly to the simple cuboidal or columnar epithelium lining the proximal convoluted tubule. The remainder of the field is occupied by proximal (P) and distal (D) convoluted tubules, cut in transverse and oblique section. The proximal tubules are more numerous, i.e., longer. One distal convoluted tubule reaches the vascular pole of a corpuscle at a macula densa (M).

Figure 13–6. Kidney, glomeruli. Injected, whole mount. *Top*, Low power. *Bottom*, Medium power.

In this preparation, *(top)* the renal artery was injected with colored colloidin and a whole mount was prepared to show an interlobular artery (I) from which branch many afferent arterioles to form glomeruli (G). Below is a higher magnification of the above, showing an afferent arteriole (A) branching from an interlobular artery to form a glomerulus (G), with an efferent arteriole (E) leaving the glomerulus. Note that the efferent arteriole is of smaller diameter than the afferent. Consequently, the glomerulus is a relatively high pressure system of capillaries.

Figure 13–7. Kidney, renal corpuscle. Masson. High power.

Both vascular (V) and urinary (U) poles are seen in this renal corpuscle. Small amounts of connective tissue (green) surround the corpuscle and tubules. The afferent arteriole (A) is seen at the vascular pole and breaks up into glomerular capillaries. Nuclei in the glomerulus are of endothelial and visceral epithelial (podocyte) cells. Thin squamous epithelium (parietal) lines Bowman's capsule and changes abruptly at the urinary pole to cuboidal epithelium of the proximal convoluted tubule (arrows). The capsular space (C—between visceral and parietal epithelium) is clearly continuous with the lumen of the proximal convoluted tubule. Note the distal convoluted tubule at the macula densa (arrowhead), with closely packed nuclei. Also present are profiles of proximal (P) and distal (D) convoluted tubules, and intertubular capillary blood vessels filled with erythrocytes (stained brown-orange).

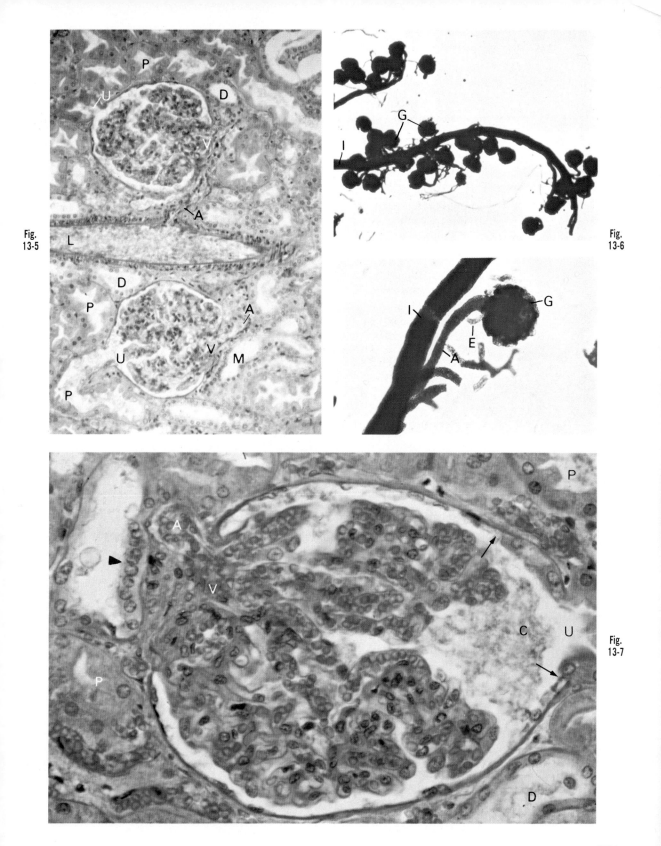

Fig.
13-5

Fig.
13-6

Fig.
13-7

Figure 13–8. Kidney, cortex. Plastic section. PAS, light green. High power.

With this stain, polysaccharides stain magenta-pink. Positive staining is seen in basal laminae surrounding tubules and the renal corpuscle and in basal laminae of the glomerular capillaries (a), some of which contain erythrocytes—here stained dark green. Positive staining (of the glycocalyx) also is seen in the brush or striated border of proximal convoluted tubules (arrows). In the renal corpuscle, note nuclei of podocytes (arrowheads), lying outside the basal laminae of glomerular capillaries, adjacent to the capsular space (s), which is continuous with the lumen of the proximal convoluted tubule. Also seen are proximal (p) and distal (d) convoluted tubules, both showing a faint basal striation (asterisks), a collecting tubule (c), and the macula densa (m).

Figure 13–9. Kidney, renal corpuscle. Plastic section. Methylene blue, basic fuchsin. Oil immersion.

At the periphery of the renal corpuscle is parietal (squamous) or capsular epithelium (c) separated by capsular space (s) from podocytes (p) of the visceral or glomerular epithelium. Major processes of podocytes (asterisks) are seen and interdigitate (arrow) between glomerular capillaries (a) containing erythrocytes. A nucleus (n) of an endothelial cell and one of a possible mesangial cell (m) are seen also. A collecting tubule appears at the right adjacent to the corpuscle. (See Figure 13–2.)

Figure 13–10. Kidney, cortex. Plastic section. Methylene blue, basic fuchsin. High power.

A renal corpuscle occupies much of the field, showing the glomerulus and the visceral and parietal epithelium; the latter is continuous (at arrowheads) with the low columnar epithelium of the proximal convoluted tubule. Capsular space is continuous with the lumen of the latter at the urinary pole (U). At the vascular pole above is a macula densa (m) and the afferent arteriole (a). Note that smooth muscle (s) in its wall changes to juxtaglomerular cells containing purple granules (arrows). Proximal (p) and distal (d) convoluted tubules and a collecting tubule (c) are seen. (See also Figure 13–11.)

Figure 13–11. Juxtaglomerular complex. Plastic section. Methylene blue, basic fuchsin. Oil immersion.

This is a higher magnification of the vascular pole of the renal corpuscle seen in Figure 13–10. Note close apposition of nuclei of cells of the macula (m), and smooth muscle (s) and granulated JG cells (arrows) in the wall of the afferent arteriole (a). The group of small, pale-staining cells with irregular nuclei (arrowheads) below the arteriole represents Lacis, or extraglomerular mesangial, cells.

Figure 13–12. Juxtaglomerular complex. Plastic section. Methylene blue, basic fuchsin. Oil immersion.

At the vascular pole of this renal corpuscle, both afferent (a) and efferent (e) arterioles are seen with smooth muscle cells (s) in their walls and juxtaglomerular, granulated cells (g) in the wall of the afferent arteriole. Extraglomerular (Lacis) cells are arrowed. Above is the macula densa (m) showing in this region of the distal tubule small cells (nuclei close together) with small, ovoid, pink-staining mitochondria. Adjacent to these cells of the macula, cells show elongated basal mitochondria (arrowhead) characteristic of the distal convoluted tubule. The glomerulus is seen at lower right and proximal convoluted tubules at left.

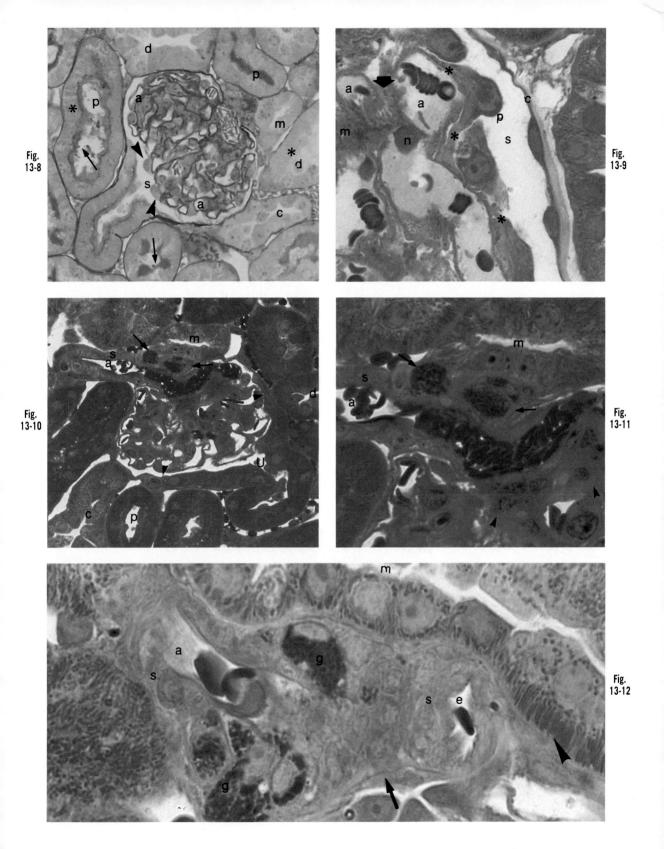

Figure 13–13. Kidney, cortex. Plastic section. Methylene blue, basic fuchsin. Medium power.

Proximal (p) and distal (d) convoluted tubules occupy most of the field, cut transversely and obliquely. The proximal convoluted tubules are lined by a simple low columnar epithelium, with brush or striated border. Nuclei are spheroidal, basal, and with prominent nucleoli, and the cytoplasm stains more darkly than that of cells of the distal tubule and shows a basal striation (asterisk). In the distal convoluted tubule, there is no brush border, nuclei are spheroidal and are located toward the lumen, and the cytoplasm shows a clear basal striation (arrowhead) as a result of elongated (orange-red) mitochondria. In collecting tubules (c), cells are small, cuboidal, and characterized by small, ovoid (red) mitochondria. Note also the intertubular capillaries (a).

Figure 13–14. Kidney, cortical tubules. Plastic section. Methylene blue, basic fuchsin. Oil immersion.

Compare the features of proximal (p) and distal (d) convoluted tubules and a collecting tubule (c). In the proximal, nuclei are spheroidal, lie near the basal lamina and often show nucleoli. The cytoplasm contains elongated (purple-staining) mitochondria forming a basal striation where cut longitudinally (asterisk). The lumen is widely patent, and the cells show a brush border (arrow). In the distal tubule, nuclei are spheroidal, lie away from the base, and may bulge into the lumen, with parallel, elongated (red-staining) mitochondria forming a prominent basal striation (arrowhead). There is no brush border. Cell outlines are not clear in either proximal or distal tubule due to complex interdigitation of cell membranes. In the collecting tubule, cells are small, cuboidal, and characterized by small, ovoid (red-staining) mitochondria. Note the prominence of intertubular capillaries (a).

Figure 13–15. Kidney, cortical tubules. Plastic section. PAS, light green. High power.

This figure shows the deep, juxtamedullary cortex with collecting tubules (c) in medullary rays on each side. The periodic acid–Schiff stains (magenta-red) the basal laminae of all tubules and, in proximal convoluted tubules (p), the brush border (arrows) and cytoplasmic lysosome-protein bodies (small granular bodies) of the endocytic process. Straight portions of the distal tubule (ascending limbs of the loop of Henle) (d) are present and, in the collecting tubules, dark or intercalated cells (arrowheads) are scattered among the clear, low cuboidal cells. Centrally there is an interlobular artery (a); thus, the adjacent halves of two lobules are seen. (See also Figure 13–4.)

Figure 13–16. Kidney, medulla. Masson. High power.

This figure is similar to Figure 13–17 from the inner stripe, outer zone of the medulla, but shows collecting ducts (C), thick ascending segments of Henle (H), and thin segments (T) in mainly longitudinal section. They lie in green-staining connective tissue of the interstitium in which are a few, elongated, fibroblast-like cells.

Figure 13–17. Kidney, medulla. Masson. High power.

This figures shows the same region as Figure 13–16, with the various tubules cut in transverse section. In the surrounding connective tissue (green), note the numerous vasa recta (V) containing erythrocytes (yellow).

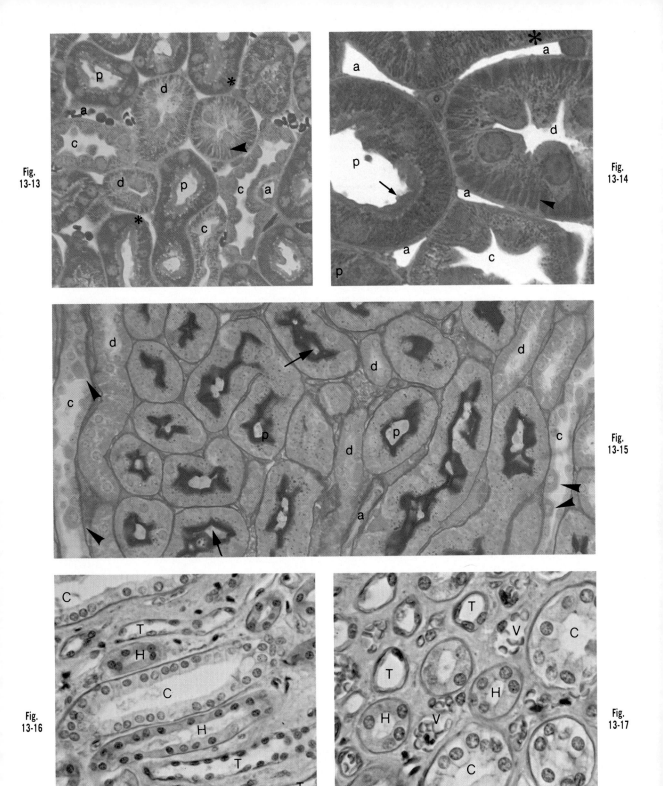

Figure 13–18. Kidney, medulla. Plastic section. H and E. High power.

Connective tissue (and basal laminae) stains dark pink with various tubules of the inner stripe, outer zone of the medulla cut in transverse section. The tubules are: collecting ducts (C = cuboidal-columnar epithelium, clear cell interfaces); thick segments of Henle or ascending portions of distal tubules (H = low, darker cuboidal); thin segments of Henle (T = squamous); and blood capillaries (V = vasa recta) lined by endothelium.

Figure 13–19. Kidney, loop of Henle. Plastic section. Methylene blue, basic fuchsin. Oil immersion.

This transverse section of the medulla (at the junction of inner and outer zones) shows thick (H) and thin (T) segments of the loop of Henle with vasa recta (V). The thick segments, or ascending, straight portions of the distal tubule, are lined by simple cuboidal epithelium with darkly (pink) staining cytoplasm showing a basal striation (arrows). Apical cytoplasm (arrowhead) is clear, and there is no brush border. The thin segment is lined by simple squamous epithelium with a wide lumen. Vasa recta are lined by endothelium that is thinner than the lining of the thin segments, some containing erythrocytes (red) with a monocyte (asterisk).

Figure 13–20. Kidney, papilla. H and E. Medium power.

This section is through the apex of a renal papilla to show main collecting tubules or excretory ducts. These ducts are lined by a pale-staining simple columnar epithelium and are formed by the union of smaller ducts, as seen here. Between ducts are parallel capillary blood vessels (V) lined by endothelium. These large ducts (of Bellini) open onto the surface of the papilla. The ducts and their openings are large and closely packed and give the papilla the appearance of a sieve, the so-called area cribrosa.

Figure 13–21. Kidney, calyx. Plastic section. H and E. High power.

The "side" of a renal papilla (left) contains tubules cut in transverse and oblique section. These are mainly collecting ducts (C) with some thick (H) and thin (T) segments of the loop of Henle and blood capillaries (V). The papilla is covered by transitional epithelium, here only two or three cells thick. Similar epithelium lines the other, pelvic aspect of the minor calyx (arrow), supported by fibroconnective tissue (A) in which are a few smooth muscle fibers (not apparent here). The lumen of the calyx is seen (arrowhead).

Figure 13–22. Fetal kidney. H and E. Low power.

This radial section of an 8-month fetal kidney shows clear distinction between cortex and medulla with a profile of an arcuate artery (A) at the junction. The medulla is pale-staining and radially striated owing to tubules cut in longitudinal section. Medullary rays extend into the cortex (arrows). The cortex is relatively thin and incompletely developed at this stage. The dark blue, spherical profiles are renal corpuscles. The juxtamedullary ones are larger and fully formed, i.e., functional, whereas those in the outer cortex appear simply as clumps of darkly staining cells and are immature. Covering the surface is a connective tissue capsule (arrowhead). The kidney is not fully developed at birth, the nephrons in the deeper layers of the cortex developing first.

Figure 13–23. Ureter. Masson. Medium power.

In transverse section, the ureter has a stellate outline. The lining epithelium is transitional, about five layers thick, and supported by a relatively dense fibroconnective tissue lamina propria, in which some blood vessels are seen. No true submucosa is recognized. The muscularis is thick with a thinner inner longitudinal layer (cut transversely) and a thicker outer circular layer (cut longitudinally). Externally is an adventitia with adipose tissue (A) and, on the anterior surface of the ureter, mesothelium of the peritoneum.

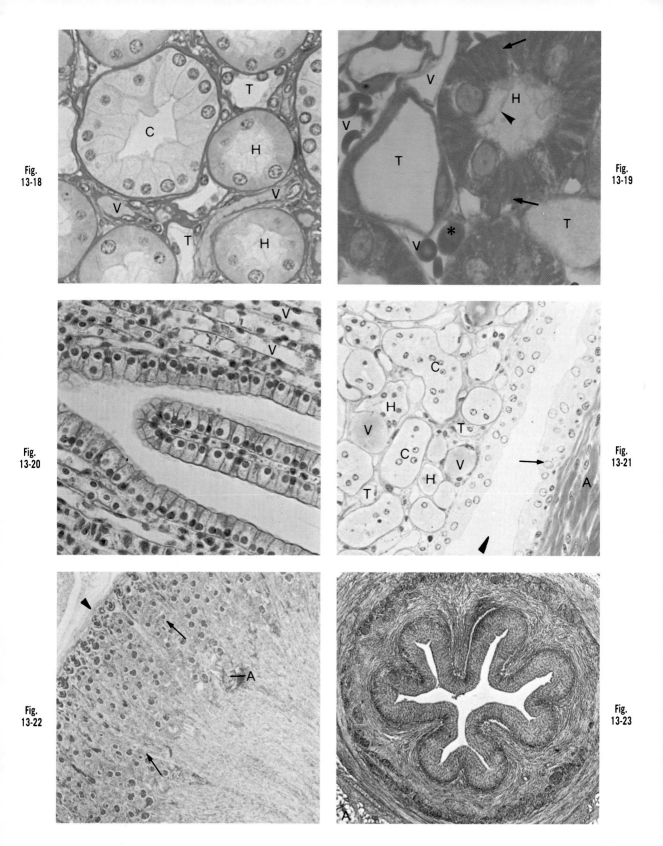

Fig.
13-18

Fig.
13-19

Fig.
13-20

Fig.
13-21

Fig.
13-22

Fig.
13-23

Figure 13–24. Ureter, transitional epithelium. Plastic section. H and E. High power.

In the ureter, the transitional epithelium is composed of five or six layers of cells. The cytoplasm of the surface cells stains more intensely than that of cells lying more deeply. These cells show a convex luminal border, and many of them are binucleate (arrows). The supporting lamina propria is relatively dense, fibroconnective tissue. (See also Figure 2–10.)

Figure 13–25. Bladder. Plastic section. H and E. Low power.

The bladder is lined by transitional epithelium, here six to eight layers thick and thrown into folds (in a contracted state). The lamina propria is thick and quite dense, its external part being somewhat loose in texture and sometimes called the submucosa. The muscularis is quite thick and consists of bundles of smooth muscle cells arranged as inner and outer longitudinal layers with a thicker middle circular layer. The full thickness is not seen here. Externally is an adventitia, with peritoneum on the superior surface only.

Figure 13–26. Female urethra. Hematoxylin, phloxin, saffranin. Low power.

This is a transverse section of the female urethra just below the bladder. Here, there is transitional epithelium supported by a lamina propria and a thick muscularis with bundles of fibers somewhat irregular in arrangement. Externally is loose connective tissue. The irregular lumen (in a contracted state) indicates a capacity for distention during voiding.

Figure 13–27. Female urethra. H and E. High power.

The lining epithelium of the inferior portion of the urethra is stratified squamous in type with an irregular junction between epithelium and connective tissue. Glandular outpocketings of the lining epithelium also are present, but are not seen here.

Figure 13–28. Penile urethra. H and E. Low power.

In the male, the terminal urethra traverses the corpus spongiosum, here cut in transverse section showing erectile (cavernous) tissue (C). The urethra is lined here by an epithelium of the stratified columnar type, continuous with branching tubular glands (of Littre), mainly on its dorsal surface (arrows). Surrounding the corpus spongiosum is dense, relatively regular connective tissue (tunica albuginea, A). (See also Figure 16–29.)

Figure 13–29. Male urethra. H and E. Medium power.

This is the terminal urethra near the tip of the penis (fossa navicularis) where the lining epithelium is stratified squamous in type. It is supported by a relatively cellular, fibroelastic connective tissue. The junction between epithelium and lamina propria is irregular.

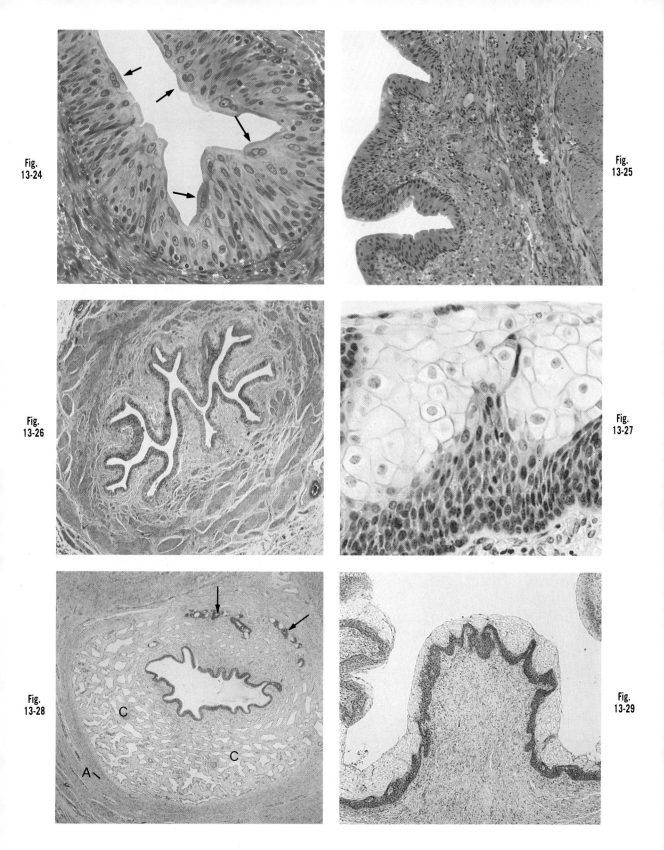

Fig.
13-24

Fig.
13-25

Fig.
13-26

Fig.
13-27

Fig.
13-28

Fig.
13-29

CHAPTER
FOURTEEN

The Endocrine System

The endocrine system is composed principally of glands that have lost connection with the parent epithelium. Since they possess no ducts and since their secretions (hormones) are released directly into the blood or lymph circulation, they are designated *ductless glands,* or *glands of internal secretion.* They have a rich blood supply that serves not only their metabolic needs but also the transport of their secretory products. Most endocrine glands are separate entities, and these—the pituitary, thyroid, parathyroid, and suprarenal glands, and the pineal body—will be considered in this chapter. Other components of the endocrine system are present as scattered masses within exocrine glands; examples are pancreatic islets and interstitial cells of the testis. These combined organs are called *mixed glands*. The liver also is a mixed gland, but here each hepatic cell exhibits both exocrine and endocrine functions. Additional endocrine elements occur as isolated cells found among the lining epithelial cells of the alimentary canal.

Although they vary in their embryological derivation, endocrine glands have a simple histological structure: they consist of either cords, plates, or clumps of cells separated by capillaries or sinusoids and supported by delicate connective tissue. Each gland secretes one or more specific *hormones*. In most glands, secretion accumulates within the cells of origin, e.g., pancreatic islets. Secretory granules, which are precursors of the actual hormones, are present within the cytoplasm of many endocrine cells, but they normally require special staining methods for their demonstration. In other glands, the secretory product is stored extracellularly in a central mass surrounded by secretory cells, thus forming a follicle; an example of this type is the thyroid gland. In the suprarenal cortex, however, secretion is released almost as rapidly as it is formed.

THE HYPOPHYSIS (PITUITARY GLAND)

The hypophysis is composed of two different tissues. The *adenohypophysis* (glandular portion) is derived from oral ectoderm and during development migrates dorsally as *Rathke's pouch* to surround partially the *neurohypophysis* (nervous portion), a ventral evagination from the floor of the midbrain. The adenohypophysis is subdivided by the residual lumen of Rathke's pouch into a large anterior portion, the *pars distalis,* and a small posterior portion, the *pars intermedia.* An extension of the pars distalis, the *pars tuberalis,* surrounds the neural stalk.

The neurohypophysis also has three components: (1) the pars nervosa, (2) the infundibular stem, and (3) the median eminence of the tuber cinereum. The latter two constitute the *neural* (infundibular) *stalk.* The *hypophyseal stalk* is composed of the neural stalk and the pars tuberalis.

In a sagittal section, two main lobes to the hypophysis can be distinguished: The *anterior lobe* refers to that portion of the gland anterior to the residual lumen—the pars distalis and pars tuberalis; the *posterior lobe* includes those portions posterior to the lumen—the pars intermedia and pars nervosa.

The parenchyma of the pars distalis is in the form of anastomosing cords and clusters of epithelial cells of two main types, *chromophils* and *chromophobes.* The latter are small cells that have little affinity for dyes. Most chromophobes are thought to be partially degranulated chromophils. The chromophils are subdivided into *acidophils* and *basophils* on the basis of the staining reactions of their cytoplasmic granules.

The cytoplasm of acidophils is crowded with small specific granules which have an affinity for either orange G or azocarmine dyes. Those that take up orange G are called orangeophils. These cells, also termed *somatotrophs,* are responsible for the secretion of growth hormone. The acidophils whose granules stain with azocarmine are called *carminophils* (or *mammotrophs*). They secrete lactogenic or luteotropic hormone (prolactin).

The basophils also are subdivided into two categories: (1) those whose granules stain with aldehyde fuchsin (beta basophils), and (2) those whose granules do not (delta basophils). Beta basophils, or *thyrotrophs,* secrete thyrotropic hormone. Delta basophils are of two types: (1) the *gonadotrophs,* which produce either follicle-stimulating hormone (FSH) or luteinizing hormone (LH), and (2) the *corticotrophs,* responsible for the synthesis of adrenocorticotropic hormone (ACTH).

Nerve cells within the supraoptic and paraventricular nuclei are neurosecretory and elaborate either *oxytocin* or *vasopressin.* This secretory material passes along the unmyelinated nerve fibers of the hypothalamohypophyseal tract to nerve terminals within the pars nervosa. Here the secretion is stored in the nerve terminals prior to discharge. Large accumulations of the stored material may be visible on light microscopy as *Herring bodies.*

THE THYROID GLAND

The thyroid gland consists of two *lateral lobes* connected by a narrow isthmus. The gland is enclosed in a capsule of connective tissue, and delicate extensions from the capsule divide the *lobes* into indefinite *lobules* that contain the structural units of the gland, the *follicles.* Each follicle consists of a layer of a simple epithelium enclosing a cavity that usually is filled with colloid, which represents a reserve of secretion.

Cells of two types are found within the epithelium. The principal cells are cuboidal in shape and have a basophil cytoplasm. They produce the *colloid,* which contains the hormones thyroxine and triiodothyronine. In addition to principal cells, the follicular epithelium contains some scattered, paler cells, the *parafollic-*

ular, or C, *cells,* characteristically located at the periphery of the follicles. These cells elaborate the hormone thyrocalcitonin.

PARATHYROID GLANDS

Two pairs of parathyroid glands lie in close relation to the thyroid gland. Each gland is composed of masses and cords of epithelial cells supported by reticular fibers and in close association with a rich network of capillaries. The epithelial cells are of two types: (1) *chief,* or *principal, cells* and (2) *oxyphil cells.* The principal cells are in the majority and they produce the parathyroid hormone. The oxyphil cells are larger than the principal cells and possess a pale cytoplasm. The function of these cells is uncertain.

SUPRARENAL (ADRENAL) GLANDS

The suprarenal (adrenal) glands show two regions that are distinct structurally, developmentally, and functionally. The outer cortex develops from epithelium (mesothelium) and is divided into three ill-defined layers: a thin outer zone, the *zona glomerulosa;* a thick middle zone, the *zona fasciculata;* and an inner zone, the *zona reticularis.* Numerous capillaries lie between the columns of cortical cells.

Three categories of hormones are elaborated within the suprarenal cortex:

1. *Mineralocorticoids,* which control electrolyte and water balance, are produced primarily in the zona glomerulosa.

2. *Glucocorticoids,* synthesized within the zona fasciculata and to some extent within the zona reticularis, participate in carbohydrate metabolism and suppress the immune response.

3. Steroid hormones of the third category, the *sex hormones,* are produced in the zona reticularis.

The inner medulla, derived from neural crest material, is composed of groups and clusters of cells, surrounded by blood capillaries. The cells, after fixation in potassium bichromate, have a granular cytoplasm that is brown in color, and are said to exhibit the *chromaffin reaction.* This reaction is due in large part to the presence of the precursors of the hormone *epinephrine.* Also present within the medulla are sympathetic ganglion cells, which occur either singly or in small groups between the chromaffin cells.

THE PINEAL BODY

The pineal body *(epiphysis cerebri)* is covered by pia mater that forms a thin capsule, from which septa extend into the organ, dividing it incompletely into lobules. The irregular lobules are composed of *epithelioid cells (pinealocytes)* and neuroglial supporting elements. The pineal body, after attaining its maximum development at about seven years of age, shows retrogressive changes. Connective tissue increases in amount, and concretions or *acervuli (corpora arenacea)* appear within the gland, principally in the septa. Although no definite function has been assigned to the gland, there is evidence to suggest that it exerts an influence upon gonadal development, particularly in the period prior to sexual maturity.

Figure 14–1. Hypophysis. H and E. Low power.

All major portions of the hypophysis are shown in this sagittal section.

The adenohypophysis, which lies to the right, has three parts. The pars distalis (D) is the largest part of the gland, and an extension from it, the pars tuberalis (T), passes superiorly, anterior to the neural stalk. The third part, the pars intermedia (I), is a thin cellular partition in which there are some small cyst-like spaces. Normally it is separated from the pars distalis by the residual lumen of Rathke's pouch (not apparent on this section).

The neurohypophysis also consists of three parts. The major portion is the pars nervosa (N) which superiorly continues into the neural stalk, the lower part of which is the infundibular stem (S). The upper part of the neural stalk, the median eminence of the tuber cinereum, is not present here. The infundibular stem and the pars tuberalis together constitute the hypophyseal stalk.

Figure 14–2. Hypophysis: pars distalis. Masson. Low power.

The parenchyma of the pars distalis is in the form of anastomosing cords and clumps of epithelial cells supported by a network of reticular fibers (not stained specifically). Large sinusoidal capillaries (arrows) occur between the parenchymal cells, which are of two main types, chromophobes and chromophils. Chromophobes (C) are small cells that often appear in groups. Chromophils are larger cells and are subdivided into acidophils and basophils on the basis of the staining reactions of their cytoplasmic granules. (See Figures 14–3 and 14–4.)

Figure 14–3. Hypophysis: pars distalis. H and E. Medium power.

Parenchymal cells form cords and clumps separated by delicate connective tissue in which lie numerous sinusoidal capillaries containing red blood cells (arrows). The small chromophobes (C) possess little cytoplasm that usually contains no specific granules. Acidophils or alpha cells (A) are larger than chromophobes, and their cell boundaries are distinct. The cytoplasm is crowded with small specific granules (deep pink). Basophils or beta cells (B) tend to be a little larger than acidophils, and their cytoplasm contains small granules that stain deeply basophil.

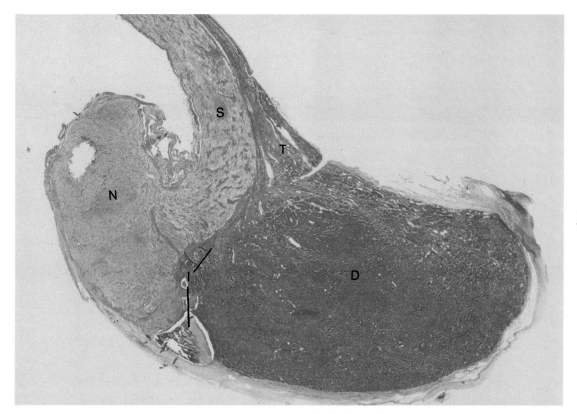

Fig.
14-1

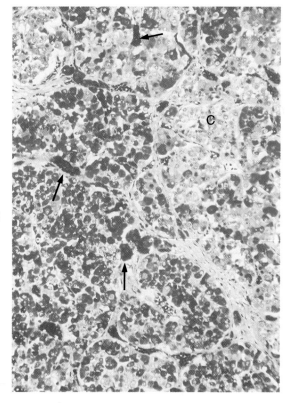

Fig.
14-2

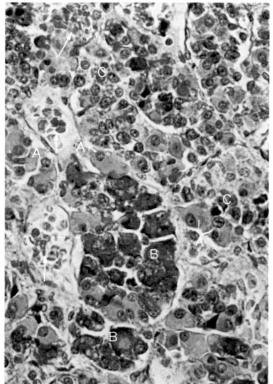

Fig.
14-3

Figure 14–4. Hypophysis: pars distalis. Masson. High power.

A portion of one clump of parenchymal cells is shown. Acidophils (A) are large cells whose cytoplasm is filled with acidophil granules. Basophils (B) tend to be larger than acidophils and less heavily granulated. The granules stain deeply basophil. Chromophobes (C) are small cells that are faintly staining. The cytoplasm is devoid of secretory granules. A large sinusoidal capillary (arrow) is closely related to the parenchymal cells.

Figure 14–5. Hypophysis: hypophyseal stalk. H and E. Medium power.

The pars tuberalis (T) contains groups or cords of cells, longitudinally oriented. The cells are small and possess little cytoplasm. They are in association with numerous blood vessels that pass down the length of the stalk, here sectioned longitudinally. The blood vessels are components of the hypophyseal portal system. The infundibular stem (S) contains numerous unmyelinated nerve fibers (pale pink), whose cell bodies lie within the supraoptic and paraventricular nuclei of the hypothalamus. Only the nuclei (pale blue) of the component cells, or pituicytes, are seen. These cells resemble neuroglial cells found elsewhere within the central nervous system.

Figure 14–6. Hypophysis: pars intermedia and pars nervosa. Mallory. Medium power.

Some large blood vessels (red) occupy the center of the field. To the left, there is a small segment of the pars distalis (D). The pars intermedia (I) is represented by a row of small irregular vesicles. The cells lining the vessels are small and pale-staining. The vesicles in life contain colloid. The pars nervosa (N) contains a few blood vessels, and, like the infundibular stem, it contains numerous unmyelinated nerve fibers and pituicytes (not apparent on this section).

Figure 14–7. Hypophysis: pars nervosa. Gomori's chrome-alum-hematoxylin. Medium power.

Two Herring bodies (H) are present within the pars nervosa. These stain deeply with hematoxylin and represent accumulations of neurosecretory material. The material is elaborated in the supraoptic and paraventricular nuclei of the hypothalamus and passes along the unmyelinated nerve fibers to the pars nervosa, where it is stored within the nerve terminals. Two small blood vessels (arrows) also are present.

Figure 14–8. Thyroid. Plastic section. H and E. Low power.

Follicles, the structural units of the gland, are crowded together with little intervening connective tissue. Each follicle consists of a layer of simple epithelium enclosing a cavity that is filled with a homogeneous material (colloid).

Figure 14–9. Thyroid. Plastic section. H and E. Low power.

Follicles vary greatly in size, as a result of the degree of distention by secretion (colloid). The follicles are separated by delicate connective tissue that supports a close net of capillaries.

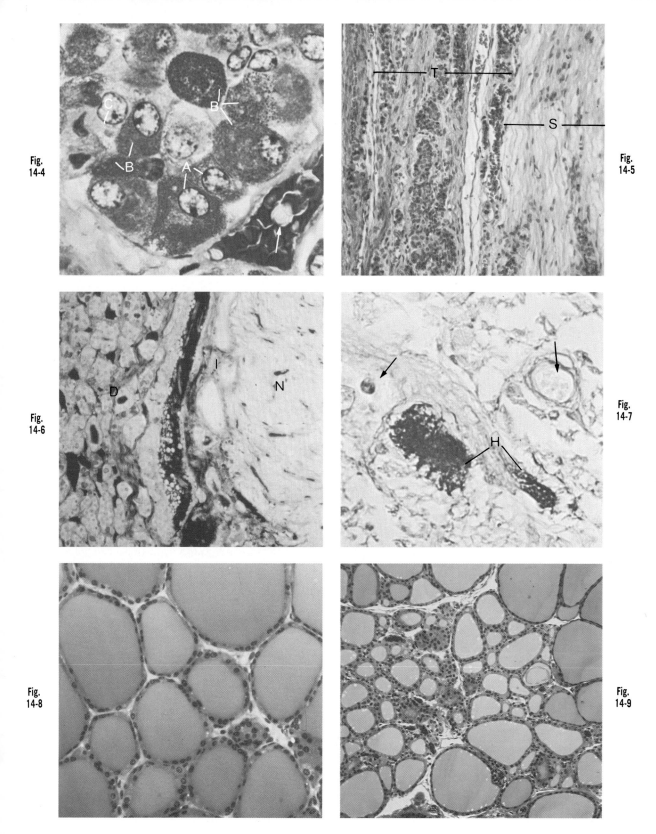

Fig.
14-4

Fig.
14-5

Fig.
14-6

Fig.
14-7

Fig.
14-8

Fig.
14-9

Figure 14–10. Thyroid. Plastic section. Toluidine blue. Medium power.

Each follicle is bounded by a simple cuboidal epithelium, and the cavities are filled with colloid, which represents a reserve of secretion. The bases of the follicular cells rest upon a delicate basal lamina (not stained specifically), and the follicles are embedded within a delicate, vascular connective tissue.

Figure 14–11. Thyroid. Plastic section. Toluidine blue. High power.

The principal cells of the follicular epithelium are irregularly cuboidal in shape and have centrally located nuclei. Many cells (arrows) possess discrete colloid droplets (darkly stained) within their cytoplasm. In addition to principal cells, the follicular epithelium contains some paler cells, the parafollicular or C cells (C), characteristically located at the periphery of the follicles. These cells elaborate thyrocalcitonin. Numerous capillaries (V) lie within the connective tissue of the gland, many in intimate relationship to follicular cells.

Figure 14–12. Parathyroid. Mallory-Azan. Low power.

Each parathyroid gland is covered by a thin capsule of connective tissue (arrows) that separates it from the thyroid gland and from the surrounding fascia. Delicate branching and anastomosing septa (blue) pass inward from the capsule and carry with them small blood vessels (red). The parenchyma of the gland is composed of masses and irregular cords of epithelial cells of two types, chief and oxyphil. Chief or principal cells are the most abundant. One group of oxyphil cells (O) is present. These cells are larger than chief cells and have a pale cytoplasm.

Figure 14–13. Parathyroid. Mallory-Azan. Medium power.

Chief or principal cells (C) occur mainly in anastomosing cords. Individual cell boundaries are not apparent. Oxyphil cell (O), present mainly in clumps, are larger than chief cells and have distinct cell boundaries. Numerous capillaries (red) occur within the delicate connective tissue between parenchymal cells.

Figure 14–14. Parathyroid. Mallory-Azan. High power.

Chief or principal cells (C) form small cords and clumps. Some possess vesicular nuclei, and others have smaller, more densely staining nuclei. Oxyphil cells (O) are larger than chief cells and have distinct cell boundaries. They possess small spherical nuclei and a considerable amount of pale-staining, finely granular cytoplasm. The parenchymal cells are embedded within delicate connective tissue (blue) that contains a close network of capillaries (red). It is claimed that all parenchymal cells abut directly against a capillary.

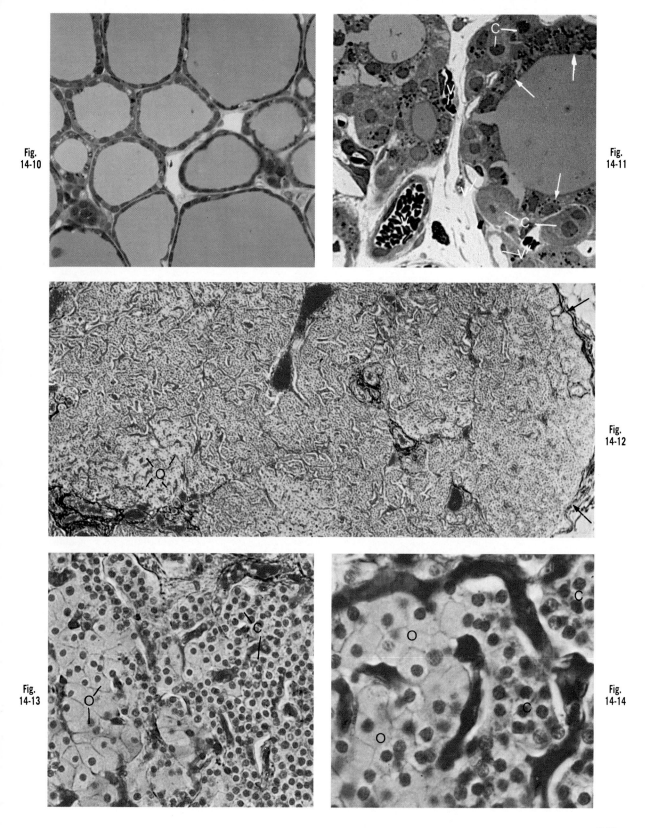

Figure 14–15. Suprarenal gland. Mallory-Azan. Low power.

The suprarenal gland is surrounded by a tough fibroelastic capsule (C), from which delicate trabeculae extend radially into the cortex of the gland. The cortex is divided into three ill-defined layers: the zona glomerulosa (ZG), immediately beneath the capsule; the zona fasciculata (ZF), the thickest layer, where cells are arranged in long cords; and the zona reticularis (ZR), the inner zone, where cell cords form an anastomosing network. The medulla (M) is composed of large cells that are ovoid and occur mainly in groups or short anastomosing cords. The gland receives a rich vascular supply. Numerous arterioles pierce the capsule and enter cortical sinusoids (red) that course between the cell cords. Other arterioles pass to the medulla and empty into a capillary plexus. Venous blood both from the cortex and from the medulla drains into venules that join to form large medullary veins (V).

Figure 14–16. Suprarenal cortex: lipid material. Sudan Black B. Medium power.

This frozen section has been stained specifically to show lipid material. The capsule (C) is unstained, and external to it there is a small group of fat cells. The outer cells of the zona glomerulosa (ZG) contain some lipid material, which appears as darkly staining droplets, but the inner cells appear devoid of lipid droplets. The remainder of the field is occupied by the zona fasciculata (ZF), the component cells of which contain numerous lipid droplets. The inner third of the zona fasciculata and the zona reticularis, not shown here, are relatively free of lipid material.

Figure 14–17. Suprarenal cortex. Plastic section. H and E. High power.

Beneath the capsule (C), the zona glomerulosa (ZG) is composed of large cells arranged in ovoid groups or arches. The cells appear vacuolated. In the zona fasciculata (ZF), of which only a small portion is shown here, cells are arranged in parallel cords, usually two cells wide, and have a spongy appearance; hence they are called spongiocytes. The cords are separated by delicate connective tissue that contains the cortical sinusoids.

Figure 14–18. Suprarenal cortex. Plastic section. Methylene blue, basic fuchsin. High power.

This section shows the inner portion of the cortex. Note the vacuolated cells of the zona fasciculata (above) and the deeply staining cytoplasm of cells of the zona reticularis (below). In the zona reticularis, the cells form an anastomosing network of cords, separated by wide sinusoidal capillaries.

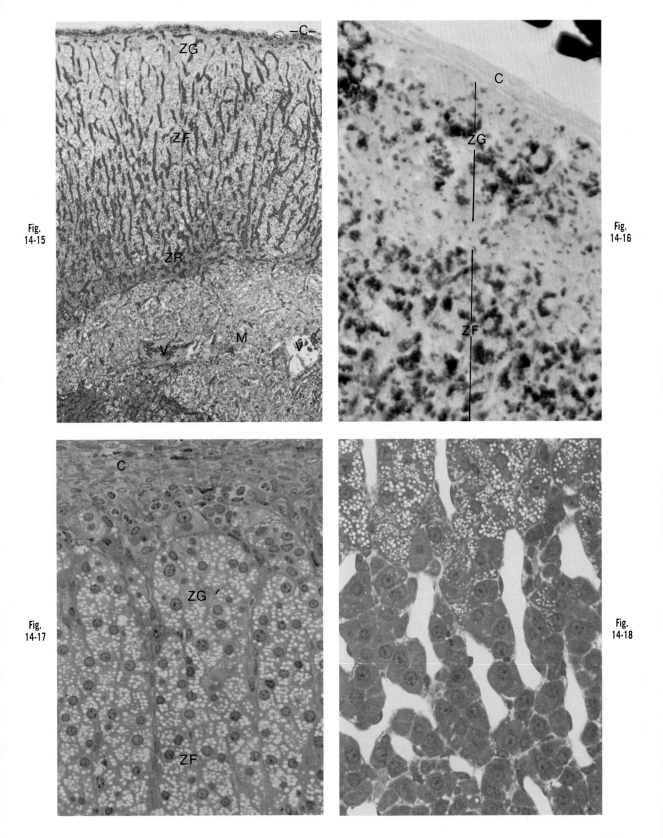

Fig.
14-15

Fig.
14-16

Fig.
14-17

Fig.
14-18

Figure 14–19. Suprarenal medulla. Chromaffin reaction. Medium power.

Cells of the medulla (M), ovoid in shape, occur mainly in small groups or short anastomosing cords. Their cytoplasm appears yellow-brown owing to the oxidation of catecholamines by fixation in potassium bichromate. Above, there is a small portion of the zona reticularis (ZR).

Figure 14–20. Suprarenal medulla. Zinc chloride. High power.

Cells of the medulla have large vesicular nuclei, and their cytoplasm contains fine granules that stain greenish-gray with zinc chloride. A small portion of the zona reticularis (ZR) also is present.

Figure 14–21. Suprarenal medulla. Plastic section. H and E. High power.

The cells, arranged in groups or anastomosing cords, are large and polyhedral. They possess large vesicular nuclei and finely granular cytoplasm. The delicate connective tissue that separates the groups and cords of cells contains numerous capillaries not visible here.

Figure 14–22. Suprarenal medulla. Mallory-Azan. High power.

The medullary (chromaffin) cells here appear pale, with scattered cytoplasmic granules. Also present are two sympathetic ganglion cells (arrows). These cells have large vesicular nuclei with distinct nucleoli and a densely staining granular cytoplasm. Note also a capillary (C) in the connective tissue between the medullary cell cords and groups.

Figure 14–23. Pineal body: juvenile. H and E. Medium power.

The pineal body consists of clumps and plates of cells separated by septa that extend into the gland from a thin capsule. Two cell types are recognized: the more common epithelioid cells, or pinealocytes, and the neuroglial supporting elements. The two cell types cannot be distinguished in this H and E preparation. The delicate septa contain numerous small blood vessels.

Figure 14–24. Pineal body: adult. H and E. Low power.

The irregular clumps of cells (or lobules) are separated by delicate connective tissue septa (pale pink). In the adult, the body is characterized by the presence of concretions or acervuli, which are black in this preparation. At high magnification, the acervuli appear lamellated.

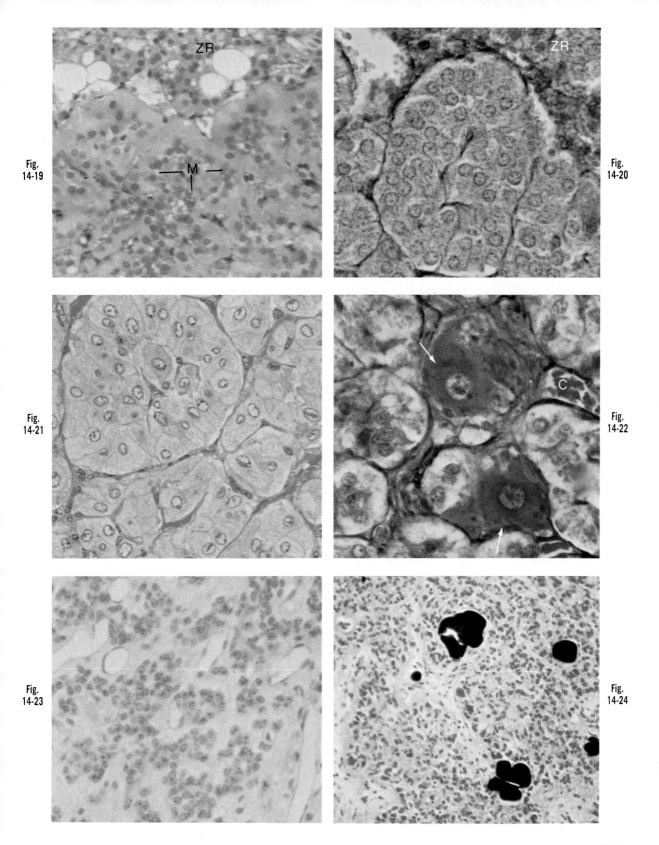

Fig. 14-19

Fig. 14-20

Fig. 14-21

Fig. 14-22

Fig. 14-23

Fig. 14-24

CHAPTER
FIFTEEN

The Female Reproductive System

The female reproductive system comprises the *ovaries,* a system of *genital ducts* (uterine tubes, uterus, and vagina), and the *external genitalia.* The mammary glands, although not genital organs, also are considered here, since they are important glands associated with the female reproductive system.

THE OVARIES

The ovaries are double glands, since functionally they are both exocrine (cytogenic) and endocrine, producing the hormones estrogen and progesterone. Each ovary exhibits an outer *cortex* and an inner *medulla.* The latter is a loose fibroelastic connective tissue with scattered strands of smooth muscle and a rich vascular supply. The cortex consists of a compact cellular stroma that contains the ovarian follicles. Before puberty, only primary, or primitive, follicles are present. Sexual maturity is characterized by the presence of growing follicles and their end products *(corpora lutea, atretic follicles).* The mature follicle is termed a *graafian follicle,* and it is believed that the process of maturation requires 10 to 14 days. The sequence of structural changes in the follicle (growth, ovulation, and the formation of a corpus luteum) is coupled with rhythmic changes in endocrine secretory activity. The latter are responsible for the cyclic changes that occur in the remainder of the reproductive tract, notably the uterus. Ovarian hormones also are involved in influencing changes in the mammary gland that result in lactation. The ovary is covered by simple *cuboidal (germinal) epithelium,* deep to which is a *tunica albuginea* of dense fibrous tissue.

GENITAL DUCTS

Fallopian (Uterine) Tubes

The fallopian (uterine) tubes extend from the ovaries to the uterus and show four distinct regions:

1. The *infundibulum* is the funnel-shaped opening into the peritoneal cavity and its margins are drawn out into numerous folds termed *fimbriae*.

2. The expanded intermediate segment, comprising two thirds of the length of the tube, is the *ampulla,* which is thin-walled.

3. This leads into the slender *isthmus* that connects with the uterus.

4. The *intramural portion* is the continuation of the canal through the uterine wall.

The wall of the tube thickens progressively toward the uterus, whereas the lumen diminishes in size in this direction. The epithelium of the mucosa is principally simple columnar, and small groups of ciliated cells alternate with groups that lack cilia.

The Uterus

The uterus is a pear-shaped organ that has two major parts: (1) an expanded upper portion, the *body,* and (2) a lower cylindrical portion, the *cervix.* The upper end of the body is referred to as the *fundus,* and the isthmus is the narrow transitional zone between the body and the cervix.

The wall of the uterus consists of three layers:

1. The *perimetrium* (outer layer) is a typical serosa consisting of a single layer of mesothelial cells supported by a thin layer of connective tissue.

2. The *myometrium* (intermediate layer) is a thick coat of smooth muscle. The muscle fibers are arranged in bundles, separated by loose connective tissue containing large blood vessels and nerves. Three layers of muscle may be distinguished, although they are ill-defined because of the presence of interconnecting bundles.

3. The *endometrium* (inner layer), or *mucosa,* possesses a surface epithelium that is simple columnar with scattered groups of ciliated cells.

Uterine glands, lined with a similar columnar epithelium, extend through the full thickness of the mucosa. The glands are separated by the *stroma,* a framework of reticular fibers and stromal cells. Lymphoid cells and granular leukocytes also are present in the stroma. It is the endometrium that is subject to cyclic changes in response to ovarian secretory activity and that contributes the maternal component to the *placenta* (decidua basalis) during pregnancy. The fetal contribution to the placenta consists of the chorionic plate and the *villi* that arise from the plate. The villi are covered by an epithelium termed the *trophoblast,* which is arranged in two layers: (1) an outer syncytial trophoblast without cell boundaries, and (2) an inner cuboidal cell layer, the *cytotrophoblast.* In the later stages of pregnancy the cellular layer progressively disappears.

The *cervix* of the uterus projects into the vagina. Inside the cervical canal, there is an abrupt transition between the simple columnar epithelium of the cervical canal and the stratified squamous epithelium that covers the lower surface of the cervix and lines the vagina.

The Vagina

The vagina is a fibromuscular sheath lined by a mucous membrane. It is continuous at its upper end with the cervix, and its lower end is bounded by the hymen, an annular fold of mucosa that separates the vagina from the vestibule. The thick stratified squamous epithelium of the mucosa rests upon a highly vascular lamina propria of dense connective tissue. The muscularis contains smooth muscle cells that are arranged principally in a longitudinal direction, although some circular fibers do occur.

EXTERNAL GENITALIA

The external genitalia, known collectively as the *vulva,* comprise the *clitoris,* the *labia majora* and *minora,* and certain glands (major and minor *vestibular glands*) that open into the vestibule.

MAMMARY GLANDS

The mammary glands are modified sweat glands that lie within the subcutaneous tissue of the pectoral region. They consist of 15 to 20 lobes, each of which is an independent gland with a separate duct system. The ducts traverse the nipple and open by a pore on the surface. There are fewer pores than ducts, owing to terminal fusion of ducts. The *areola,* an area of skin extending outward from the nipple, is pigmented and contains specialized areolar glands. At puberty, the mammary glands enlarge rapidly in the female, principally as a result of development of adipose and other connective tissue. The glands remain incompletely developed until pregnancy occurs, when extensive changes take place. After cessation of lactation, the glands undergo retrogressive changes and return to a resting state.

Figure 15–1. Ovary and endometrium.

This diagram illustrates the interrelations of the ovary and the endometrium during a menstrual cycle. (Modified from Schroder.)

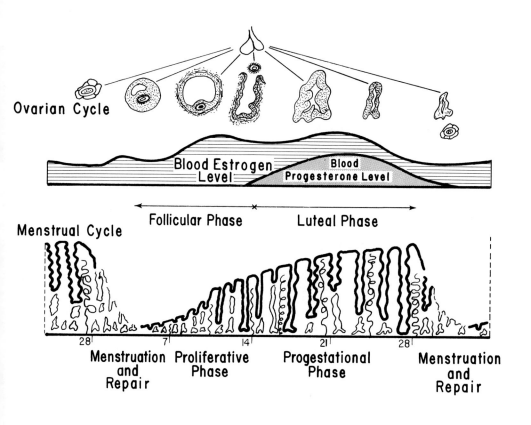

Ovarian Cycle

Blood Estrogen Level

Blood Progesterone Level

Follicular Phase   Luteal Phase

Menstrual Cycle

28   7   14   21   28

Menstruation   Proliferative   Progestational   Menstruation
and   Phase   Phase   and
Repair   Repair

Figure 15–2. Ovary. Mallory-Azan. Low power.

The ovary is attached at the hilum (H) to a fold of peritoneum, the mesovarium, that continues to the broad ligament. Two zones may be distinguished within the ovary. The inner zone, the medulla (M), is loose connective tissue that merges into the core of the mesovarium at the hilum. It contains numerous large blood vessels. The outer zone, the cortex (C), is a compact cellular stroma that contains the ovarian follicles. One large follicle (F) shows an antrum cavity. Also present is a degenerating corpus luteum (CL).

Figure 15–3. Ovary: cortex. Plastic section. Methylene blue, azure A, basic fuchsin. Low power.

The free surface of the ovary is covered by a layer of cuboidal cells, the germinal epithelium. Beneath this, there is a zone of dense connective tissue, the tunica albuginea (TA). The underlying cortex consists of a compact, cellular stroma that contains three growing follicles. The follicular cells form a stratified layer around the ovum (seen in two follicles) and are separated from it by the zona pellucida (arrows).

Figure 15–4. Ovary: germinal epithelium. Plastic section. Methylene blue, azure A, basic fuchsin. High power.

The germinal epithelium is composed of a single layer of cuboidal cells. At the hilum, this layer is continuous with the mesothelial (peritoneal) covering of the mesovarium. Beneath the epithelium is the dense, irregular connective tissue of the tunica albuginea.

Figure 15–5. Ovary: cortex. Plastic section. H and E. Medium power.

The cortical stroma is markedly cellular and contains spindle-shaped cells with elongated nuclei. Embedded within the stroma are primary (P) and growing (G) follicles. The former consist of an immature ovum surrounded by a single layer of flattened follicular cells. In growing follicles, the follicular cells assume a cuboidal shape and later produce a stratified layer around the ovum. A refractile, deeply staining membrane—the zona pellucida (arrows)—is interposed between the ovum and the follicular cells.

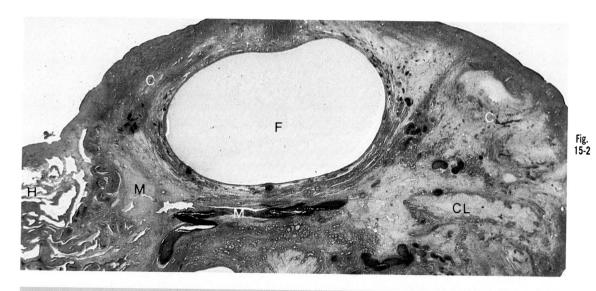

Fig.
15-2

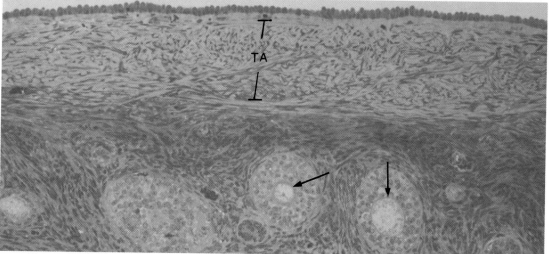

Fig.
15-3

Fig.
15-4

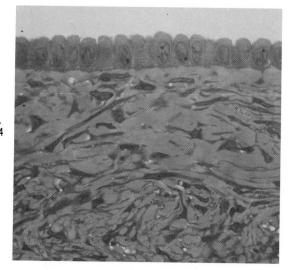

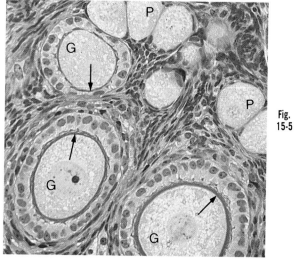

Fig.
15-5

Figure 15–6. Ovary: primary follicles. Plastic section. H and E. High power.

Two primary follicles are present within the cellular cortical stroma. Each follicle contains an immature ovum (primary oocyte) with a large vesicular nucleus. The nucleus of the upper oocyte also shows a prominent nucleolus. The oocytes are surrounded by a single layer of flattened follicular cells.

Figure 15–7. Ovary: growing follicle. Plastic section. H and E. High power.

The large immature ovum shows a pale vesicular nucleus with a distinct nucleolus and an opaque and finely granular cytoplasm. It is surrounded by a refractile membrane, the zona pellucida, that separates it from the stratified layer of cuboidal follicular cells. The surrounding stromal cells are condensing to form a capsule, the theca folliculi (arrows), around the follicle.

Figure 15–8. Ovary: growing follicle. Plastic section. Methylene blue, basic fuchsin. Medium power.

This follicle shows greater stratification of the follicular cells than that seen in Figure 15–7 and early development of the antral cavity (A). It is filled with a clear fluid, the liquor folliculi. A capsule of follicular cells, the theca folliculi (arrows), surrounds the follicle.

Figure 15–9. Ovary: graafian follicle. Plastic section. H and E. Medium power.

The cortical stroma contains a row of primary follicles (top) and an almost mature graafian follicle. The primary oocyte of the latter, with a vesicular nucleus and a prominent nucleolus, is surrounded by the zona pellucida and by a group of follicular cells, the corona radiata. The whole mound of tissue, the cumulus oophorus, projects into the antral cavity (A). A stratified layer of follicular cells forms a continuous irregular layer, the membrana granulosa (MG), around the antral cavity. A well-defined theca folliculi (arrows) surrounds the membrana granulosa.

Figure 15–10. Ovary: early corpus luteum. H and E. Low power.

Following ovulation, the wall of the follicle collapses and becomes transformed into a temporary glandular structure, the corpus luteum. The central portion of the follicle, initially filled with blood, is replaced by a primitive type of connective tissue (C). The granulosa cells of the follicle differentiate into granulosa lutein cells that form a thick, folded layer (G) around the remains of the follicular cavity.

Figure 15–11. Corpus luteum. H and E. Low power.

The corpus luteum appears pale owing to the large size of the component granulosa lutein cells. Delicate connective tissue septa (arrows), containing blood vessels, pass from the theca (dark red) into the interior of the corpus luteum.

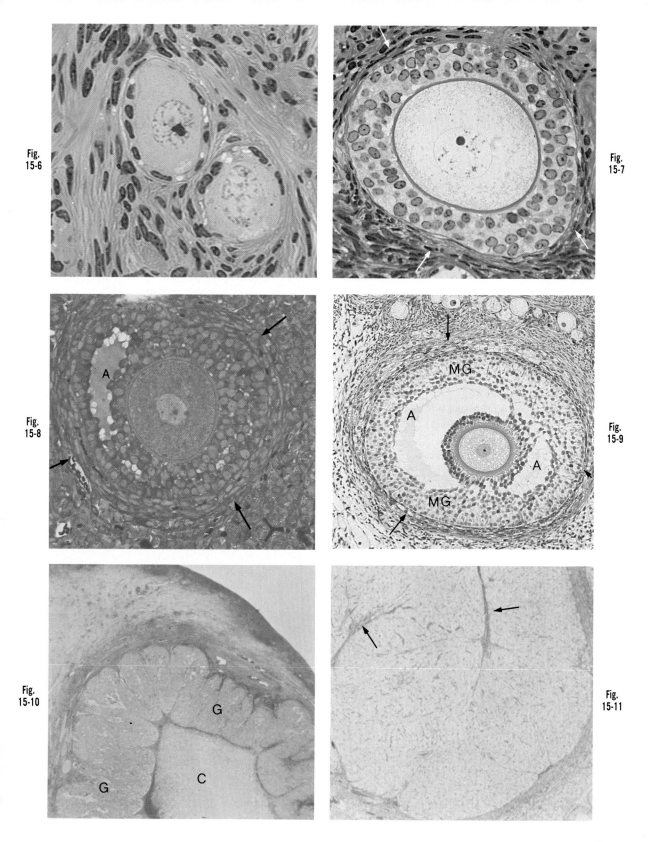

Fig. 15-6

Fig. 15-7

Fig. 15-8

Fig. 15-9

Fig. 15-10

Fig. 15-11

Figure 15–12. Corpus luteum. Plastic section. H and E. High power.

The majority of the field is occupied by granulosa lutein cells. They are large, pale-staining cells with the vesicular nuclei and abundant cytoplasm that appears vacuolated owing to the removal of lipid material during preparation. Fine connective tissue strands containing capillaries run between the cells. The corpus luteum is bounded by cells of the theca externa (arrows), which retain their fusiform shape.

Figure 15–13. Corpus luteum. Plastic section. Methylene blue, azure A, basic fuchsin. High power.

A group of granulosa lutein cells is shown. Many cells exhibit nuclei with distinct nucleoli. The extensive cytoplasm is finely granular and contains numerous vacuoles. The appearance is typical of a steroid-producing endocrine gland. Numerous capillaries lie between component cells.

Figure 15–14. Early corpus albicans. H and E. Low power.

As a corpus luteum commences to degenerate, the former rich vascularization declines and component cells decrease in size and undergo a fatty degeneration. Hence the body appears pale-staining. It is surrounded by more densely staining ovarian stroma. Later, the body becomes hyalinized and transformed into a white scar, the corpus albicans.

Figure 15–15. Atretic follicle. Azan. Medium power.

At any time during development of a follicle, the process may be arrested and the follicle replaced by a mass of connective tissue, the atretic follicle. Here, a portion of an atretic follicle resulting from the degeneration of a graafian follicle is shown. The center (C) is occupied by connective tissue that has replaced the follicular cells. The thecal margins of the original follicle remain as a thick hyalinized band, here stained blue. Ovarian stroma surrounds the atretic follicle.

Figure 15–16. Fallopian tube: ampulla. Mallory-Azan. Low power.

The mucosal lining is thrown into longitudinal folds, here sectioned transversely, that branch to divide the lumen (L) into a labyrinth of spaces. The epithelium is simple columnar and rests upon a markedly cellular lamina propria that contains numerous large blood vessels (red). The surrounding muscularis, not shown here, consists of a broad inner circular layer and a thin outer longitudinal layer.

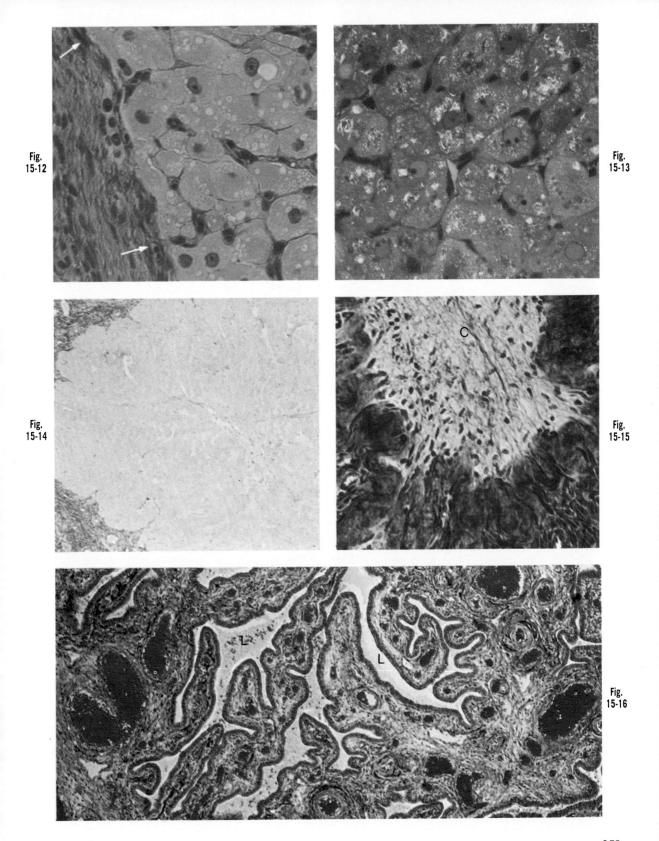

Fig.
15-12

Fig.
15-13

Fig.
15-14

Fig.
15-15

Fig.
15-16

Figure 15–17. Fallopian tube: ampulla. Plastic section. H and E. High power.

A short mucosal fold occupies the majority of the field. The simple columnar epithelium, here sectioned slightly obliquely, contains two cell types, ciliated and nonciliated. The ciliated cells, which occur in groups, have numerous cilia and show basal bodies that are visible as dense, closely opposed granules in the apical cytoplasm (arrows). The nonciliated cells generally are narrow and peg-shaped, with blebbing of the apical cytoplasm. These cells are thought to be secretory in nature. The core of the mucosal fold consists of a cellular lamina propria (LP).

Figure 15–18. Fallopian tube: ampulla in pregnancy. Plastic section. Methylene blue, azure A, basic fuchsin. High power.

The base of a mucosal fold is shown. During pregnancy, the simple columnar epithelium is low (compare with Figure 15–17). It is still contains two cell types, ciliated and nonciliated. There usually is an increase in the number of nonciliated, peg-shaped cells in pregnancy, but it is not apparent here.

Figure 15–19. Uterus: early proliferative phase. H and E. Low power.

The endometrium, or uterine mucosa, consists of an epithelial lining and an endometrial stroma. The epithelial lining (E) is a simple columnar epithelium from which uterine glands (G) extend through the full thickness of the mucosa. These are simple tubules that may branch toward their basal ends. The glands are separated by a connective tissue stroma that is highly cellular. Beneath the endometrium, a small portion of myometrium (M), containing large, empty blood vessels, is shown.

Figure 15–20. Uterus: secretory phase. H and E. Low power.

Only the superficial layers of the endometrium are shown. The endometrium is thick (compare with Figure 15–19) and the glands are markedly coiled and lie within a stroma that appears pale because of the presence of edema fluid within it. Once the structural changes associated with the secretory phase become apparent, three endometrial zones can be recognized. The narrow surface zone, or compact layer (C), contains the straight necks of the glands. The tortuous portions of the glands occupy the middle zone, or spongy layer (S). These two layers together constitute the functional layer that is lost at menstruation. The blind ends of the glands lie in the deepest zone, or basal layer, not shown here. (See Figure 15–21.)

Figure 15–21. Uterus: secretory phase. Mallory-Azan. Medium power.

Only the deeper layers of the endometrium are shown. In the spongy layer (S), the glands are tortuous and lie within a stroma that is markedly cellular, containing stromal cells and wandering lymphoid cells and granular leukocytes. The basal layer (B) contains the blind ends of the uterine glands, which participate little in the cyclic changes and are not lost at menstruation.

Figure 15–22. Uterus: early menstrual phase. Van Gieson. Low power.

The surface layers of the endometrium (right) have been lost, and the remaining glands lie within a dense, avascular stroma that is heavily infiltrated with leukocytes. The basal layer (lower left) is intact and contains extravasated blood (red) within its stroma. A small portion of the myometrium (M) also is present.

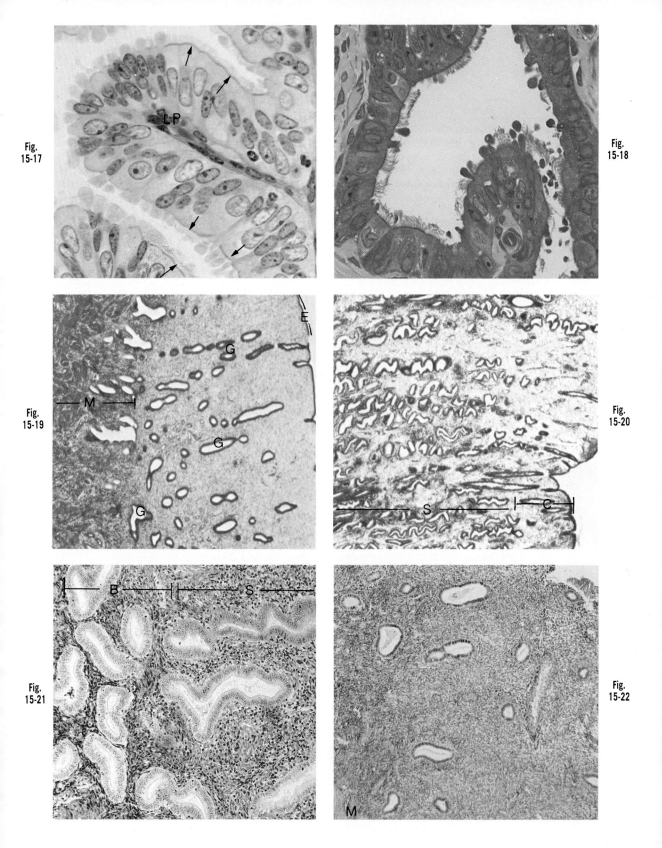

Fig.
15-17

Fig.
15-18

Fig.
15-19

Fig.
15-20

Fig.
15-21

Fig.
15-22

261

Figure 15–23. Umbilical cord. H and E. Low power.

The umbilical cord is covered by a single-layered epithelium of the enveloping chorion and has a core of mucous connective tissue (see Figure 3–15). Within the cord are two umbilical arteries (A) and a single umbilical vein (V). Each artery has a thick muscular coat, or tunica media. The vein is unusual in that its wall, unlike that of most veins, consists principally of a tunica media. The tunica adventitia is difficult to define and merges into the surrounding mucous connective tissue.

Figure 15–24. Umbilical artery. Plastic section. Methylene blue, azure A, basic fuchsin. Medium power.

The umbilical artery, here sectioned transversely, is unusual in that it possesses a media composed of two thick muscular layers: an inner longitudinal layer (L) and an outer circular layer (C). It also lacks an internal elastic membrane. A portion of the lumen, darkly staining, lies to the left. The artery lies within a delicate, mucous connective tissue, covered externally by chorion (arrow).

Figure 15–25. Placental villi (8th month). H and E. High power.

Each villus has a core of loose connective tissue containing fetal capillaries (arrows) and a covering of trophoblast. At this stage, the trophoblast consists only of syncytial trophoblast, which shows dense nuclei and a dense, acidophil cytoplasm. Intercellular boundaries cannot be distinguished. Earlier during pregnancy, a layer of cytotrophoblast is interposed between the syncytial trophoblast and the connective tissue core of the villi. The space between villi is the intervillous space that contains maternal blood.

Figure 15–26. Placental villi (9th month). Plastic section. Methylene blue, azure A, basic fuchsin. High power.

Each villus is covered by an attenuated layer of syncytial trophoblast. Many of the fetal capillaries, lying within the core of loose connective tissue, are closely opposed to the syncytial trophoblast (arrows). A portion of the chorionic plate, containing a mast cell, is present above.

Figure 15–27. Uterine cervix and vagina. Masson trichrome. Medium power.

The portio vaginalis is shown here. The cervical canal (C) appears irregular in outline owing to the glandular invagination of the lining epithelium, which is simple tall columnar in nature. Immediately beneath the epithelium, the lamina propria is cellular, but its deeper layers contain closely packed collagenous fibers (green). The thick epithelium (left), which covers the portion of the cervix that projects into the vagina, is stratified squamous nonkeratinizing in type. The junction between the two types of epithelium is not shown here, but it would occur just below the section.

Figure 15–28. Cervical canal. Plastic section. H and E. High power.

The mucous membrane of the cervical canal (C) consists of an epithelium and a lamina propria. The simple columnar epithelium is composed of tall, mucus-secreting cells. The ovoid nuclei lie at the bases of the cells and the apical cytoplasm is pale, owing to the presence of secretory material. Numerous long, branching clefts, the plicae palmatae, extend from the epithelium into the lamina propria, which is a delicate, cellular, and vascular connective tissue.

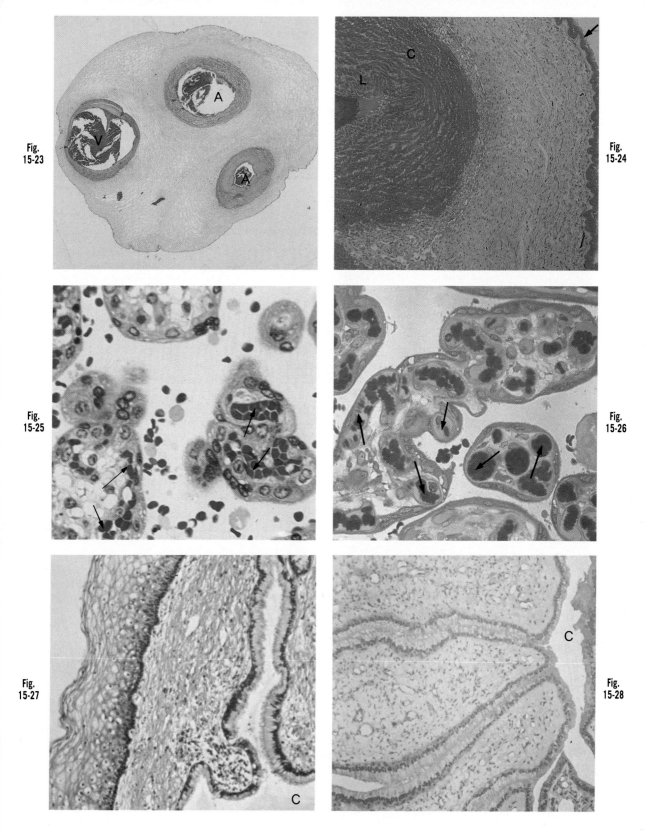

Fig. 15-23

Fig. 15-24

Fig. 15-25

Fig. 15-26

Fig. 15-27

Fig. 15-28

Figure 15–29. Vagina. H and E. Medium power.

The mucosa is lined with thick stratified squamous epithelium that is nonkeratinizing. Component cells are loaded with glycogen and thus appear vacuolated in this preparation. The underlying lamina propria is relatively dense connective tissue that contains numerous lymphocytes and polymorphonuclear leukocytes and blood vessels (arrows). The junction between epithelium and lamina propria is irregular because of the presence of connective tissue papillae.

Figure 15–30. Nipple: areolar gland. Azocarmine. Low power.

This section shows the epidermis (above) and one large areolar gland (below). The epidermis of the areolar skin is relatively thick and exhibits marked cornification (red). The underlying dermis (blue) contains an areolar gland (gland of Montgomery), which is a branched gland of the apocrine type. Large, vacuolated secretory cells lie at the periphery of the gland, and centrally a narrow coiled duct (arrow) extends toward the surface epidermis.

Figure 15–31. Mammary gland: prepubertal. H and E. Low power.

Prior to puberty, ducts are the principal epithelial elements of the gland. Here a small duct, lined by a simple cuboidal epithelium, lies embedded within interlobular connective tissue that is dense and contains small amounts of adipose tissue.

Figure 15–32. Mammary gland: pregnancy. H and E. Low power.

During pregnancy, ducts within the lobules of each lobe proliferate and form buds that enlarge into alveoli. Lobules expand and interlobular connective tissue and fat decrease in amount. Here, portions of several lobules are shown. The lobules contain groups of alveoli and scattered, wide intralobular ducts. The epithelial elements of each lobule are embedded within a loose, cellular connective tissue. Interlobular connective tissue is relatively dense and contains some fat cells.

Figure 15–33. Mammary gland: pregnancy. H and E. Medium power.

A portion of one lobule is shown. Alveoli vary in size and are lined by a simple cuboidal epithelium. A layer of myoepithelial cells (not visible here) occurs between the alveolar epithelium and the basal lamina. The lumina of many alveoli contain acidophil secretory material. Intralobular ducts histologically appear similar to alveoli, and functionally they are true secretory ducts that also possess myoepithelial elements. The embedding intralobular connective tissue is cellular, whereas the surrounding interlobular connective tissue is relatively dense.

Figure 15–34. Mammary gland: lactation. H and E. Medium power.

Portions of two lobules are shown. Alveoli are dilated and may appear as saccules. The lumina of some contain pale-staining secretory material. The alveolar lining is a simple cuboidal epithelium; myoepithelial cells are not apparent in this section. The surrounding intralobular connective tissue is condensed and appears markedly cellular owing to infiltration with lymphocytes. The interlobular connective tissue (IL) also is condensed and consists principally of collagenous fibers.

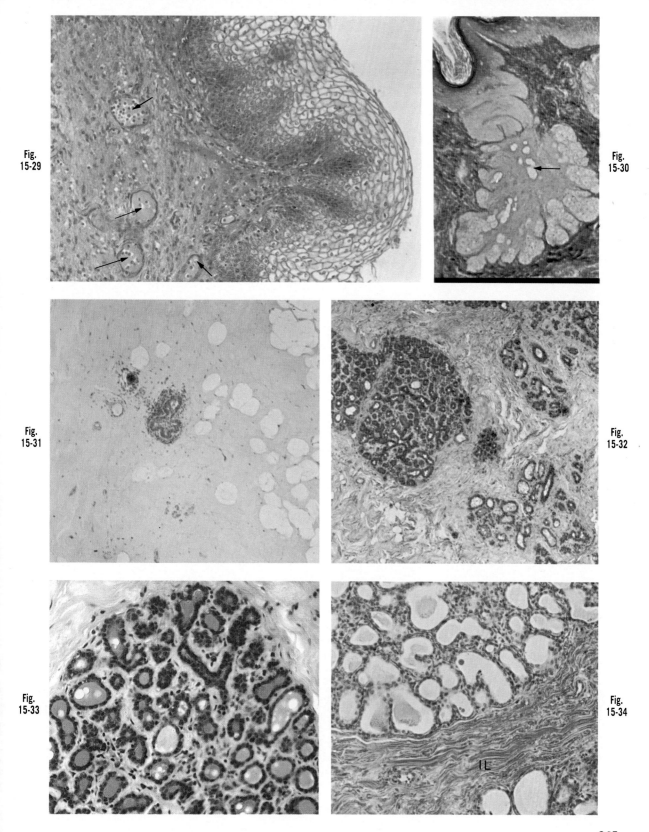

Fig.
15-29

Fig.
15-30

Fig.
15-31

Fig.
15-32

Fig.
15-33

Fig.
15-34

265

SIXTEEN

The Male Reproductive System

The male reproductive system comprises the testes, the ducts of the testes, the auxiliary glands associated with them, and the penis.

THE TESTIS

The testis is a double gland because functionally it is both exocrine and endocrine. The exocrine component is a compound tubular gland, and the product is chiefly the sex cells; thus the testis may be referred to as a cytogenic gland. The endocrine product is an internal secretion elaborated by certain specialized cells, the interstitial cells (of Leydig). The testis is covered by the mesothelium of the visceral layer of the *tunica vaginalis testis,* deep to which is a thick connective tissue capsule, the *tunica albuginea.* This thickens posteriorly to form the *mediastinum testis,* an area where the ducts, blood vessels, and nerves enter or leave the testis. Thin fibrous partitions radiate from the mediastinum testis to the capsule and divide the interior into about 250 pyramidal compartments, the *lobuli testis.* Each lobule contains one to four seminiferous tubules and the interstitial cells that are located in the interstices between the tubules. The tubules are highly convoluted and are lined by the germinal or seminiferous epithelium. This epithelium contains cells of two distinct types: (1) spermatogenic cells, and (2) supporting cells (of Sertoli).

Spermatogenic Cells

The spermatogenic cells differentiate progressively from the basal region of the tubule to the lumen (spermatogenesis), and those nearest the lumen transform into spermatozoa (spermiogenesis) and detach from the epithelium to lie free within the lumen. Cells composing the seminiferous epithelium are allocated special names. Spermatogonia lie on the basal lamina of the tubule and contain 23 pairs (a total of 46) of chromosomes. These cells divide mitotically to produce daughter cells, each with 23 pairs of chromosomes, that either persist as spermatogonia or differentiate into primary spermatocytes. Primary spermatocytes are the largest of maturing germ cells and they divide meiotically to give rise to secondary spermatocytes. As a result of the meiotic division, 23 chromosomes (22 autosomes plus one sex chromosome, either X or Y) pass to each secondary spermatocyte. The division also is peculiar in that cytokinesis is incomplete and the two resulting secondary spermatocytes remain connected by a bridge of protoplasm. Secondary spermatocytes are smaller than primary spermatocytes and they are seen infrequently, since they divide mitotically after a very brief interphase to give rise to spermatids. The latter cells remain in a syncytial cluster because cytokinesis again is incomplete. Spermatids, each with 23 chromosomes, do not divide but through a cellular transformation become mature spermatozoa. The head of the mature spermatozoon consists of a condensed spermatid nucleus covered anteriorly by the acrosome that is contributed to by the Golgi apparatus. Other organelles and components of the spermatid contribute to the flagellum of the spermatozoon.

Sertoli Cells

The supporting cells of Sertoli are tall, pillar-like cells that are attached peripherally to the basal lamina of the seminiferous tubule. They provide mechanical and nutritional support to spermatids and to maturing spermatozoa, and they participate in the release of mature spermatozoa into the lumen. Where Sertoli cells border on each other, the contiguous surfaces show complex occluding junctional specializations. These junctions form a barrier (the blood-testis barrier) that divides the seminiferous epithelium into basal and adluminal compartments. The specialized junctions represent strong adhesive sites between Sertoli cells and between Sertoli cells and germ cells, and spermatocytes must cross this barrier to gain access to the adluminal compartment.

GENITAL DUCTS

After release from the seminiferous epithelium, mature spermatozoa pass into the *tubuli recti,* the straight terminations of the seminiferous tubules that are lined only with Sertoli cells. Tubuli recti open into the *rete testis,* a network of anastomosing channels within the mediastinum testis. Ten to 15 *ductuli efferentes* connect the rete testis to the single *ductus epididymidis,* a highly convoluted tube that continues distally into the *ductus deferens.* The ductus passes to the prostatic urethra and, as it does so, the lumen increases in size and the muscular coat thickens. Immediately prior to its entry into the urethra, it dilates to form the *ampulla.* The *ejaculatory duct,* formed by the junction of ampulla and seminal vesicle, pierces the prostate to open into the urethra.

AUXILIARY GLANDS

The auxiliary glands associated with the duct systems of the testes are:
1. The *seminal vesicles*.
2. The *prostate*.
3. The *bulbourethral glands*.

Each seminal vesicle is a tortuous, elongated diverticulum off the ductus deferens. The lumen is irregular and honeycombed by high branching folds of the mucosa.

The prostate gland encircles the urethra near the neck of the bladder and is an aggregate of 30 to 50 small, compound tubuloalveolar glands that drain into the prostatic urethra by 15 to 30 small excretory ducts. The glands are embedded within a fibromuscular stroma and are enclosed within a fibrous capsule that contains a plexus of veins.

The bulbourethral glands (of Cowper) are paired bodies that lie within the connective tissue behind the membranous urethra. Each is a compound tubuloalveolar gland whose duct enters the posterior portion of the cavernous segment of the urethra.

THE PENIS

The penis serves as the common outlet for urine and seminal fluid and is the copulatory organ. It is formed by three cylinders of erectile tissue: the paired *corpora cavernosa penis* dorsally and the single *corpus cavernosum urethrae (corpus spongiosum)* ventrally. The latter encloses the cavernous portion of the urethra. Erectile tissue is composed of wide irregular spaces lined by endothelium and separated by a connective tissue that contains smooth muscle fibers. The skin covering the penis is thin and delicate, and terminally it reduplicates over the glans penis (the bulbous enlargement of the corpus spongiosum) as a fold, the *prepuce*.

Figure 16–1. Segment of a human seminiferous tubule.

This diagrammatic representation illustrates the process of spermatogenesis.

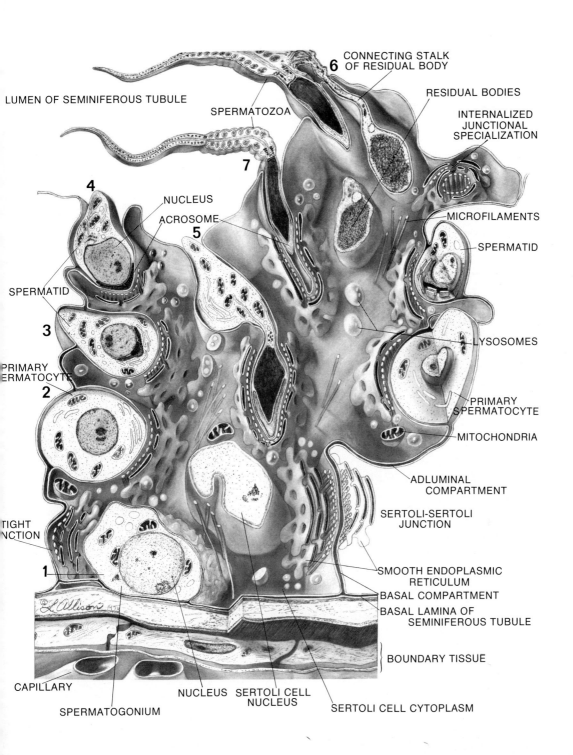

CONNECTING STALK
OF RESIDUAL BODY

6

RESIDUAL BODIES

INTERNALIZED
JUNCTIONAL
SPECIALIZATION

LUMEN OF SEMINIFEROUS TUBULE

SPERMATOZOA

7

MICROFILAMENTS

SPERMATID

4

NUCLEUS

ACROSOME

5

LYSOSOMES

SPERMATID

3

PRIMARY
SPERMATOCYTE

PRIMARY
SPERMATOCYTE

MITOCHONDRIA

2

ADLUMINAL
COMPARTMENT

SERTOLI-SERTOLI
JUNCTION

TIGHT
JUNCTION

1

SMOOTH ENDOPLASMIC
RETICULUM

BASAL COMPARTMENT

BASAL LAMINA OF
SEMINIFEROUS TUBULE

BOUNDARY TISSUE

CAPILLARY

NUCLEUS

SERTOLI CELL
NUCLEUS

SERTOLI CELL CYTOPLASM

SPERMATOGONIUM

Figure 16–2. Testis. Iron hematoxylin, aniline blue. Low power.

The testis is enclosed within a thick fibrous capsule, the tunica albuginea (TA). On the inner aspect of the tunica albuginea, dense connective tissue is replaced by a loose connective tissue containing numerous blood vessels, the tunica vasculosa testis (arrows). Connective tissue septa that extend inward from the capsule to divide the testis into pyramidal compartments, the lobuli testis, are not apparent on this section. The seminiferous tubules, since they are convoluted, are cut in various planes.

Figure 16–3. Testis. Iron hematoxylin, aniline blue. Medium power.

Portions of the tunica albuginea (TA) and of the tunica vasculosa testis (TV) are present above. Beneath the capsule, sectioned seminiferous tubules, separated by interstitial connective tissue, generally show wide lumina, some containing spermatozoa. The seminiferous epithelium, composed principally of sex cells, is stratified and is surrounded by the boundary tissue (arrows). The latter contains connective tissue fibers and cells and some smooth muscle cells. The interstitial tissue is a loose connective tissue containing epithelioid cells, the interstitial cells of Leydig (L).

Figure 16–4. Testis. Plastic section. H and E. Medium power.

In this material, seminiferous tubules appear closely packed and generally their lumina are wide and empty. The boundary tissue around each tubule is acidophil (pink), and there is little intervening interstitial tissue between the tubules.

Figure 16–5. Testis. Plastic section. H and E. High power.

A portion of the tunica albuginea (TA) lies to the right. The seminiferous tubules are surrounded by the boundary tissue and separated by a narrow interstitial space (arrows) containing blood vessels. The seminiferous epithelium contains two distinct types of cells—supporting cells and germ or spermatogenic cells. Nuclear characteristics distinguish supporting cells (of Sertoli) from spermatogenic elements. Nuclei of Sertoli cells (arrowheads) are pale and ovoid, with the long axis of each generally directed radially, and each possesses a distinct nucleolus. Spermatogenic cells differentiate progressively from the basal region to the lumen. The densely staining heads of spermatozoa are present close to the lumen.

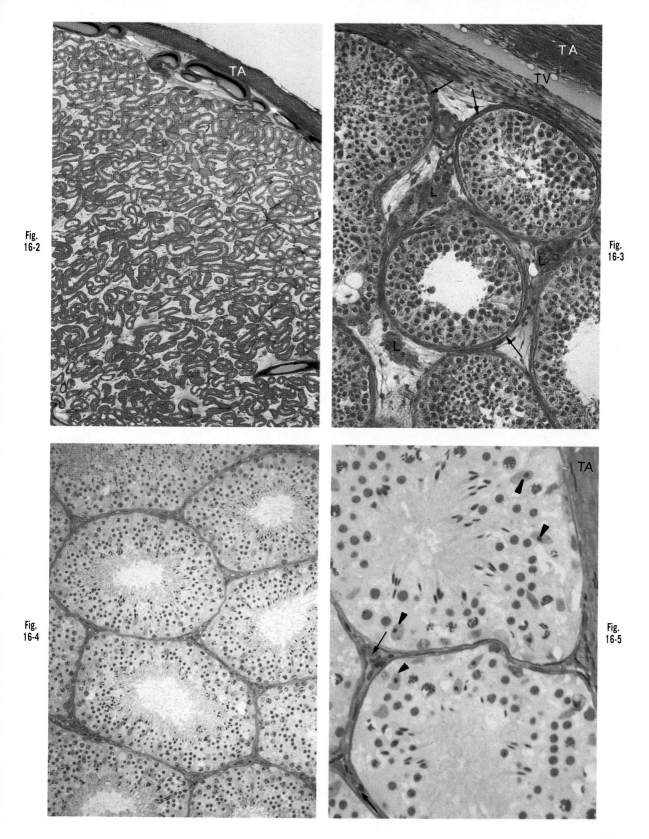

Fig. 16-2

Fig. 16-3

Fig. 16-4

Fig. 16-5

Figure 16–6. Testis. Plastic section. Methylene blue, azure A, basic fuchsin. Medium power.

The testicular capsule lies above. It is composed of three tunics: the tunica vaginalis (arrowheads), a single layer of attenuated mesothelial cells; the tunica albuginea (TA), a thick layer of fibroelastic connective tissue that also contains smooth muscle cells (not apparent here); and tunica vasculosa (TV), containing numerous blood vessels. In relation to the latter are groups of interstitial cells of Leydig (darkly staining). Portions of two seminiferous tubules, surrounded by boundary tissue (arrows), underlie the testicular capsule.

Figure 16–7. Testis: seminiferous epithelium. Plastic section. H and E. High power.

Portions of two seminiferous tubules, separated by their basal laminae and boundary tissue (arrows), are shown. Sertoli cells (S), with their characteristic nuclei, lie close to the basal lamina of each tubule. Spermatogonia (G) are located directly above the basal lamina and show spherical or ovoid nuclei. Primary spermatocytes (P) lie in the next layer, immediately above the spermatogonia, and are the largest germ cells. Their nuclei show condensed chromatin. Spermatids (T) form one or more layers close to the lumen; they are the smallest of the germ cells. Sperm heads are densely staining, and tails project into the lumen (L).

Figure 16–8. Testis: seminiferous epithelium. Plastic section. H and E. Oil immersion.

A portion of one seminiferous tubule, surrounded by boundary tissue (arrow) is shown. Sertoli cells (S), with their distinctive nuclei, show indefinite cell boundaries. The apical cytoplasm of one of them is closely associated with sperm heads. A spermatogonium (G) lies immediately in relation to the basal lamina. The next layer contains primary spermatocytes (P), above which are spermatids (T). Secondary spermatocytes are not present; they are seen rarely, since they rapidly divide to produce spermatids.

Figure 16–9. Testis: Leydig cells. Plastic section. H and E. High power.

The tunica albuginea (TA), covered by the mesothelium of the visceral layer of the tunica vaginalis testis (arrow), lies above, and below is a portion of a seminiferous tubule. Between the two, there is a group of interstitial cells of Leydig (L). These are large, epithelioid cells that show spherical nuclei with distinct nucleoli and a finely granular cytoplasm.

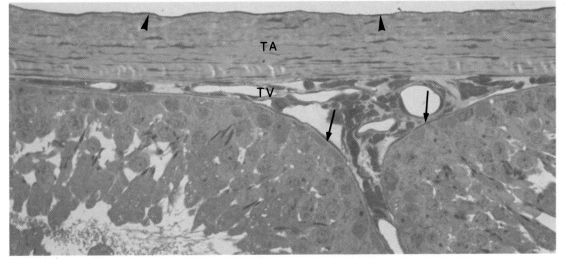

Fig. 16-6

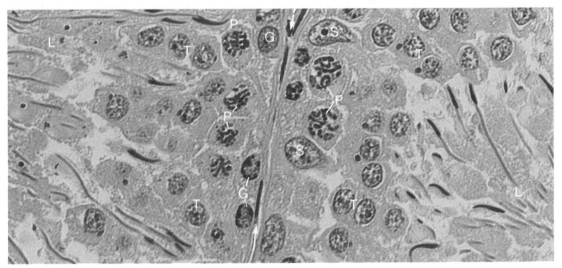

Fig. 16-7

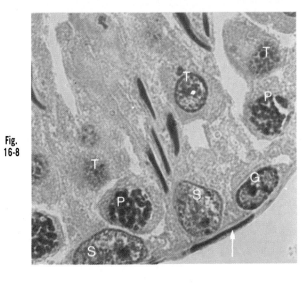

Fig. 16-8

Fig. 16-9

275

Figure 16–10. Testis: Leydig cells. Plastic section. Toluidine blue. Oil immersion.

The interstitium contains a large group of Leydig cells, characterized by the presence within their cytoplasm of numerous lipid droplets (dark blue). Nuclei are vesicular and contain distinct nucleoli. Also present within the interstitium are small connective tissue cells, principally fibroblasts, and a capillary (C) containing red blood cells. A portion of a seminiferous tubule (T) lies above right.

Figure 16–11. Testis: Leydig cell. Iron hematoxylin, aniline blue. High power.

A portion of a seminiferous tubule, surrounded by boundary tissue, lies to the left. Within the loose connective tissue of the interstitium (right), there is one large Leydig cell. The cytoplasm is finely granular and deep staining, and within it pale, rod-shaped crystalloids of Reinke are apparent.

Figure 16–12. Testis: pampiniform plexus. Plastic section. H and E. Low power.

This section of the external region of the mediastinum testis shows a branch of the testicular artery (A) surrounded by an extensive plexus of small veins, the pampiniform plexus. The plexus precools the arterial blood entering the testis by a countercurrent heat exchange mechanism.

Figure 16–13. Rete testis. Plastic section. H and E. Medium power.

The rete testis is a network of anastomosing channels within the dense connective tissue of the mediastinum testis. The irregular channels are lined by a simple epithelium that generally is simple cuboidal. The surrounding connective tissue contains a few small blood vessels.

Figure 16–14. Ductuli efferentes. Plastic section. H and E. Medium power.

The spirally wound efferent ductules within the head of the epididymis here are sectioned transversely. The ductules are lined by a simple layer of epithelium, mostly simple columnar, which is ciliated. A thin band of circularly arranged smooth muscle cells (nuclei of which are arrowed) surrounds each ductule. The presence of spermatozoa within the lumina is unusual.

Figure 16–15. Ductus epididymidis. Plastic section. H and E. Medium power.

The ductus epididymidis is highly tortuous and forms the body and tail of the epididymis. In sections through these regions, the duct is cut numerous times. The epithelium is uniform in height and is pseudostratified, with scattered basal cells and tall columnar cells. The latter possess ovoid nuclei, situated either basally or centrally within the cells. The apical cytoplasm is acidophil and the cells bear stereocilia on the free surface. The lumen may be empty or it may contain large concentrations of spermatozoa. The duct is surrounded by a basal lamina and by a thin layer of smooth muscle cells (arrows), and is embedded within a loose connective tissue.

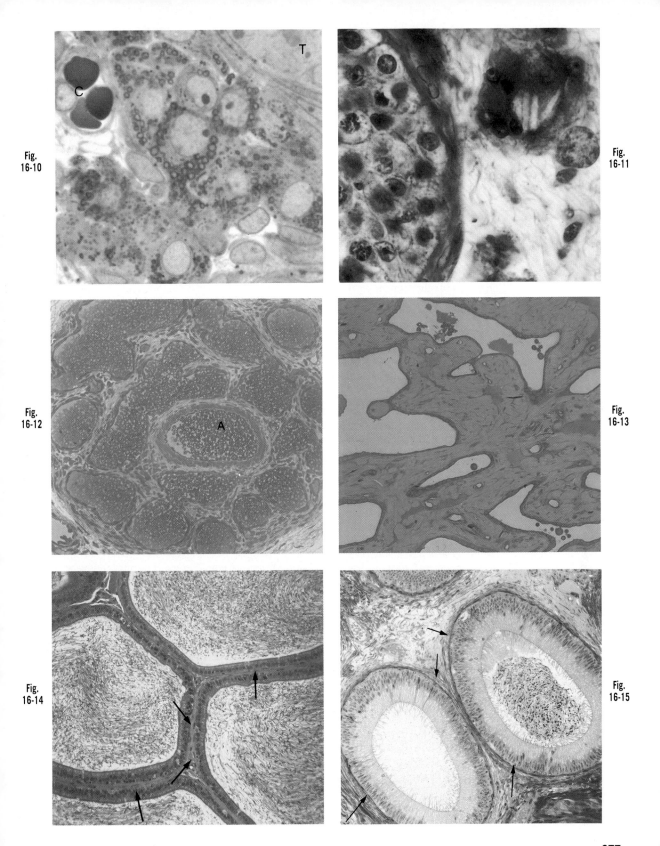

Fig.
16-10

Fig.
16-11

Fig.
16-12

Fig.
16-13

Fig.
16-14

Fig.
16-15

Figure 16–16. Ductus epididymidis. Plastic section. H and E. High power.

The regular height of the pseudostratified columnar epithelium lining the duct is clearly apparent. Scattered small basal cells, with small spherical nuclei, lie immediately in relation to the basal lamina. The ovoid nuclei of the tall columnar cells lie either basally or more centrally within the cells. The apical cytoplasm is pale and vacuolated, and long stereocilia project into the lumen. A thin layer of circularly arranged smooth muscle cells (arrows) surrounds the duct, which is embedded within a loose, cellular connective tissue.

Figure 16–17. Ductus epididymidis. PAS, light green. Medium power.

Portions of two segments of the duct are shown. The apical cytoplasm of the tall columnar cells lining the duct contains secretory droplets (pink, arrows) and the stereocilia exhibit a positive reaction with periodic acid–Schiff (PAS). The lumen is packed with spermatozoa.

Figure 16–18. Ductus epididymidis: stereocilia. Plastic section. H and E. High power.

The nuclei of the tall columnar cells are ovoid, and the apical cytoplasm is finely granular and vacuolated. On their luminal surface, the cells bear tufts of stereocilia (long, slender branching microvilli that are nonmotile). A layer of circularly arranged smooth muscle cells (arrows) surrounds the duct.

Figure 16–19. Ductus deferens. Iron hematoxylin, aniline blue. Low power.

Relatively, the wall of the duct is thick and the lumen narrow. The epithelium is pseudostratified and is surrounded by a delicate lamina propria. The mucosa rises into short longitudinal folds, here sectioned transversely. Beneath the mucosa, there is a narrow band of submucosa (arrows), composed principally of collagenous fibers. The muscular coat is thick and contains bundles of smooth muscle fibers oriented into three layers: a thin layer of longitudinal bundles (IL), a broad middle circular layer (C), and an outer longitudinal layer (OL). A fibrous adventitia (A) surrounds the muscle coat.

Figure 16–20. Ductus deferens: ampulla. Plastic section. H and E. Medium power.

As the ampulla of the duct is approached, the lumen becomes wider and the mucosal folds are more marked. The epithelium is pseudostratified columnar, and the mucosal folds contain a core of delicate lamina propria. A narrow zone of submucosal connective tissue (SM) separates the mucosa from the underlying muscle coat (M).

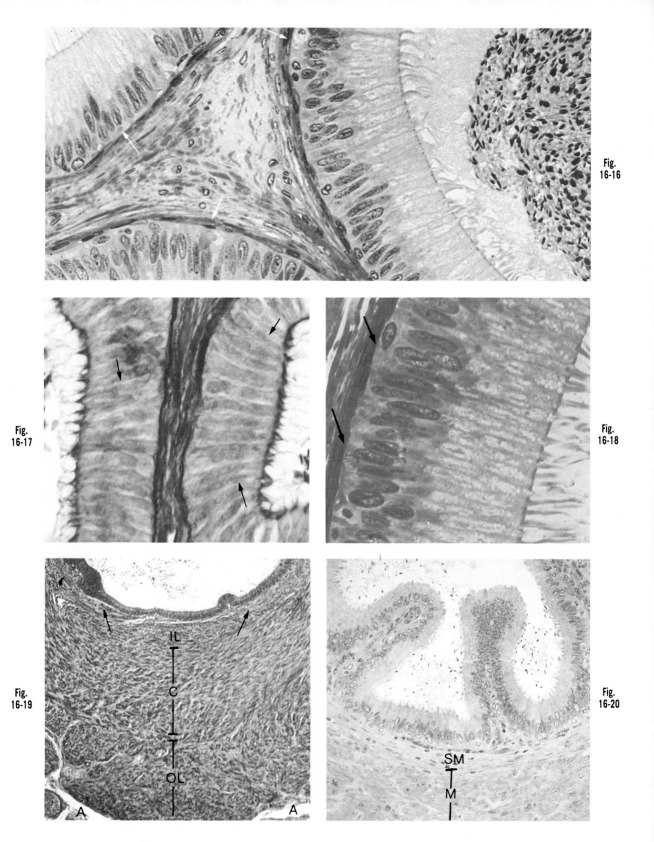

Fig. 16-16

Fig. 16-17

Fig. 16-18

Fig. 16-19

Fig. 16-20

Figure 16–21. Seminal vesicle. Mallory. Low power.

The seminal vesicle is a highly tortuous, elongated diverticulum off the terminal portion of the ductus deferens. Two segments of the vesicle are shown here. The mucosa is markedly folded. High primary folds (1) branch into secondary and tertiary folds that project far into the lumen (L) and frequently merge with one another. Thus, the lumen appears to be divided into numerous compartments, although all do communicate freely. The mucosa is surrounded by a thick muscle coat (M) in which most of the bundles of smooth muscle fibers are circularly arranged, although peripheral bundles tend to be more longitudinal in their orientation. The surrounding adventitia contains coarse collagenous fibers.

Figure 16–22. Seminal vesicle. Mallory. Medium power.

The bases of several mucosal folds that extend into the lumen (L) are shown. The lumen contains some densely staining masses of secretion. The epithelium generally is pseudo-stratified columnar and the folds contain a core of delicate connective tissue continuous with that of the underlying lamina propria (LP). The smooth muscle fibers in the surrounding muscle coat (M) are circularly arranged.

Figure 16–23. Seminal vesicle. Plastic section. H and E. High power.

A branching mucosal fold occupies the majority of the field. Although the epithelium of the seminal vesicle typically is pseudostratified, it shows many variations. Here it is simple columnar, with distinct cell boundaries. It rests upon a delicate, cellular connective tissue (arrows) that forms the core of the mucosal folds.

Figure 16–24. Seminal vesicle. Plastic section. H and E. High power.

The bases of several mucosal folds extend superiorly into the lumen, which contains some densely staining secretion. The epithelium here is simple columnar, and the apical cytoplasm appears vacuolated as a result of the presence of lipid droplets associated with some small pigment granules. The mucosa lies upon a thick muscle coat in which most smooth muscle fibers are circularly arranged.

Figure 16–25. Prostate gland. H and E. Low power.

The prostate gland is an aggregate of numerous small compound tubuloalveolar glands of different sizes. The smallest glands lie within the mucosal layer of the urethra, the next largest within the submucosal layer, and the largest (shown here) within the prostatic stroma. The secretory alveoli and tubules vary in size and are very irregular, and the lining epithelium is folded and cuboidal to columnar in type. The glands are embedded within the stroma, which is a fibroelastic connective tissue that contains numerous strands of smooth muscle fibers.

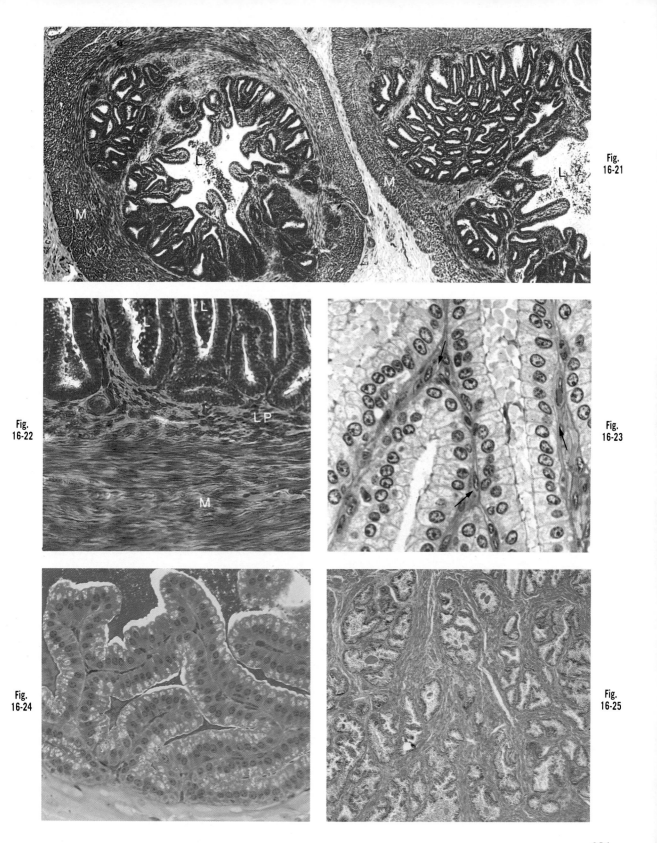

Fig.
16-21

Fig.
16-22

Fig.
16-23

Fig.
16-24

Fig.
16-25

Figure 16–26. Prostate gland. H and E. Medium power.

Several alveoli, irregular in shape, are embedded within a cellular stroma that is fibromuscular. The alveoli are lined by an epithelium that is simple cuboidal to simple columnar in type. The lumina of several alveoli contain acidophil condensations of secretory material—the prostatic concretions, or corpora amylacea.

Figure 16–27. Prostate gland. Plastic section. Methylene blue, azure A, basic fuchsin. High power.

Two large alveoli, irregular in shape, are embedded within a cellular stoma that contains numerous small bundles of smooth muscle fibers (arrows). The lining epithelium of the alveoli is simple columnar and the apical cytoplasm stains palely. A prostatic concretion, exhibiting concentric layering, is present in one alveolus.

Figure 16–28. Penis. Van Gieson. Low power.

This transverse section passes through the base of the glans penis at its junction within the shaft. The paired corpora cavernosa (C) appear small, since they are sectioned through their conical ends. They are surrounded by a thick fibrous sheath, the tunica albuginea (T), and are separated by a common pectiniform septum (S). The corpus spongiosum (U), which lies in the groove between the corpora cavernosa, contains the cavernous urethra, which exhibits an irregular, crescent-shaped lumen. The subcutaneous tissue surrounding the erectile tissue is delicate and devoid of fat. The skin covering the organ is thin, and terminally it reduplicates over the glans as the prepuce (P). Portions of the space between the prepuce and the glans may be seen in two locations (arrows).

Figure 16–29. Penis: corpus spongiosum. Iron hematoxylin, aniline blue. Low power.

The urethra is lined by a stratified or pseudostratified columnar epithelium, beneath which there is a loose connective tissue lamina propria (light blue). The entire mucosa appears irregular, and invaginations of epithelium extend deeply to terminate in mucous urethral glands (of Littre, arrows). The mucosa is surrounded by erectile tissue of the corpus spongiosum, bounded by a sheath of collagenous fibers, the tunica albuginea (T).

Figure 16–30. Penis: helicine arteries. Iron hematoxylin, aniline blue. Medium power.

Erectile tissue is supplied by helicine arteries, which are longitudinal vessels that are directed distally. In the quiescent state, these vessels have a spiral course, their media is thick, and their intima is thrown into longitudinal folds, here sectioned transversely (arrows): thus their lumina appear crescentic. These vessels open directly into the sinuses of the erectile tissue, and during erotic stimulation they straighten out and their lumina dilate. Also present is a mucous urethral gland of Littre (G).

Figure 16–31. Penis: erectile tissue. Masson. Medium power.

Erectile tissue is composed of a framework of irregular trabeculae, consisting of collagenous (green), elastic, and smooth (brown) muscle fibers, which are extensions of the tunica albuginea. Within this framework are irregular endothelium-lined spaces, the blood sinuses (S). During erotic stimulation, the engorgement of these sinuses with blood results in erection of the penis.

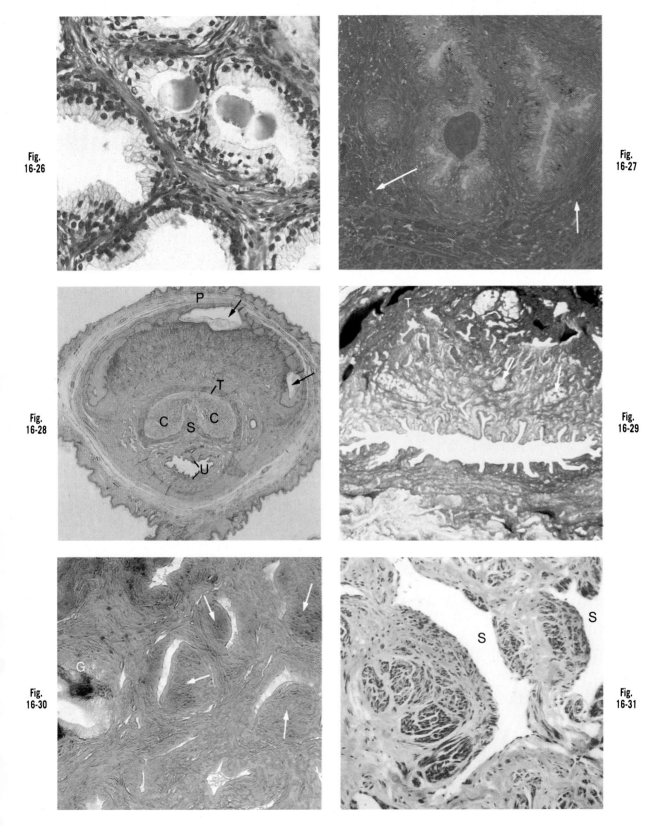

Fig.
16-26

Fig.
16-27

Fig.
16-28

Fig.
16-29

Fig.
16-30

Fig.
16-31

CHAPTER
SEVENTEEN

Organs of Special Sense

SENSORY RECEPTORS

Sense organs receive stimuli from the body and from the external environment and transmit information to the central nervous system. General sense organs are distributed widely in epithelium, connective tissue, muscle, and tendon. Special receptors occur in limited areas associated with sensations of smell, taste, sight, hearing, and balance. Receptors generally are nerve endings or specialized cells on which nerve endings terminate. The actual mechanism whereby action potentials are generated is poorly understood.

Various classifications of receptors are used, e.g., *thermoreceptors* (sensitive to temperature change), *mechanoreceptors* (touch, pressure), *chemoreceptors* (chemical change), and *osmoreceptors* (changes in osmotic pressure). Receptors can also be classified on the origin of the stimulus, e.g., *exteroreceptors* (stimuli from the exterior), *proprioceptors* (deep body sensation) and *interoreceptors* (viscera and blood vessels).

Morphologically, receptors can be grouped into *free*, or *naked*, *endings* and *encapsulated endings*. Some of the receptors have been described where appropriate in previous chapters. Examples of free and encapsulated endings will be described in this chapter, although most of the text is concerned with the eye and the ear.

THE EYE

The *eyeball* and *optic nerve*, together with accessory organs such as eyelids and lacrimal glands, are located in the bony orbit. The eyeball itself is a complex photosensitive organ, but consists of three basic coats:
1. The fibrous (outer) coat.
2. The vascular (uveal) coat.
3. The nervous coat (retina).

The outer coat is fibrous and is formed by the *sclera* and *cornea.* The sclera is tough, white fibrous tissue and covers the posterior five-sixths of the globe. The anterior one-sixth is formed by the cornea, which is transparent and curved more acutely than the sclera (a radius of 8 mm, compared with one of 12 mm for the sclera), and thus it bulges slightly. At the corneoscleral junction is a sulcus from which conjunctiva is reflected from the eyeball onto the interior surfaces of the eyelids.

The middle, or uveal, coat is a vascular, nutrient layer with three components. Posteriorly is the *choroid,* which merges just posterior to the corneoscleral junction with the *ciliary body.* In addition to blood vessels, the ciliary body contains smooth muscle fibers for lens accommodation, and ciliary processes where aqueous humor is formed. More anteriorly, the uveal coat reflects internally as the *iris,* diverging from the cornea. The iris is a diaphragm with a central aperture, the *pupil,* that can be varied in diameter with light intensity.

The inner nervous coat, the *retina,* is divided into two distinct portions. Over just more than the posterior half of the globe it contains the photoreceptors and other nervous elements and is multilayered, this part being connected by the optic nerve to the central nervous system. Just posterior to the ciliary body, the retina becomes thin, and this non-nervous layer lines the internal surface of the ciliary body and continues anteriorly on the posterior surface of the iris. The junction between nervous and non-nervous portions of the retina is termed the *ora serrata.*

The *lens* is biconvex, lies immediately behind the iris, and is held in place by a suspensory ligament attached circumferentially to the ciliary body. The narrow space between lens and iris is the *posterior chamber,* which communicates freely through the pupil with the *anterior chamber,* this being the space between the iris posteriorly and the cornea anteriorly. Both anterior and posterior chambers contain a clear fluid, the *aqueous humor.* Behind the lens, the entire cavity of the globe is filled by a transparent gel, the *vitreous humor.* Thus, there is between the sensory retina and the exterior, i.e., the pathway for light, a series of transparent refractive media consisting of cornea, aqueous humor, lens, and vitreous body.

Just below and to the nasal side of the posterior pole of the eye, the optic nerve exits from the globe. Blood vessels enter the eye with the optic nerve (the central artery) to supply the retina and through the sclera to reach the choroid.

THE EAR

The organs of both hearing and balance are contained in the ear, divided anatomically into three parts:

External Ear. The external ear is formed by the *auricle,* or *pinna,* the *external auditory canal,* and the *tympanic membrane.* The auricle has a core of elastic cartilage covered by skin, while the canal is held patent by elastic cartilage in the outer third, continuous with that of the auricle, and by bone in the inner two thirds. It is lined by modified skin with hairs, sebaceous glands, and modified sweat, or *ceruminous,* glands. The canal is closed deeply by the tympanic membrane, which has a core of connective tissue and is covered externally by very thin skin and internally by the cuboidal epithelium lining the middle ear cavity.

Middle Ear. The middle ear, or *tympanic* cavity, is small and in the shape of a biconcave lens. Externally is the tympanic membrane separating it from the auditory canal, and anteriorly a narrow canal, the auditory tube, connects with the nasopharynx. This tube equalizes pressure on both sides of the tympanic membrane. Posteriorly, the middle ear cavity communicates with air cells in the mastoid bone. Medially is the outer wall of the inner ear and crossing the cavity is a chain of three articulated small bones:

1. The *malleus,* attached to the inner aspect of the tympanic membrane.
2. The *incus.*
3. The *stapes,* which fits into the foramen ovale of the inner ear.

These bones transmit vibrations of the eardrum to the perilymph of the inner ear (scala vestibuli of the cochlea). Also associated with the middle ear are two small muscles (tensor tympani and stapedius).

Inner Ear. The inner ear is a system of canals and cavities within the petrous temporal bone, the *osseous labyrinth,* within which is a system of smaller canals, the *membranous labyrinth.* The osseous labyrinth is filled with a fluid called *perilymph,* and the membranous labyrinth with *endolymph,* the two fluids thus separated by the wall of the membranous labyrinth. The osseous labyrinth is complex in shape, with a large central cavity (the vestibule) located medial to the tympanic cavity. Opening into its posterior aspect are three semicircular canals (anterior, posterior, and lateral), each with a dilatation, or *ampulla,* near one opening into the vestibule. Although there are three *semicircular canals,* there are only five openings into the vestibule, the nonampullated ends of the posterior and anterior canals fusing to form a single opening. Anteriorly the vestibule opens into the *cochlea,* a coiled tube that winds for 2¾ turns around a bony axial stem, the *modiolus* (like the central pillar of a spiral staircase). The membranous labyrinth lies within the bony labyrinth and has a similar conformation except that the vestibule is occupied by two separate cavities, a *utricle* posteriorly and a *saccule* anteriorly. The utricle communicates posteriorly with the five openings of the semicircular canals and anteriorly with the saccule, which in turn connects with the cochlea. Sensory areas are located in the ampullae of the semicircular canals *(cristae ampullares)* and in the utricle and saccule *(maculae utriculi and sacculi),* and these subserve static and kinetic senses (gravity and head movement, for balance). The organ of hearing, the spiral *organ of Corti,* is located along the length of the *cochlear duct.*

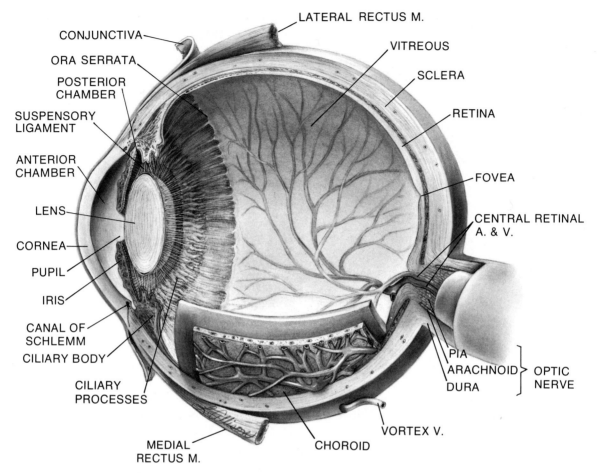

Figure 17–1. The eye.

In this diagram the eye is sectioned horizontally.

Figure 17–2. Lens, posterior surface.

This scanning electron micrograph shows part of the posterior surface of the lens (L). Attached to it are zonular fibers (Z) of the suspensory ligament that pass to the ciliary body (C) and region of the ora serrata (O). (Courtesy of Dr. D. H. Dickson.)

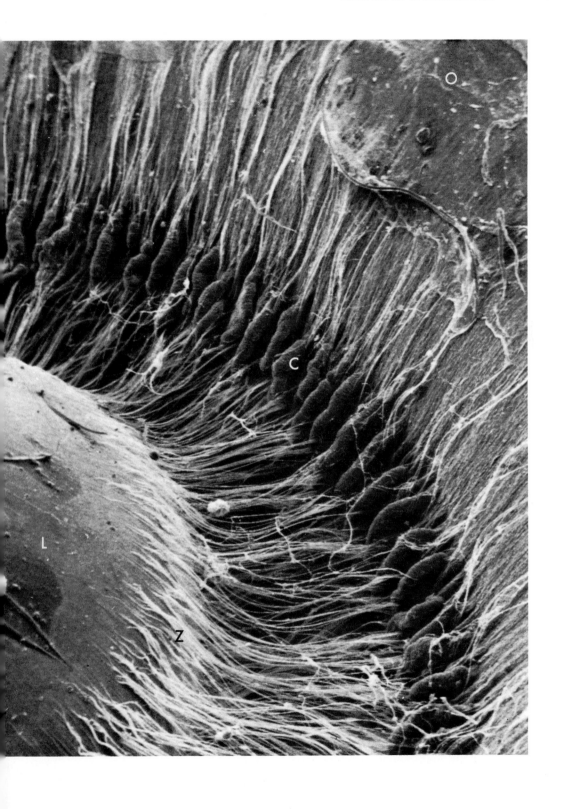

Figure 17–3. Diagram of cochlea and the organ of Corti.

Shown here is a single turn of the spiral bony (osseous) labyrinth in transverse section. Centrally lies the cochlear duct (scala media) containing the organ of Corti and filled with endolymph. Above is the scala vestibuli and below the scala tympani, both filled with perilymph.

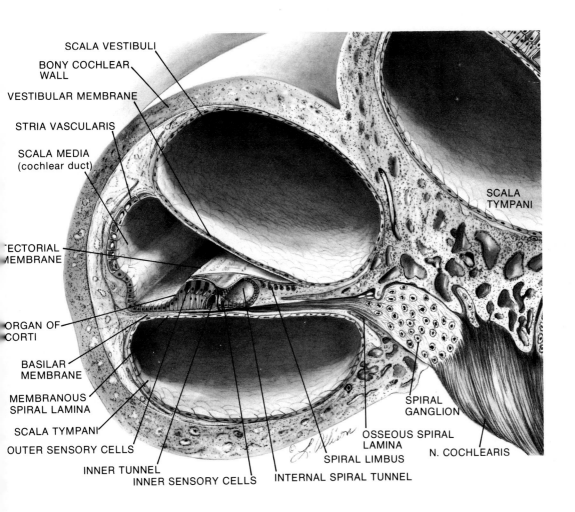

SCALA VESTIBULI

BONY COCHLEAR WALL

VESTIBULAR MEMBRANE

STRIA VASCULARIS

SCALA MEDIA (cochlear duct)

TECTORIAL MEMBRANE

ORGAN OF CORTI

BASILAR MEMBRANE

MEMBRANOUS SPIRAL LAMINA

SCALA TYMPANI

OUTER SENSORY CELLS

INNER TUNNEL

INNER SENSORY CELLS

INTERNAL SPIRAL TUNNEL

SPIRAL LIMBUS

OSSEOUS SPIRAL LAMINA

SPIRAL GANGLION

N. COCHLEARIS

SCALA TYMPANI

Figure 17–4. Free nerve endings. Golgi. Medium power.

In this section of dermis, a small nerve fiber (N) branches, with thin, terminal nerve fibers (black) passing to a hair follicle (H = hair shaft). The nerve fibers lie both longitudinally (center) and around follicles (top right, arrowhead) to terminate mainly in the glassy membrane of the dermal root sheath. They are called peritrichial nerve endings and are stimulated by movement of the hair, appreciating the sensation of touch. One nerve fiber usually supplies many follicles. Similar nerve endings are found in connective tissue elsewhere and in epithelia such as the epidermis, cornea, and glands.

Figure 17–5. Neurotendinous organ. Gold chloride. High power.

Neurotendinous organs (Golgi tendon organs) are located in tendons near muscle-tendon junctions. Here, a bundle of tendon fibers (F) is ensheathed in a thin connective tissue capsule and a bundle of myelinated nerve fibers (N) penetrates the capsule, divides into three main branches, and terminates in numerous small club-shaped endings (arrows). Muscle fibers (M) also are present. Similar organs are found in joint capsules and ligaments and are proprioceptive.

Figure 17–6. Meissner's corpuscle. Golgi. Medium power.

A Meissner corpuscle (arrowheads) and its nerve (N) are located in a dermal papilla of skin (E = epidermis). The corpuscle is ovoid with layers of disc-like, transversely disposed cells (yellow) between which the terminal nerve fibers (arrows) ramify, the whole with a thin connective tissue capsule. These corpuscles are sensitive to touch and are particularly numerous in skin of digits, lips, nipples, and genitalia.

Figure 17–7. Vater-Pacini corpuscle. H and E. Low power.

These are large, up to 2 mm in diameter by 4 mm in length, and ovoid. The corpuscle is seen in transverse section. In the core runs a nerve fiber (N) and surrounding it are lamellae of connective tissue, usually about 60 layers, composed of flattened cells, bilaterally arranged with two longitudinal clefts, the whole enveloped in a sheath (C) of flat cells with prominent basal lamellae between the layers of cells. These corpuscles are found in subcutaneous tissues, in joints, periosteum, mesentery, and ligaments, and register position and movement, responding to pressure and vibration. (See Figures 17–8 and 10–3.)

Figure 17–8. Vater-Pacini corpuscle. H and E. Medium power.

In longitudinal section, this corpuscle shows the nerve-containing core (arrow), the surrounding lamellae (L), and the peripheral capsule (C) or sheath of closely packed flattened cells.

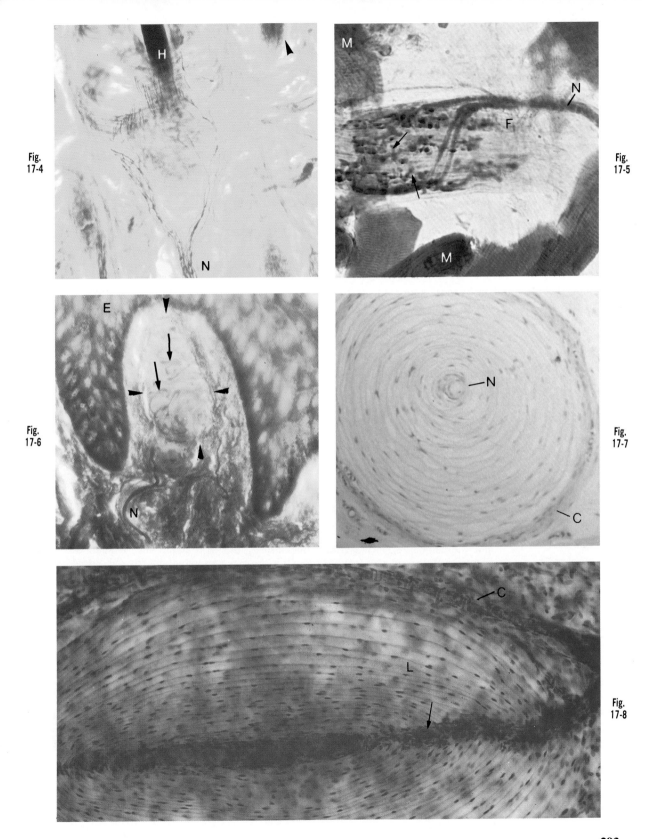

Fig. 17-4

Fig. 17-5

Fig. 17-6

Fig. 17-7

Fig. 17-8

Figure 17–9. Cornea. H and E. Low power.

Five layers are recognized in the cornea, the anterior surface to the right. Most anteriorly is the corneal epithelium (E), stratified squamous in type and five or six cells thick, lying upon Bowman's membrane (B), a thin, structureless membrane not seen clearly here. The bulk of the cornea is composed of the substantia propria (P), formed by lamellae of collagen with fibroblasts or keratocytes between lamellae. Deeply is another structureless membrane composed of atypical collagen, Descemet's membrane (D), and then corneal endothelium (M). The endothelium is a single layer of low cuboidal cells in contact with aqueous humor in the anterior chamber.

Figure 17–10. Cornea. Plastic section. Methylene blue, azure A, basic fuchsin. Medium power.

The corneal epithelium (left) is supported by Bowman's membrane (arrow), not seen clearly here, but there are no nuclei immediately beneath the epithelium. In the substantia propria are the slender, elongated processes (p) and nuclei (n) of keratocytes (fibroblasts) with lamellae of collagen fibers (c). Descemet's membrane (D) is structureless and the endothelium (E) is thin, formed by near-squamous cells in this rat cornea.

Figure 17–11. Corneal epithelium. Plastic section. H and E. Oil immersion.

A mitotic figure (arrowhead) is seen in the epithelium, indicative of its regenerative powers. The epithelium is six or seven layers thick and lies upon the thin, structureless, and acellular Bowman's membrane (B). Part of the substantia propria is seen (right) with nuclei of keratocytes (arrow). The cornea is avascular, and its epithelium is highly sensitive and contains numerous free nerve endings.

Figure 17–12. Sclera, choroid. Plastic section. Methylene blue, basic fuchsin. High power.

The sclera (S) is formed by dense fibrous tissue with flat, thick bundles of collagen fibers (c). Externally is the episcleral tissue (e) of looser fibroelastic tissue and, internally, the lamina fusca (f) has smaller collagen bundles (arrow), more elastic tissue, and some melanocytes (arrowhead). The choroid (C) shows large vessels (v), the choriocapillaris (l), and the lamina elastica (Bruch's membrane, b), with numerous, pigment-containing processes of melanocytes (m). At top left is the pigment epithelium (p) and outer segments of photoreceptors (rods, r). (See also Figures 17–15, 17–16, and 17–27.)

Figure 17–13. Choroid. Plastic section. H and E. Oil immersion.

Most of the thickness of the choroid is seen with larger vessels (v) and melanocytes (m) forming its bulk. Internally are capillaries of the choriocapillaris (l), separated from the pigment epithelium of the retina (p) by the lamina elastica or Bruch's membrane (b), a shiny homogeneous layer only 1 to 4 μm thick. (See also Figure 17–14.)

Figure 17–14. Choroid. Plastic section. Hematoxylin, light green. Oil immersion.

Only the inner portion of the choroid is seen with vessels (v) of the vessel layer and capillaries (l) of the choriocapillaris. The lamina elastica (b) beneath the pigment epithelium (p) is stained only faintly. Melanocytes in the choroid are stellate with several slender cytoplasmic processes, their nuclei (n) nearly obscured by pigment (melanin) granules that fully occupy the cytoplasm. Melanin has a role in the absorption of light rays.

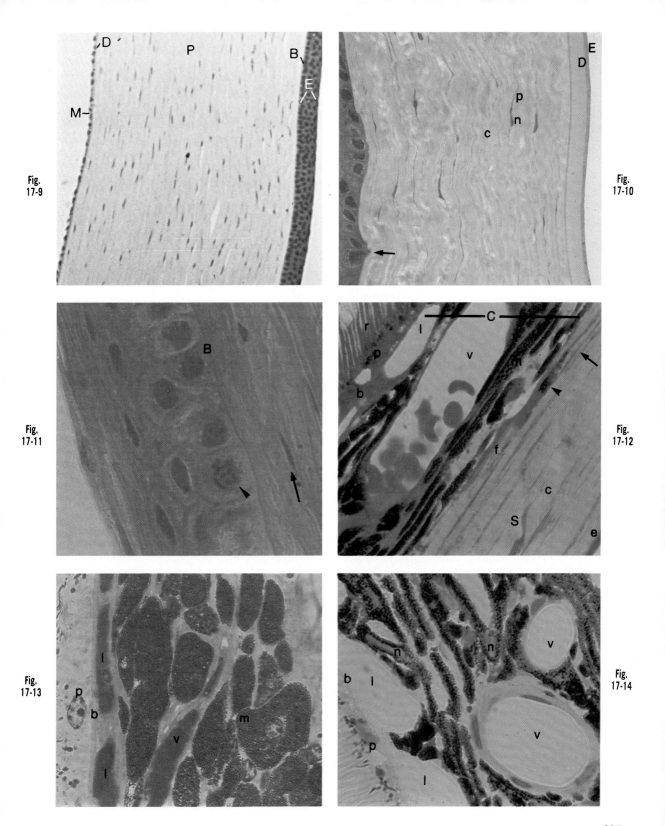

Fig.
17-9

Fig.
17-10

Fig.
17-11

Fig.
17-12

Fig.
17-13

Fig.
17-14

Figure 17–15. Corneoscleral junction. Mallory. Low power.

A small part of the sclera (S) joins the cornea (C) at the corneoscleral junction or limbus (L), the lumbus being a transition zone. The sclera terminates internally in the scleral spur (arrow). The posterior extremity of Descemet's membrane is called the ring of Schwalbe (arrowhead), and fibers of the trabecular network (T) pass from here posteriorly to the scleral spur and ciliary body (B). External to the meshwork is the canal of Schlemm (A). The ciliary epithelium on the internal surface of the ciliary body is formed by two layers of cuboidal cells. The outer layer is pigmented (P) and continuous with that of the retina; the inner is nonpigmented and represents the forward prolongation of the entire thickness of the sensory retina. Both layers continue forward on to the posterior surface of the iris (I), where both layers are heavily pigmented. Melanocytes (M, black) are seen between muscle fibers of the ciliary body.

Figure 17–16. Ora serrata, ciliary body, sclera. Plastic section. Methylene blue, azure A, basic fuchsin. Low power.

The ora serrata (please see Fig. 17–1), the junction between nervous (R) and non-nervous (C) portions of the retina, is seen (arrow) and at this region in the uveal coat, choroid continues into ciliary body (B), which is somewhat thicker. Its inner surface (against the vitreous) is covered by the ciliary (non-nervous) portion of the retina and is irregular showing shallow grooves or striae (s) passing forward from the ora serrata and deeper, radial grooves and ridges anteriorly. These are the ciliary processes (P). Situated externally is the sclera (S). The ciliary processes are illustrated in Figure 17–19 at higher magnification.

Figure 17–17. Ciliary body, iris. H nd E. Low power.

This is similar to Figure 17–15, with identical labeling. Note ciliary processes (P); in the ciliary body (B), there is ciliary muscle (pink) with melanocytes (black). The root of the iris shows posterior pigmented epithelium and an anterior surface that, in fact, is discontinuous and formed by fibroblasts and melanocytes supported by delicate connective tissue.

Figure 17–18. Ciliary body. H and E. High power.

This shows ciliary muscle (pink) with melanocytes (M) in the ciliary body, ciliary epithelium with outer pigmented layer and inner nonpigmented layer covering ciliary processes (P), and the root of the iris where both layers of epithelium are heavily pigmented (arrow).

Figure 17–19. Ciliary body and processes. Plastic section. Methylene blue, azure A, basic fuchsin. High power.

This is a higher magnification of Figure 17–16, showing the ciliary body (B) below, here with melanocytes and numerous blood vessels (the vascular layer). Above, toward the vitreous, it shows the ciliary processes, covered by the ciliary epithelium or non-nervous layer of the retina. This epithelium has an outer, pigmented layer (p) continuous with the pigmented epithelium of the retina and an inner, nonpigmented layer (n). The connective tissue core of the processes contains numerous vessels (v), the probable site of formation of aqueous humor.

Figure 17–20. Ciliary processes. Plastic section. Methylene blue, azure A, basic fuchsin. Oil immersion.

The inner layer of cuboidal cells of the ciliary epithelium (top) is nonpigmented, and the outer layer is heavily pigmented, these cells being filled with pigment (melanin) granules. In the core of the ciliary process are numerous capillaries filled with erythrocytes (red pink), this probably being the site of formation of aqueous humor.

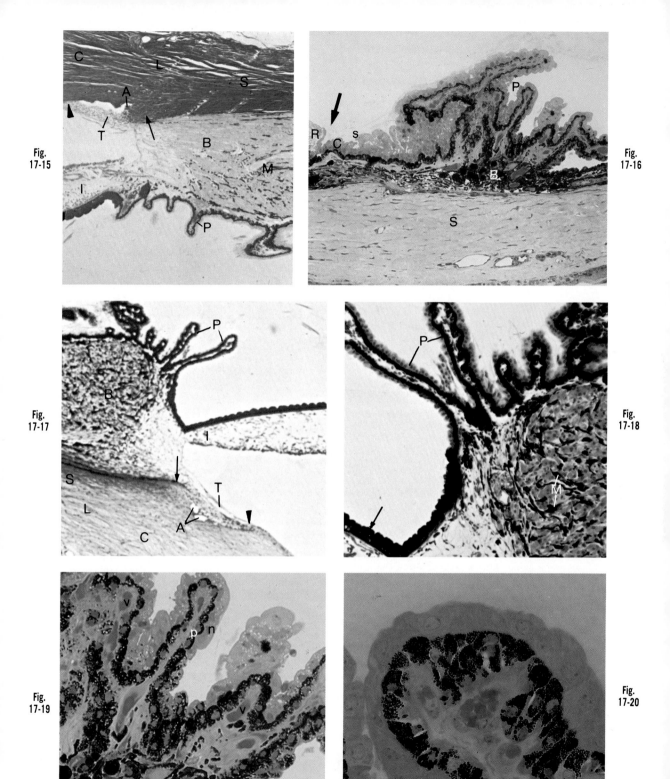

Fig. 17-15

Fig. 17-16

Fig. 17-17

Fig. 17-18

Fig. 17-19

Fig. 17-20

Figure 17–21. Iris. Plastic section. Methylene blue, azure A, basic fuchsin. Low power.

The pupillary margin is to the right, and the full thickness is seen of the central, pupillary zone of the iris. The anterior surface (above) is irregular (and incomplete) (please see Figure 17–22). The posterior surface (below) is uniformly black, formed by two layers of pigmented cells. In the stroma are bundles of smooth muscle cells (m) of the sphincter papillae muscle, here cut transversely, and some melanophores (black). The number of melanophores and their content of pigment determine eye color. Here, they are few in a blue eye (they arc much more numerous in a brown eye). Also present are blood vessels (arrowheads) that run radially, but in a spiral manner, hence, the appearance of staggered oblique/transverse profiles. This permits the vessels to accommodate to change in length with change in pupil diameter.

Figure 17–22. Iris, dilator pupillae. Plastic section. H and E. Medium power.

Anteriorly (above) there is no definite cellular membrane, but fibroblasts (pink) and pigmented cells (black) form a discontinuous layer with collagen fibers in the intercellular spaces. In the delicate connective tissue stroma are blood vessels (v) and stellate melanophores (M), numerous in this brown eye (compare with Fig. 17–21). Posteriorly (below) there is the pigmented epithelium—two layers of heavily pigmented cells. The anterior or basal layer is made up of myoepithelial cells with their basal processes (pink, arrowheads) forming the dilator pupillae muscle. This is a section of the peripheral ciliary zone, where the iris is relatively thin near its root.

Figure 17–23. Iris, sphincter and dilator pupillae. Plastic section. H and E. High power.

This is a section near the pupillary margin of the iris. The stroma contains blood vessels (v) and bundles of smooth muscle fibers of the sphincter pupille (M), here cut transversely. The pigment cells (p) here have been called "clump" cells, differing from the melanophores that lie more anteriorly and peripherally. These clump cells are spherical, have fewer processes, lie near the pupillary margin, and are phagocytic. Posteriorly (below) is the pigmented epithelium: the posterior (1) layer heavily pigmented, the anterior or basal layer (2) of myoepithelial, pigmented cells, their basal processes (pink, arrowheads) forming the dilator pupillae.

Figure 17–24. Lens. H and E. Low power.

The lens is enclosed by the lens capsule, thicker on the anterior surface (above), and is homogeneous and structureless. Beneath it on the anterior surface only is the subcapsular epithelium (e), a simple cuboidal epithelium. Toward the equator (L), the cells become taller and transform into lens fibers. The lens fibers, which form the lens substance, are elongated cells in the shape of a six-sided prism, closely packed and concentrically arranged parallel to the surface. The younger, external fibers retain their nuclei (n), which are lost from the older cells of the inner nucleus of the lens. The lens is biconvex, elastic, and avascular. Ciliary processes also are seen at top right.

Figure 17–25. Lens, equator. Plastic section. H and E. High power.

The lens capsule is thicker anteriorly (arrow) than posteriorly (arrowhead). The fine, pink fibrils seen attaching to it (asterisks) are zonular fibers of the suspensory ligament. At the equator (L), the cells of the subcapsular epithelium (e) become taller and transform into lens fibers (f). Individual, elongated lens fibers can be seen (open arrow).

Figure 17–26. Lens. H and E. High power.

Lens fibers, here cut transversely, show a regular hexagonal pattern accounting for the crystalline nature of the lens. No nuclei are seen. Anteriorly is lens epithelium (E) covered by the homogeneous lens capsule (C).

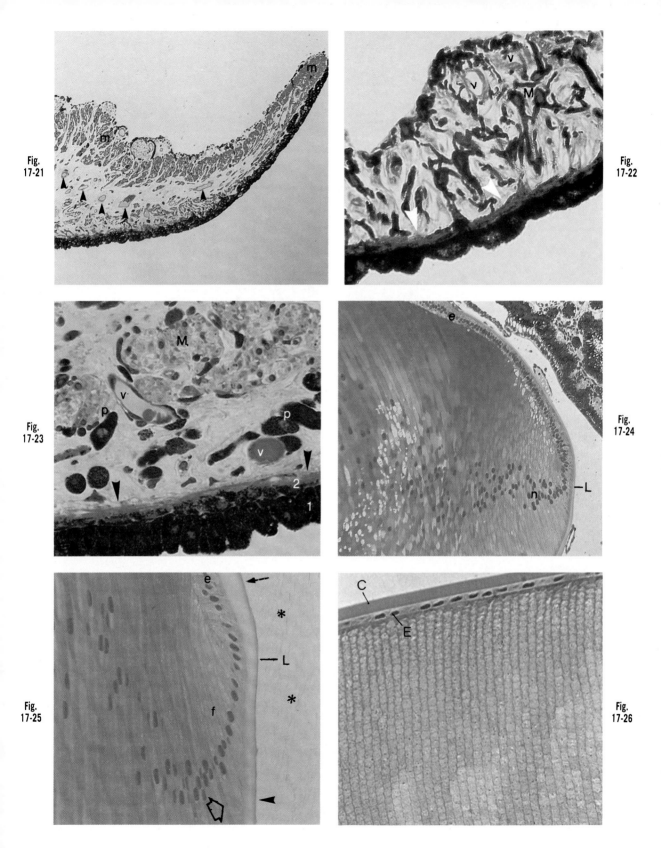

Fig. 17-21

Fig. 17-22

Fig. 17-23

Fig. 17-24

Fig. 17-25

Fig. 17-26

Figure 17–27. Retina. Mallory. Low power.

Collagen stains blue and demonstrates the thickness of the sclera (S). A large quantity of pigment is found in the choroid (C), in melanocytes. This layer also contains numerous blood vessels. Owing to collapse of the vessels, this layer appears thinner than it is in life. The nervous retina (R) shows a regular, lamellated appearance, the layers being seen better at higher magnification in the following figures. Note the pigment epithelium (1).

Figure 17–28. Retina. Plastic section. Methylene blue, azure A, basic fuchsin. High power.

Below is part of the choroid containing numerous melanocytes with the choriocapillaris (c) beneath the retina. All layers of the retina are seen. They are: 1, pigment epithelium with pigment (melanin) granules; 2, layer of photoreceptors with outer (o) and inner (i) segments; 3, external limiting membrane; 4, outer nuclear layer (nuclei of photoreceptors); 5, outer plexiform layer, where photoreceptors synapse with bipolar cells; 6, inner nuclear layer of bipolar nerve cell bodies; 7, inner plexiform layer, where bipolar cells synapse with ganglion cells; 8, ganglion cell layer, composed of cell bodies of ganglion cells; 9, optic nerve fiber layer, formed by the central processes of ganglion cells passing posteriorly to form the optic nerve; and 10, internal limiting membrane separating the retina from the vitreous body (above). Note that this is peripheral retina; basically then, the photoreceptors are rods, there are comparatively few ganglion cells, and the nerve fiber layer is thin. The darker cytoplasmic strands passing radially (arrowheads) are of Müller's supporting cells.

Figure 17–29. Retina. Iron hematoxylin. High power.

This is similar to the previous figure with the same labeling. Cones are clearly distinguishable from rods in layer 2, the cones being shorter, darker, and thicker, with their nuclei in a single row in layer 4 just internal to the internal limiting membrane. Rods are paler, thinner, and longer. Rods clearly show inner (R, arrowhead) and outer (R, arrow) segments, as do cones (outer—C, arrow; inner—C, arrowhead). Apart from direct conducting neurons, i.e., bipolar and ganglion cells, nuclei of other cells are present but not distinguishable. These are of association and centrifugal neurons, such as horizontal and amacrine cells with nuclei in layer 6, and of supporting cells, such as the cells of Müller and other glial cells. The retina has a very rich vascular supply, although blood vessels are not apparent in this figure.

Figure 17–30. Retina, squirrel. Plastic section. H and E. Oil immersion.

Erythrocytes (blue) are seen in capillaries of the choriocapillaris (C). This animal has only cones, and in layer 2 these clearly show pale-staining inner (I) and dark-staining outer (O) segments. Between the outer segments are apical processes (arrows) of retinal pigment epithelial cells (1) containing melanin granules. Nuclei of cones lie in the outer nuclear layer (4), just internal to the external limiting membrane (3). Also seen are outer cone fibers (arrowheads) passing through the external limiting membrane (3) to connect cones with their perikarya in the outer nuclear layer, and inner cone fibers (asterisk) passing to the outer plexiform layer (5).

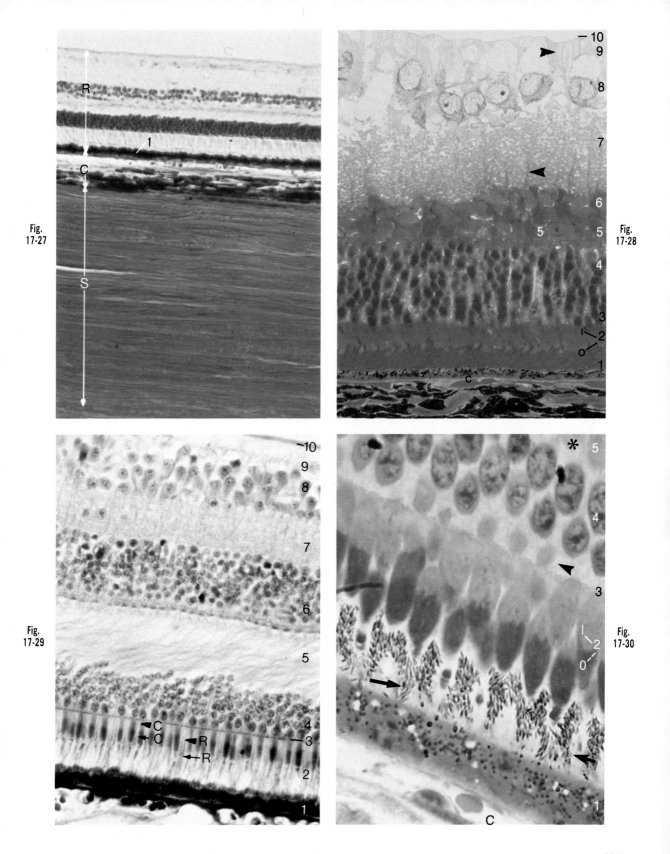

Fig.
17-27

Fig.
17-28

Fig.
17-29

Fig.
17-30

Figure 17–31. Retina, fovea centralis. Iron hematoxylin. Low power.

Seen here are sclera (S) traversed by a large blood vessel, choroid (C), and the retina at the fovea centralis, a shallow pit where the retina is modified. The pigment epithelium (1) is seen, and at the fovea the inner layers of the retina (outer plexiform to optic nerve fiber layer) are virtually absent. Photoreceptors here all are elongated cones, i.e., slender and resembling rods, and these synapse with bipolar cells located at the margin of the fovea. Thus, inner cone fibers slant out to the margin. This is the region of clearest vision and maximal visual acuity.

Figure 17–32. Optic nerve. Mallory. Low power.

The optic nerve is a tract of the central nervous system, not a true peripheral nerve, connecting retinal ganglion cells and the midbrain. The nerve is covered by meninges (blue-staining) that merge with sclera at the eyeball. Extending into the nerve from pia mater, the innermost layer of meninges, are septa (S) carrying blood vessels. These septa divide the nerve into bundles. Centrally located are profiles of the central artery (A) and vein (V) of the retina.

Figure 17–33. Eyelid. H and E. Low power.

This is a section through the lower eyelid, covered anteriorly (above) by thin skin with fine hairs (h), sweat (s), and sebaceous glands (b) with a supporting dermis (d) of delicate connective tissue. At the lid margin (left), there are two or three rows of long, stiff hairs or eyelashes (e), with associated sebaceous glands (arrowheads). Beneath the skin is striated muscle (m) of the orbicularis oculi, posterior to which is dense connective tissue (c) of the septum orbitale, thickéned as the tarsal plate (not seen here). Contained in this layer is a single row of tarsal (Meibomian) glands (t)—large sebaceous glands opening by ducts (arrow) at the lid margin. Posteriorly (below) is the conjunctiva.

Figure 17–34. Tarsal (Meibomian) glands. Plastic section. H and E. High power.

The secretory alveoli or sacculi of the tarsal glands are lined by a single row of low cuboidal cells (arrows) in which mitoses occur. As cells pass to the center of an alveolus, they become larger and accumulate lipid, becoming vacuolated (v). Later, the entire cell (asterisk) breaks down (holocrine secretion) to form the secretory material, the nuclei of these dying cells becoming pyknotic (arrowheads). These glands drain via ducts to the lid margin, the glands lying in dense connective tissue (c) of the septum orbitale and tarsal plate.

Figure 17–35. Conjunctiva. Plastic section. H and E. High power.

This mucous membrane lines the inner surface of the eyelids from which it is reflected on to the eyeball, being continuous with corneal epithelium at the corneal margin and with skin at the lid margins. It is a stratified epithelium, about four layers thick, and scattered among the epithelial cells are pale-staining, mucus-secreting goblet cells. It is supported by a cellular lamina propria.

Figure 17–36. Lacrimal gland. H and E. Medium power.

Parts of several lobules of the gland are seen with an interlobular duct (D) in an interlobular septum, and an intralobular duct (L). Secretory acini are serous in type. The main lacrimal gland, located in the superolateral corner of the orbit, is a compound, tubuloalveolar serous gland with prominent myoepithelial cells, not discernible at this magnification.

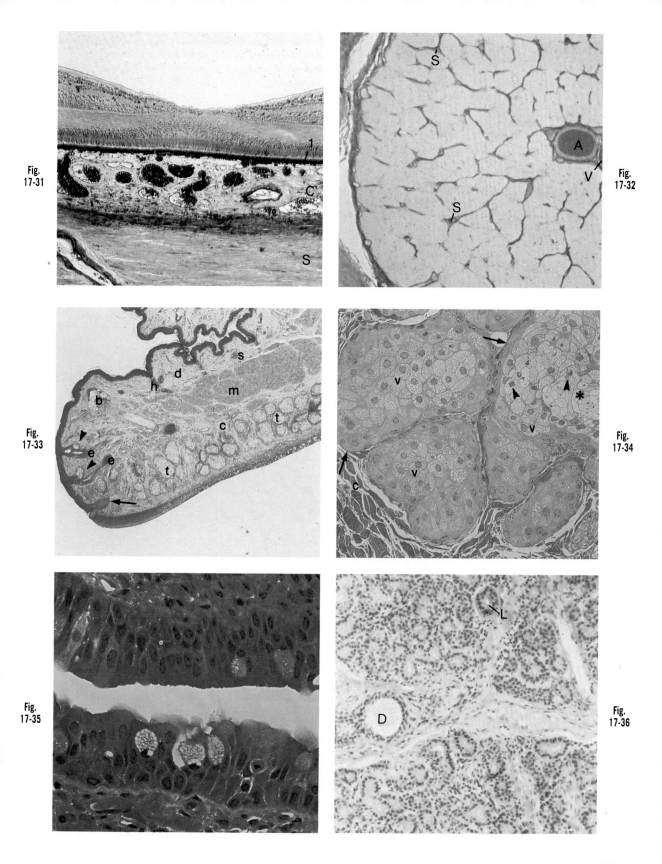

Fig.
17-31

Fig.
17-32

Fig.
17-33

Fig.
17-34

Fig.
17-35

Fig.
17-36

Figure 17–37. Auricle. H and E. Low power.

The auricle or pinna shows a core of elastic cartilage (E); here it is sectioned near its edge, with a perichondrium (p) in which elastic fibers are predominant. On each surface is thin skin, with epidermis and dermis. As in skin elsewhere, the dermis contains hairs (h) and sebaceous (b) and sweat (s) glands, although in general these are poorly developed.

Figure 17–38. Middle ear. H and E. Low power.

This is an oblique horizontal section of the right middle ear cavity as seen from above. It shows the deepest portion of the external auditory meatus (E) extending deeply to the tympanic membrane (T). In the middle ear cavity, anteriorly the cavity continues as the pharyngotympanic tube (A); posteriorly located is a profile of bone of the head of the incus (I); and medially the stapes (S) shows a base plate (arrow) fitting into the fenestra ovalis. Also in the medial wall is the promontory (P) formed by the basal turn of the cochlea and the fenestra rotunda (round window), and closed by the secondary tympanic membrane (arrowhead). In the inner ear, spaces—the scala vestibuli (V) and the scala tympani (S)—are occupied by perilymph. Just posterior to the fenestra ovalis (oval window) is the canal for the facial (VIIth) nerve (F).

Figure 17–39. Semicircular canal. H and E. Medium power.

This section of part of the petrous temporal bone shows an ovoid cavity of a semicircular canal (bony labyrinth) containing a canal of the membranous labyrinth. This is eccentric, the convexity of the semicircular canal closely apposed to bone on one side and with thin, connective tissue trabeculae traversing the wide perilymph space between bony and membranous labyrinths. The membranous canal is filled with endolymph.

Figure 17–40. Semicircular canal, ampulla. Plastic section. Methylene blue, azure A, basic fuchsin. Medium power.

The ampulla of each semicircular canal contains a crista or crest lying transversely across the long axis of the canal: here, it is cut in cross section. The lining of the membranous semicircular canal itself is squamous or low cuboidal epithelium (arrows) supported by thin connective tissue, and the canal contains endolymph. The crista has a core of delicate connective tissue containing blood vessels (v) and nerves (arrowheads), branches of the vestibular portion of the eighth cranial nerve. At its base, the lining epithelium changes to a complex neuroepithelium that is covered by the homogeneous, gelatinous cupula (C). Below is bone (b) of the surrounding bony labyrinth. (See also Figure 17–41.)

Figure 17–41. Crista ampullaris. H and E. High power.

The connective tissue core of the crista contains blood vessels and nerves (not seen). The epithelium at the base is simple cuboidal, but changes toward the tip into a taller, columnar type with two distinct rows of nuclei. One cell type is tall, slender, and with ovoid nuclei near the basal lamina. This is the sustentacular cell (S). The second type has pale-staining cytoplasm, is flask-shaped, and has a dark spherical nucleus in the second "row": this is the sensory hair cell (H), with apical hair-like processes extending into a gelatinous, noncellular, eosinophil membrane called the cupula (C). The hair cells actually are of two types, not distinguishable here, and are stimulated by a change in rotational velocity.

Figure 17–42. Macula utriculi. Plastic section. Methylene blue, azure A, basic fuchsin. Medium power.

Maculae of both utricle and saccule show three cell types. The sustentacular cells (S) are tall columnar, darkly staining, and with basally located nuclei and apical microvilli. Hair (sensory) cells (H) are of two types, one piriform (type I) and the other cylindrical (type II), poorly distinguished here, but both with pale-staining cytoplasm and large, vesicular, spherical nuclei. Apically, both have a sensory hair bundle (arrowheads) composed of 30 to 100 stereocilia and a single kinocilium. This bundle passes to the otolithic membrane (O), a gelatinous membrane containing many small crystalline bodies, the otoconia or otoliths, here stained dark purple. In the connective tissue beneath the neuroepithelium are numerous blood vessels (v) and nerve fibers (n) of the vestibular nerve. The maculae detect change in position of the head.

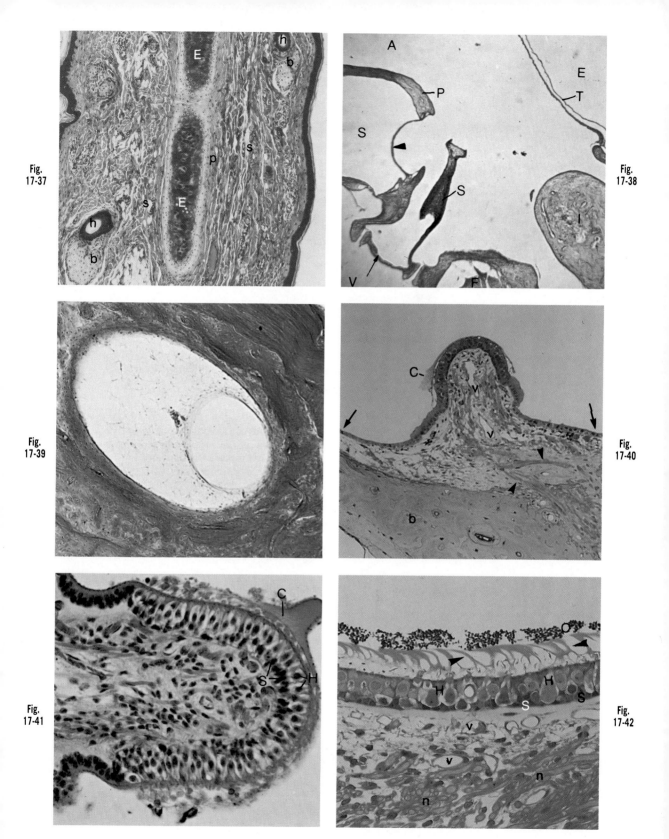

Fig.
17-37

Fig.
17-38

Fig.
17-39

Fig.
17-40

Fig.
17-41

Fig.
17-42

Figure 17–43. Cochlea. H and E. Low power.

This section is through the length of the cochlea of a guinea pig with the apex or helicotrema (H) to the left. The axial stem or modiolus (M) contains the auditory (cochlear) nerve (N). The cochlea shows three turns (1, 2, 3) in a spiral around the modiolus, the basal turn of greater diameter. In each turn, there is a small triangular mass (G) adjacent to the modiolus; this is the spiral ganglion. A thin basilar membrane extends outward from the region of the spiral ganglion to a thickening of periosteum (K) called the spiral ligament, in the outer wall. A second thin membrane, the vestibular membrane, also crosses the cavity so that in each turn there are three cavities. (Please see Figures 17–44 through 17–47.)

Figure 17–44. Cochlea, spiral ganglion. Plastic section. Methylene blue, azure A, basic fuchsin. Medium power.

The spiral ganglion occupies the spiral canal of the modiolus (bone, B) and consists of bipolar nerve cells. The bipolar form is well seen in the cell labeled "N." The peripheral processes (dendrites) of these cells pass to inner and outer hair cells of the organ of Corti, the latter passing across the central tunnel (of Corti). Two types of bipolar cells have been described, types I and II, respectively, supplying inner and outer hair cells.

Figure 17–45. Cochlea. H and E. Medium power.

Parts of three turns of the cochlea are seen. Central in the modiolus is the cochlear nerve (N) and collections of ganglion cells (G) of the spiral ganglion. A spur of bone, the spiral lamina (L) projects outward, really in the form of the thread of a screw as it spirals around the modiolus. Attached to it is the basilar membrane (B) passing out to the spiral ligament (K), a periosteal thickening of the outer wall. A thinner vestibular membrane (V) passes from the spiral lamina to the outer wall. These two membranes divide each turn of the cochlea into scala vestibuli (S) and scala tympani (T), filled with perilymph, with the central cochlear duct (C) filled with endolymph. The organ of Corti lies on the basilar membrane and is seen better at higher magnification.

Figure 17–46. Organ of Corti. H and E. High power.

Centrally situated is the cochlear duct (C), separated by the thin vestibular membrane (V) from the scala vestibuli (S), and by the basilar membrane (B) from the scala tympani (T). Externally is the thickened periosteum of the spiral ligament (K), over which the lining epithelium of the cochlear duct is thickened to a low columnar type with blood vessels beneath it as the stria vascularis (arrow)—the probable site of formation of endolymph. Lying on the basilar membrane is the organ of Corti (see Fig. 17–3). The central tunnel of triangular outline (arrowhead) lies between inner and outer pillar cells and the basilar membrane. Above the tunnel is the tectorial membrane (X) extending outward from the limbus. (Please see Figure 17–47.) (Additional labels appear in Figure 17–45.)

Figure 17–47. Organ of Corti. H and E. Oil immersion.

The tectorial membrane (X) here is artificially raised from the hair cells. The vestibular (V) and basilar (B) membranes are seen bounding the cochlear duct. On the basilar membrane are inner (P_1) and outer (P_2) pillar cells bounding the tunnel with nuclei of a single row of inner (H_i) and three rows of outer (H_o) cells. Other cells seen are border cells (asterisk), phalangeal cells (C), and cells of Hensen (D) and Claudius (E).

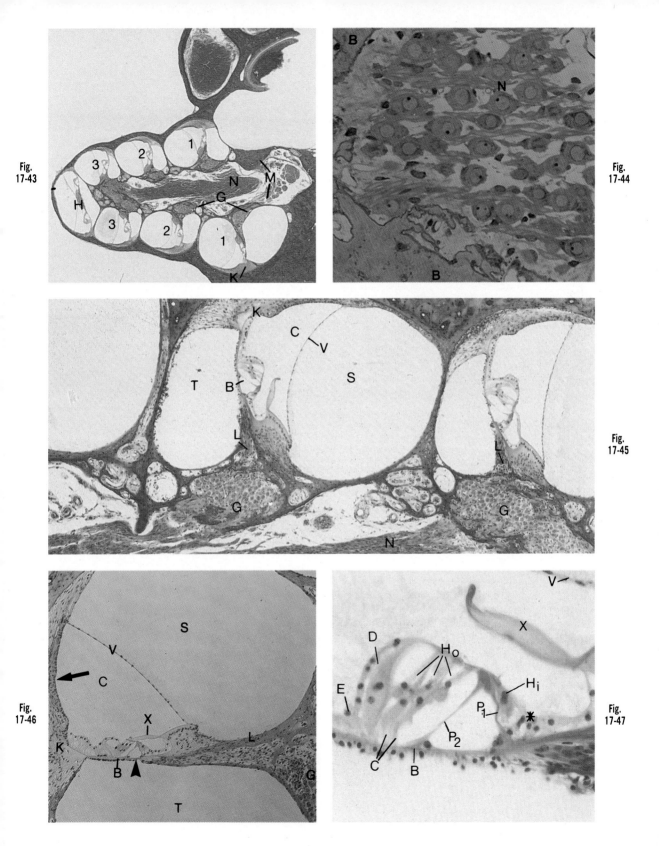

Fig.
17-43

Fig.
17-44

Fig.
17-45

Fig.
17-46

Fig.
17-47

INDEX

Page numbers in *italics* indicate illustrations.